FUNDAMENTALS OF
CLINICAL NUTRITION

FUNDAMENTALS OF
CLINICAL NUTRITION

SECOND EDITION

with 57 illustrations and 41 color illustrations

EDITOR

SARAH L. MORGAN, MD, RD, FADA, FACP
Associate Professor and Director
Division of Clinical Nutrition and Dietetics
Departments of Nutrition Sciences and Medicine
Schools of Health Related Professions, Medicine, and Dentistry
University of Alabama at Birmingham
Birmingham, Alabama

ASSISTANT
EDITOR

ROLAND L. WEINSIER, MD, DrPH, FACP
C.E. Butterworth Jr. Professor and Chair
Department of Nutrition Sciences
Professor, Departments of Medicine and Nutrition Sciences
Schools of Health Related Professions, Medicine, and Dentistry
University of Alabama at Birmingham
Birmingham, Alabama

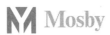 Mosby

A Harcourt Health Sciences Company

St. Louis   London   Philadelphia   Sydney   Toronto

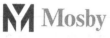

A Harcourt Health Sciences Company

Editor: Michael Brown
Developmental Editor: Linda Caldwell
Editorial Assistant: Brandyce Briggs
Project Manager: Carol Sullivan Weis
Production Editor: Rick Dudley
Designer: Jen Marmarinos
Manufacturing Supervisor: Karen Lewis
Cover Photograph: © Photo Researchers, Inc.

Mosby, Inc.
11830 Westline Industrial Drive
St. Louis, Missouri 63146

Library of Congress Cataloging-in-Publication Data

Fundamentals of clinical nutrition / editor, Sarah L. Morgan,
   assistant editor, Roland L. Weinsier. — 2nd ed.
     p.   cm.
   Includes bibliographical references and index.
   ISBN 0-8151-9669-5
   1. Dietetics. 2. Diet therapy. 3. Nutrition. I. Morgan, Sarah
L. II. Weinsier, Roland L.
   [DNLM: 1. Diet Therapy. 2. Nutrition. 3. Nutrition Disorders.
WB 400 F981 1998]
RM216.F95   1998
615.8′54—dc21
DNLM/DLC   97-19137

00 01 02 03 04 / 9 8 7 6 5 4 3 2

Contributors

Jaime Aranda-Michel, M.D.
Fellow, Clinical Nutrition and Dietetics
Departments of Nutrition Sciences and Medicine
Schools of Medicine, Health Related Professions, and Dentistry
University of Alabama at Birmingham
Birmingham, Alabama

Joseph E. Baggott, Ph.D.
Assistant Professor
Division of Nutritional Biochemistry and Molecular Biology
Departments of Nutrition Sciences and Medicine
Schools of Medicine, Health Related Professions, and Dentistry
University of Alabama at Birmingham
Birmingham, Alabama

Pi-Ling Chang, Ph.D.
Assistant Professor
Division of Nutritional Biochemistry and Molecular Biology
Departments of Nutrition Sciences and Medicine
Schools of Medicine, Health Related Professions, and Dentistry
University of Alabama at Birmingham
Birmingham, Alabama

Cathy Crawford, R.D., C.D.E.
University of Alabama Health Services Foundation/Kirklin Clinic
Clinical Dietitian for Endocrinology and Cardiology
Birmingham, Alabama

Reinaldo Figueroa, M.D.
Assistant Professor of Pediatrics and Nutrition Sciences
Division of Pediatric Gastroenterology and Nutrition
School of Medicine
University of Alabama at Birmingham
Birmingham, Alabama

Frank A. Franklin, Jr, M.D., Ph.D.
Professor of Pediatrics and Nutrition Sciences, Director GI/Nutrition
Departments of Pediatric Gastroenterology and Nutrition
School of Medicine
University of Alabama at Birmingham
Birmingham, Alabama

Patricia S. Goode, M.D.
Division of Geriatrics
Department of Medicine
School of Medicine
University of Alabama at Birmingham
Birmingham, Alabama

Michael Goran, Ph.D.
Associate Professor and Director
Division of Physiology and Metabolism
Department of Nutrition Sciences
Schools of Medicine, Health Related Professions, and Dentistry
University of Alabama at Birmingham
Birmingham, Alabama

Douglas C. Heimberger, M.D., M.S., F.A.C.P.
Associate Professor
Departments of Nutrition Sciences and Medicine
Schools of Medicine, Health Related Professions, and Dentistry
University of Alabama at Birmingham
Birmingham, Alabama

Donald D. Henrud, M.D., M.P.H.
Assistant Professor of Preventive Medicine and Nutrition
Divisions of Preventive Medicine and Endocrinology/Metabolism
Mayo Medical School
Mayo Clinic
Rochester, Minnesota

Juan M. Navia, Ph.D.
Professor Emeritus
Departments of Comparative Medicine and Nutrition Sciences
School of Medicine
University of Alabama at Birmingham
Birmingham, Alabama

Christopher M. Reinold, M.P.H., R.D.
Senior Nutrition Coordinator
Jefferson County Department of Health
Birmingham, Alabama

Christine S. Ritchie, M.D., M.P.H.
Assistant Professor of Medicine
Division of Gerontology/Geriatric Medicine
School of Medicine
University of Alabama at Birmingham
Birmingham, Alabama

Howerde E. Sauberlich, Ph.D.
Professor
Department of Nutrition Sciences
Schools of Medicine, Health Related Professions, and Dentistry
University of Alabama at Birmingham
Birmingham, Alabama

Charles B. Stephensen, Ph.D.
Associate Professor and Interim Director
Division of Public Health Nutrition
Departments of International Health and Nutrition Sciences
Schools of Public Health and Nutrition Sciences
University of Alabama at Birmingham
Birmingham, Alabama

Glen A. Thompson, Pharm.D.
Division Director
Department of Pharmacy
University of Alabama Hospitals
Birmingham, Alabama

Adrian H. Thurstin, Ph.D.
Associate Professor
Division of Geriatric Psychiatry
Department of Psychiatry and Behavioral Neurobiology
School of Medicine
University of Alabama at Birmingham
Birmingham, Alabama

Nedra P. Wilson, M.S., R.D.
Associate Professor
Division of Clinical Nutrition and Dietetics
Department of Nutrition Sciences
Schools of Health Related Professions, Medicine, and Dentistry
University of Alabama at Birmingham
Birmingham, Alabama

Nancy Wooldridge, M.S., R.D.
Assistant Professor
Pediatric Pulmonary Center
Departments of Pediatrics and Nutrition Sciences
School of Medicine
University of Alabama at Birmingham
Birmingham, Alabama

Preface

As physician-nutritionists, our backgrounds include training in both internal medicine and clinical nutrition. In the past, so-called nutrition specialists were in reality gastroenterologists, hematologists, or pediatricians who just happened to profess some knowledge of nutrition as it related to their field of practice. What was a nutritionist anyway? What procedures would he or she use? With what organ or body system would he or she be identified? At least one could identify with and imagine the role of the cardiologist, the endocrinologist, or the nephrologist.

However, times and medical practice have changed. More than half of the leading causes of death in this country are nutrition-related. Half of the health-promoting behaviors recommended by physicians in practice are nutrition-related. They include recommendations on the type and amount of dietary fat intake, salt consumption, cholesterol intake, and vitamin use. In response to the rapidly growing need for physicians who are well trained in nutrition as clinicians, researchers, and teachers, more and more residents and fellows are looking for and receiving specialization in clinical nutrition.

Most readers of this book will be medical students and residents in training, and for most of them this book will represent their main exposure to nutrition.

Unfortunately, many medical schools in the United States require no formal instruction in nutrition. Whether your school does or not, this monograph should accomplish the following two objectives: (1) it should complement your medical training by emphasizing the relevance of nutrition to your medical practice, and (2) it should heighten your awareness of nutrition as a medical specialty that is vitally important for both disease prevention and the treatment of diseases of essentially every organ system. If this book achieves either or both of these aims, it has been a worthwhile endeavor.

Sarah L. Morgan, MD, RD, FADA, FACP

Roland L. Weinsier, MD, DrPH, FACP

Acknowledgments

This book is a publication of the Department of Nutrition Sciences of the University of Alabama at Birmingham. This work was supported by 1R29 AR42674 through the National Institutes of Arthritis and Musculoskeletal and Skin Diseases and the Office of Dietary Supplements and in part by the National Institutes of Health Department of Research Resources Clinical Research Center grant RR-32-31S1.

We deeply appreciate the clerical and administrative assistance of Ms. Debra Richardson.

Contents

FUNDAMENTALS OF
CLINICAL NUTRITION

Part

1

LIFESTYLE, DIET, AND DISEASE

1

Dietary Trends

Americans have a wide variety of foods from which to choose. This variety is constantly expanding as new products are developed and additional agricultural sites are identified worldwide. With our improved transportation system, *seasonal food* is almost an antiquated term. Locally produced foods will always be favored, but strawberries and other such seasonal foods are increasingly available year-round, even in small-town grocery stores. However, Americans are not necessarily eating a healthful diet. Most diets are too high in calories, salt, and fat and too low in fiber and complex carbohydrates.

A nutritious diet is clearly an important aspect of achieving wellness. Scientists find it difficult to name certain foods that affect risk of a specific disease, but there is no debate that food plays an important role in wellness and health. It is clear that diet is only one component of a healthy lifestyle, with heredity and environmental factors playing important roles as well.

A concentrated effort to improve our population's diet began in 1988 with the release of *The Surgeon General's Report on Nutrition and Health*. It outlined ways to improve health by changing food intake. The National Research Council responded a year later and issued similar guidelines for reducing health risks in a report entitled *Diet and Health*. The U.S. Department of Health and Human Services applied these recommendations to an official strategy for improving our nation's health, published as *Healthy People 2000: National Health Promotion and Disease Prevention Objectives. The Dietary Guidelines for Americans* were issued by the U.S. Department of Agriculture (USDA) and the Department of Health and Human Services as an approach to improve food consumption to help meet these health objectives. The dietary recommendations focused on achieving a healthy weight and reducing disease risks through reducing fat and cholesterol, increasing carbohydrate and fiber, limiting sodium and sugar, and consuming alcohol in moderation, while maintaining adequate intakes of calcium and fluoride. The guidelines that follow help in promoting good health and reducing risk for several medical conditions and diseases such as coronary heart disease, hypertension, stroke, osteoporosis, some cancers, and obesity.

These guidelines are designed for all Americans over age 2.

DIETARY GUIDELINES FOR AMERICANS

- Eat a variety of foods.
- Balance the food you eat with physical activity—maintain or improve your weight.
- Choose a diet with plenty of grain products, vegetables, and fruits.
- Choose a diet low in fat, saturated fat, and cholesterol.
- Choose a diet moderate in sugars.
- Choose a diet moderate in salt and sodium.
- If you drink alcoholic beverages, do so in moderation.

These guidelines can be met by choosing more foods from grains, vegetables, and fruits; moderate amounts of low-fat dairy products, lean meats, fish, and poultry; and less foods that contain large amounts of fats and sugar.

The Food Guide Pyramid in Fig. 1-1 graphically presents these seven guidelines.

The Food Guide Pyramid groups foods according to their nutrient content. It promotes variety and balance for a healthful diet. Foods from the base should be eaten more frequently and should provide the greatest percentage of calories. The bread, cereal, rice, and pasta group provides complex carbohydrates and dietary fiber. The fruit and vegetable level of the pyramid provides fiber, vitamins such as A, C, and folate, and essential minerals. The milk group is an important source of calcium, vitamin D, riboflavin, protein, and other nutrients. The meat group also contributes protein and minerals such as zinc and iron.

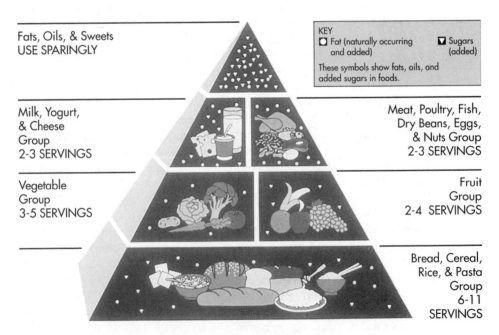

Fig. 1-1   The Food Guide Pyramid.

The recommended number of daily servings of different foods for adults is as follows (see Fig. 1-1):

Breads, cereals, grains, and pasta	6-11 servings
Fruits	2-4 servings
Vegetables	3-5 servings
Meat, poultry, fish, and legumes	2-3 servings
Dairy products	2-3 servings
Fats, oils, and sweets	Use sparingly

Examples of one serving of a food are as follows:

Breads, Cereals, Grains, and Pasta: 1 slice bread or ½ cup rice or pasta, 1 ounce ready-to-eat cereal

Fruits: 1 medium piece fruit or ¾ cup fruit juice, ¼ cup dried fruit

Vegetables: ½ cup cooked or chopped raw vegetables, 1 cup leafy raw vegetables

Meat: 2½ to 3 ounces of meat, poultry, or fish (the amount equivalent to the size of one deck of playing cards); one egg counts as 1 ounce of meat

Dairy: 1 cup of low-fat milk or of low-fat yogurt, 1½ ounces of low-fat cheese

Within each of the groups are foods that should be consumed only occasionally. They are foods with added salt and sugar, such as many processed foods; those highly refined, therefore lacking in fiber; and those made with whole milk, for example, cheese with more than 5 g of fat per ounce.

Calories from food fuel the body. As people age, fewer calories are needed. Therefore the nutrient quality of the diet should be carefully considered. Those foods that are the most nutrient dense include whole grains, fruits, and vegetables. If the base for a person's diet comes from these foods, the following general guidelines for a healthful daily diet can be met:

60% to 65% of calories from carbohydrates

20% to 25% of calories from fat (7% to 10% of calories from saturated fat)

12% to 15% of calories from protein

2400 to 3000 mg sodium

Less than 300 mg cholesterol

UNDERSTANDING FOOD LABELS

The current food label, called *Nutrition Facts,* makes choosing healthful foods much easier (Fig. 1-2). Comparisons can be made, resulting in better decisions. The % Daily Value seems to be the most difficult for consumers to understand. It simply shows how a food fits in the overall daily diet. If a label states that a food only contributes 5% of the total sodium recommended for a day, it is obvious that food would be a good choice compared with one that contributed 30% or more, such as a serving of canned soup. The % Daily Value column is based on 2000 kcal and tells the consumer if the food is high or low in the nutrients of interest. A person's need may be more or less, but the numbers are still quite useful in making comparisons.

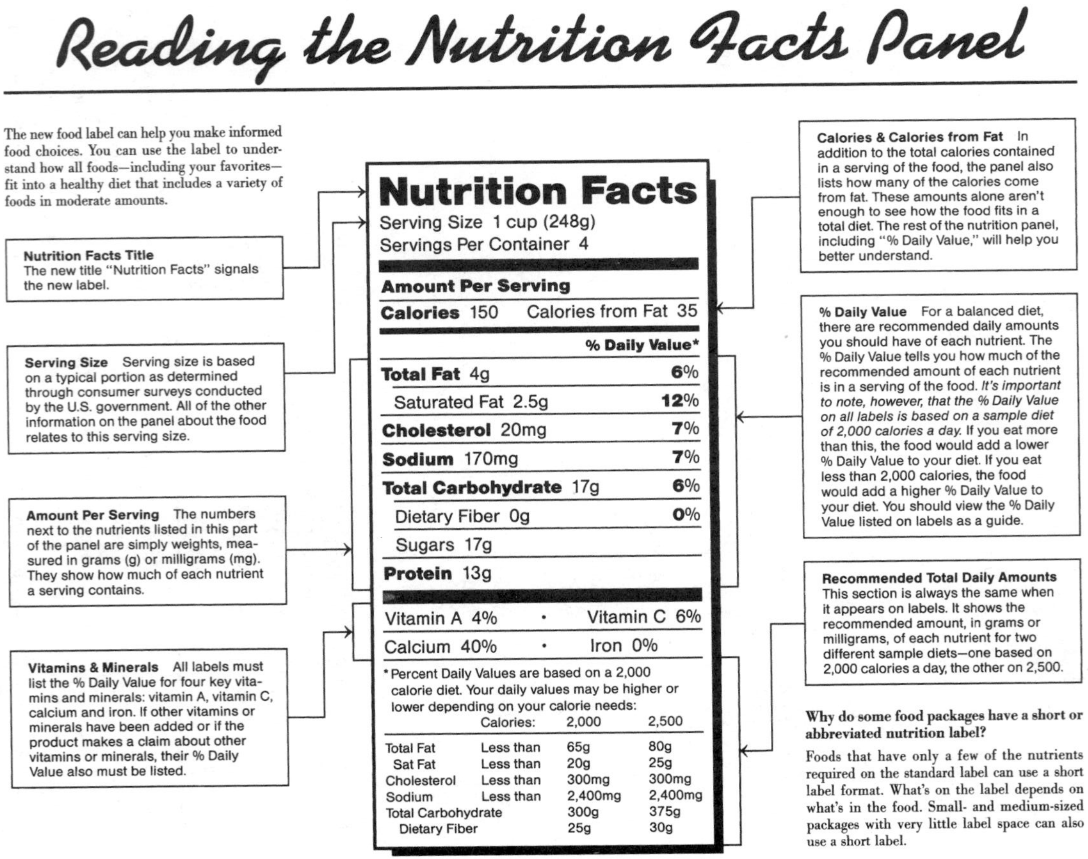

Reading the Nutrition Facts Panel

The new food label can help you make informed food choices. You can use the label to understand how all foods—including your favorites—fit into a healthy diet that includes a variety of foods in moderate amounts.

Nutrition Facts Title The new title "Nutrition Facts" signals the new label.

Serving Size Serving size is based on a typical portion as determined through consumer surveys conducted by the U.S. government. All of the other information on the panel about the food relates to this serving size.

Amount Per Serving The numbers next to the nutrients listed in this part of the panel are simply weights, measured in grams (g) or milligrams (mg). They show how much of each nutrient a serving contains.

Vitamins & Minerals All labels must list the % Daily Value for four key vitamins and minerals: vitamin A, vitamin C, calcium and iron. If other vitamins or minerals have been added or if the product makes a claim about other vitamins or minerals, their % Daily Value also must be listed.

Calories & Calories from Fat In addition to the total calories contained in a serving of the food, the panel also lists how many of the calories come from fat. These amounts alone aren't enough to see how the food fits in a total diet. The rest of the nutrition panel, including "% Daily Value," will help you better understand.

% Daily Value For a balanced diet, there are recommended daily amounts you should have of each nutrient. The % Daily Value tells you how much of the recommended amount of each nutrient is in a serving of the food. *It's important to note, however, that the % Daily Value on all labels is based on a sample diet of 2,000 calories a day. If you eat more than this, the food would add a lower % Daily Value to your diet. If you eat less than 2,000 calories, the food would add a higher % Daily Value to your diet. You should view the % Daily Value listed on labels as a guide.*

Recommended Total Daily Amounts This section is always the same when it appears on labels. It shows the recommended amount, in grams or milligrams, of each nutrient for two different sample diets—one based on 2,000 calories a day, the other on 2,500.

Why do some food packages have a short or abbreviated nutrition label?

Foods that have only a few of the nutrients required on the standard label can use a short label format. What's on the label depends on what's in the food. Small- and medium-sized packages with very little label space can also use a short label.

Nutrition Facts

Serving Size 1 cup (248g)
Servings Per Container 4

Amount Per Serving

Calories 150   Calories from Fat 35

	% Daily Value*
Total Fat 4g	6%
Saturated Fat 2.5g	12%
Cholesterol 20mg	7%
Sodium 170mg	7%
Total Carbohydrate 17g	6%
Dietary Fiber 0g	0%
Sugars 17g	
Protein 13g	

Vitamin A 4%	•	Vitamin C 6%
Calcium 40%	•	Iron 0%

*Percent Daily Values are based on a 2,000 calorie diet. Your daily values may be higher or lower depending on your calorie needs:

Calories:	2,000	2,500
Total Fat	Less than	65g	80g
Sat Fat	Less than	20g	25g
Cholesterol	Less than	300mg	300mg
Sodium	Less than	2,400mg	2,400mg
Total Carbohydrate		300g	375g
Dietary Fiber		25g	30g

Fig. 1-2 New food label.

The Reference Daily Intake represents the highest Recommended Dietary Allowance (RDA) for nutrients (Tables 1-1 and 1-2), notably iron for women, so that all individuals are covered. Reference Daily Intakes replace the U.S. Recommended Dietary Allowances.

There are specific requirements for product labels and terms used on the labels. These terms, which are descriptors, can help in making better food choices:

Free: an amount that is "nutritionally insignificant" and can be labeled as zero

Calorie-free: fewer than 5 kcal per serving

Sugar-free: less than 0.5 g per serving

Sodium-free: less than 5 mg of sodium per serving

Fat-free: less than 0.5 g of fat per serving, provided that it has no added ingredient that is fat or oil

Cholesterol-free: Less than 2 mg of cholesterol per serving and 2 g or less of saturated fat per serving

Percent fat-free: refers to the actual fat-free weight of a food and may only describe foods that meet the definition established by the Food and Drug Administration (FDA) for low-fat or fat-free products; the higher the fat-free percent, the better choice the product is

Low: would allow frequent consumption of a food low in a nutrient without exceeding the dietary guidelines

Low-sodium: no more than 140 mg of sodium per serving

Low-fat: no more than 3 g of fat per serving

Low in saturated fat: may be used to describe a food that contains 1 g or less of saturated fat per serving

Low in cholesterol: 20 mg or less of cholesterol per serving and the product can only have 2 g or less of saturated fat per serving

High: is 20% or more of the Daily Value; a Good Source is 10% to 19% of the Daily Value

More: this term means that a serving of food, whether altered or not, contains a nutrient that is at least 10% of the Daily Value more than the reference food

Reduced: this term means that a nutritionally altered product contains 25% less of a nutrient or of calories than the regular or reference product

Reduced-fat: must contain at least 25% less of the fat of the reference food (e.g., Reduced fat, 25% less fat than our regular brownie. Fat content has been reduced from 8 g to 6 g.)

Reduced saturated fat: must contain at least 25% less of the saturated fat of the reference food

Reduced-cholesterol: 25% less cholesterol per serving than its comparison food. The reduction in cholesterol must exceed 20 mg per serving. All claims of cholesterol content are prohibited when a food contains more than 2 g of saturated fat per serving. The label of a food containing more than 11.5 g of total fat per serving or per 100 g of the food must disclose those levels immediately after any cholesterol claim.

Reduced-sodium: the food must contain at least 25% less sodium than the regular product

Table 1-1   Recommended Dietary Allowances.[1] Food and Nutrition Board, National Academy of Sciences—National Research Council, revised 1989. Designed for the maintenance of good nutrition of practically all healthy people in the United States

Category	Age (years) or condition	Weight[2] (kg)	Weight[2] (lb)	Height[2] (cm)	Height[2] (in)	Pro-tein (g)	Vita-min A (μg RE)[3]	Vita-min D (μg)[4]	Vita-min E (mg α-TE)[5]	Vita-min K (μg)	Vita-min C (mg)
Infants	0.0-0.5	6	13	60	24	13	375	7.5	3	5	30
	0.5-1.0	9	20	71	28	14	375	10	4	10	35
Children	1-3	13	29	90	35	16	400	10	6	15	40
	4-6	20	44	112	44	24	500	10	7	20	45
	7-10	28	62	132	52	28	700	10	7	30	45
Males	11-14	45	99	157	62	45	1000	10	10	45	50
	15-18	66	145	176	69	59	1000	10	10	65	60
	19-24	72	160	177	70	58	1000	10	10	70	60
	25-50	79	174	176	70	63	1000	5	10	80	60
	51+	77	170	173	68	63	1000	5	10	80	60
Females	11-14	46	101	157	62	46	800	10	8	45	50
	15-18	55	120	163	64	44	800	10	8	55	60
	19-24	58	128	164	65	46	800	10	8	60	60
	25-50	63	138	163	64	50	800	5	8	65	60
	51+	65	143	160	63	50	800	5	8	65	60
Pregnant						60	800	10	10	65	70
Lactating	1st 6 months					65	1300	10	12	65	95
	2nd 6 months					62	1200	10	11	65	90

[1]The allowances, expressed as average daily intakes over time, are intended to provide for individual variations among most normal persons as they live in the United States under usual environmental stresses. Diets should be based on a variety of common foods to provide other nutrients for which human requirements have been less well defined.
[2]Weights and heights of Reference Adults are actual medians for the U.S. population of the designated age, as reported by NHANES II. The median weights and heights of those under 19 years of age were taken from Hamill PW, Drizd TA, Johnson CL, et al: Physical growth: National Center for Health Statistics percentiles, *Am J Clin Nutr* 32:607-629, 1979. The use of these figures does not imply that the height-to-weight ratios are ideal.

Less: This term means that a food, whether altered or not, contains 25% less of a nutrient or calories than the reference food (e.g., potato chips that have 25% less fat than regular potato chips could carry a *less* claim). *Fewer* is an acceptable synonym.

Lite/light: this descriptor can mean two things. First, that a nutritionally altered product contains one-third fewer calories or half the fat of the reference food. If the food derives 50% or more of its calories from fat, the reduction must be 50% of the fat. Second, that the sodium content of a low-calorie, low-fat food has been reduced by 50%. In addition, *light in sodium* may be used on food in which the sodium content has been reduced by at least 50%. The term *light* still can be used to describe such properties as texture and color as long as the label explains the intent; for example, *light brown sugar* and *light and fluffy.*

Water-soluble vitamins						Minerals						
Thia-min (mg)	Ribo-flavin (mg)	Niacin (mg NE)[6]	Vita-min B_6 (mg)	Fol-ate (μg)	Vita-min B_{12} (μg)	Cal-cium (mg)	Phos-phorus (mg)	Mag-nesium (mg)	Iron (mg)	Zinc (mg)	Iodine (μg)	Sele-nium (mg)
0.3	0.4	5	0.3	25	0.3	400	300	40	6	5	40	10
0.4	0.5	6	0.6	35	0.5	600	500	60	10	5	50	15
0.7	0.8	9	1.0	50	0.7	800	800	80	10	10	70	20
0.9	1.1	12	1.1	75	1.0	800	800	120	10	10	90	20
1.0	1.2	13	1.4	100	1.4	800	800	170	10	10	120	30
1.3	1.5	17	1.7	150	2.0	1200	1200	270	12	15	150	40
1.5	1.8	20	2.0	200	2.0	1200	1200	400	12	15	150	50
1.5	1.7	19	2.0	200	2.0	1200	1200	350	10	15	150	70
1.5	1.7	19	2.0	200	2.0	800	800	350	10	15	150	70
1.2	1.4	15	2.0	200	2.0	800	800	350	10	15	150	70
1.1	1.3	15	1.4	150	2.0	1200	1200	280	15	12	150	45
1.1	1.3	15	1.5	180	2.0	1200	1200	300	15	12	150	50
1.1	1.3	15	1.6	180	2.0	1200	1200	280	15	12	150	55
1.1	1.3	15	1.6	180	2.0	800	800	280	15	12	150	55
1.0	1.2	13	1.6	180	2.0	800	800	280	10	12	150	55
1.5	1.6	17	2.2	400	2.2	1200	1200	320	30	15	175	65
1.6	1.8	20	2.1	280	2.6	1200	1200	355	15	19	200	75
1.6	1.7	20	2.1	260	2.6	1200	1200	340	15	26	200	75

[3]Retinol equivalents. 1 retinol equivalent = 1 μg retinol or 6 μg β-carotene.
[4]As cholecalciferol. 10 μg cholecalciferol = 400 IU of vitamin D.
[5]α-Tocopherol equivalents. 1 mg d-α tocopherol = 1 α-TE.[6]1 NE (niacin equivalent) is equal to 1 mg of niacin or 60 mg of dietary tryptophan.
From the National Academy of Sciences: *Recommended Dietary Allowances,* ed 10, 1989, National Academy Press.

Fresh: can only be linked to raw food that has never been frozen or heated, or that contains no preservatives

Lean and extra lean: This describes the fat content of meat, poultry, seafood, and game. Lean means less than 10 g of fat, 4.5 g or less of saturated fat, and less than 95 mg of cholesterol per serving. Extra lean means less than 5 g of fat, less than 2 g of saturated fat, and less than 95 mg of cholesterol per serving.

ALTERNATE FOOD PLANS

More Americans are choosing vegetarian diets for health reasons or because of their cultures or beliefs. The Dietary Guidelines and the Recommended Dietary Allowances for nutrients can be met through a vegetarian diet (Fig. 1-3). Variety in food choices is the key to a nutritious vegetarian diet. Vegans, those who only

Table 1-2 Estimated safe and adequate daily dietary intakes of selected vitamins and minerals*

Category	Age (years)	Vitamins		Trace elements†				
		Biotin (µg)	Pantothenic acid (mg)	Copper (mg)	Manganese (mg)	Fluoride (mg)	Chromium (µg)	Molybdenum (µg)
Infants	0-0.5	10	2	0.4-0.6	0.3-0.6	0.1-0.5	10-40	15-30
	0.5-1	15	3	0.6-0.7	0.6-1.0	0.2-1.0	20-60	20-40
Children and adolescents	1-3	20	3	0.7-1.0	1.0-1.5	0.5-1.5	20-80	25-50
	4-6	25	3-4	1.0-1.5	1.5-2.0	1.0-2.5	30-120	30-75
	7-10	30	4-5	1.0-2.0	2.0-3.0	1.5-2.5	50-200	50-150
	11+	30-100	4-7	1.5-2.5	2.0-5.0	1.5-2.5	50-200	75-250
Adults		30-100	4-7	1.5-3.0	2.0-5.0	1.5-4.0	50-200	75-250

*Because there is less information on which to base allowances, these figures are not given in the main table of RDA and are provided here in the form of ranges of recommended intakes.

†Since the toxic levels for many trace elements may be only several times usual intakes, the upper levels for the trace elements given in this table should not be habitually exceeded.

Modified from the National Academy of Sciences: *Recommended Dietary Allowances*, ed 10, Washington, DC, 1989, National Academy Press.

eat food of plant origin and do not consume dairy products or eggs, will need to supplement their diets with vitamin B_{12}. Calcium and vitamin D supplementation will likely be needed, especially for growing children. Vegans must also give careful attention to iron, zinc, and riboflavin. Fortified breakfast cereals and whole grains are especially useful in meeting the needs for these nutrients.

The vegetarian diet is generally a healthy approach to eating, but it is not magical. It requires careful food selections but not to the extreme that was once thought. It is now known that complementary incomplete proteins do not have to be consumed at the same meal. A variety of foods that contain amino acids, such as grains, legumes, and breads, eaten throughout the day will supply the body with the necessary protein.

The vegetarian pyramid differs from the USDA Food Guide Pyramid in its emphasis on plant sources of the nutrients most likely to be missed when animal foods are not included. For example, soy milk with added calcium, vitamin B_{12}, and vitamin D is listed in the milk group and a specific recommendation is given to consume at least 3 teaspoons of added vegetable oil each day.

VITAMIN AND MINERAL SUPPLEMENTS

Making smart food choices can eliminate the need for vitamin supplements for most people. However, many people choose to take supplements and need to understand that high levels of some vitamins and minerals, notably the fat-soluble vitamins, can have toxic effects.

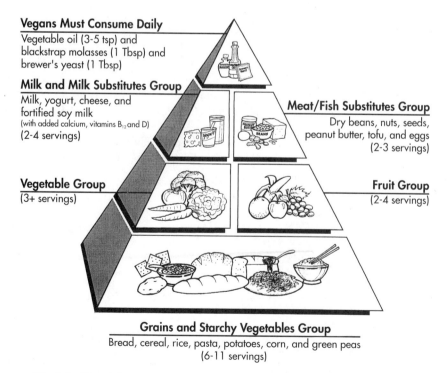

Vegans Must Consume Daily
Vegetable oil (3-5 tsp) and blackstrap molasses (1 Tbsp) and brewer's yeast (1 Tbsp)

Milk and Milk Substitutes Group
Milk, yogurt, cheese, and fortified soy milk
(with added calcium, vitamins B_{12} and D)
(2-4 servings)

Meat/Fish Substitutes Group
Dry beans, nuts, seeds, peanut butter, tofu, and eggs
(2-3 servings)

Vegetable Group
(3+ servings)

Fruit Group
(2-4 servings)

Grains and Starchy Vegetables Group
Bread, cereal, rice, pasta, potatoes, corn, and green peas
(6-11 servings)

Fig. 1-3 Vegetarian pyramid. (Courtesy A Sparks, New York Medical College.)

Foods contain all of the vitamins and minerals that most people need. Some individuals might benefit from nutritional supplementation in amounts consistent with the following definitions for replacement or supplemental vitamins and minerals. They include: habitual dieters of long duration, people who are ill and have experienced loss of appetite or impaired nutrient absorption, pregnant and lactating women, infants on formula not using a fluoridated water supply, and people with certain high-risk conditions such as anorexia nervosa.

A physician may prescribe supplements from the following categories:

1. Replacement or supplemental vitamins and minerals. These generally contain 50% to 150% of the RDA for the nutrients provided. Replacement vitamins are best used as supplements in patients at risk for the development of vitamin deficiency.
2. Therapeutic vitamins and minerals. These should not exceed 2 to 10 times the RDA for the nutrients included. Fat-soluble vitamins generally are present at 2 times or less the RDA. Therapeutic vitamins should be used for treatment of deficiency states or in situations where absorption and utilization of vitamins are reduced or requirements are increased.

RESOURCE LIST

The following resources offer free and low-cost nutrition information:

1. The American Dietetic Association Center for Nutrition and Dietetics, (800) 366-1655. Recorded nutrition messages available at all times. Registered dietitians available Monday to Friday 8 AM to 8 PM (ET).
2. USDA Food Survey Nationwide, 4700 River Road, Unit 83, Riverdale, MD, 20737, (301) 734-8457.
3. USDA Meat and Poultry Hotline, (800) 535-4555. Recorded food safety messages available at all times. Home Economists available Monday to Friday 9 AM to 5 PM (ET).
4. National Heart, Lung and Blood Institute, National High Blood Pressure Education Program Information Center, P.O. Box 30105, Bethesda, MD 20824-0105; (301) 251-1222.
5. Regional FDA offices. To receive information or to combat nutrition fraud and misinformation. Call district FDA for referrals on questions that local FDA cannot answer.

SUGGESTED READINGS

Achterberg C, McDonnel E, Bagny R: How to put the Food Guide Pyramid into practice, *J Am Diet Assoc* 94:1030-1035, 1994.

Food and Drug Administration: An FDA consumer special report: focus on food labeling, *FDA Consumer,* May 1993.

Healthy People 2000: national health promotion and disease prevention objectives, US Department of Health and Human Services, Public Health Service, DHHS Pub No (PHS) 91-50213, Washington, DC, 1990, US Government Printing Office.

Kritchevsky D: Dietary guidelines—the rationale for intervention, *Cancer Suppl* 72:1011-1114, 1993.

Nutrition and your health: dietary guidelines for Americans, ed 4, Washington, DC, 1995, US Department of Agriculture and US Department of Health and Human Services.

Rock CL, Jacob RA, Bowen PE: Update on the biological characteristics of the antioxidant micronutrients: vitamin C, vitamin E, and the carotenoids, *J Am Diet Assoc* 96:693-702, 1996.

2

Diseases of Modern Society With Nutritional Correlates

Obesity and body composition
Diabetes mellitus
Nutrition and cardiovascular disease
Nutrition and hypertension
Cancer
Oral diseases
Osteoporosis
Nutritional anemias
Eating disorders
Effects of alcohol on nutritional status

OBESITY AND BODY COMPOSITION

Overview—obesity as a health risk

Obesity is probably the most important nutritional problem in this country today. In the short time frame between 1976 to 1980 and 1988 to 1991, the prevalence of significantly overweight adults rose 33%. Currently over 20% of adolescent children and approximately one third of U.S. adults are overweight, and certain populations are disproportionately affected—nearly 50% of African-American women are overweight.

It is not clear if obesity is a direct risk to health, but it unquestionably increases the risk of other diseases, including coronary artery disease, diabetes, hypertension, and certain cancers. The overall economic cost of obesity is estimated to be over $100 billion a year. This problem has demanded a heightened focus in the health care practices of physicians on the comorbidities of obesity and their prevention.

Factors predisposing to obesity

It is almost certain that obesity has multiple causes and that there are different types of obesity. Although the mechanisms causing obesity are not completely understood, their net effect is an imbalance of energy intake and expenditure.

Genetic factors. Discovery of the ob gene in the mouse model has raised hopes that a gene or a gene product might be found that will directly help humans. This important discovery in inbred mice has important implications for our understanding of the causation of obesity; however, to date no genetic mutations

13

have been found that directly explain obesity in humans. Given the right environmental conditions, it has been clearly established in humans that certain familial traits contribute to one's predisposition to obesity, but these traits do not themselves account for the development of obesity (Fig. 2-1). It is also unclear how such genetic or familial factors predispose to weight gain. Currently, there is no firm data to indicate that an individual who is lean but genetically predisposed to obesity will have certain characteristics, such as specific taste preferences, metabolically efficient muscle fiber types, or reduced maintenance energy requirements. Having a genetic predisposition for or against obesity does not preclude an overriding environmental influence. In fact, regardless of one's familial or genetic predisposition, environmental factors such as increased requirements for routine physical activity or unavailability of energy-dense foods can prevent the development of obesity.

Neuroendocrine syndromes. Neuroendocrine abnormalities (Box 2-1) cause obesity in less than 1% of cases, and those that are more likely to cause obesity (e.g., hypothyroidism, Cushing's syndrome, polycystic ovary syndrome) rarely cause severe degrees of obesity. Thus markedly obese persons are least likely to have an underlying neuroendocrine disorder.

Abnormalities of energy metabolism. To contribute to weight gain, an abnormality in energy metabolism would have to cause a reduction in maintenance energy requirements. Thus, assuming that energy intake and voluntary physical activity remained the same, the metabolic disorder would have to reduce daily energy expenditure. There are three main components of energy expenditure: resting energy expenditure, thermic effect of food, and activity-related energy expenditure (Box 2-2).

Resting and total daily energy expenditures are somewhat variable among individuals, even when they are of the same size. Nevertheless, on average, energy requirements increase in proportion to the amount of weight gained, and heavier persons almost invariably have higher daily energy needs. Thus there is currently no consistent, convincing evidence that reduced energy requirements contribute meaningfully to the tendency of some individuals to gain weight.

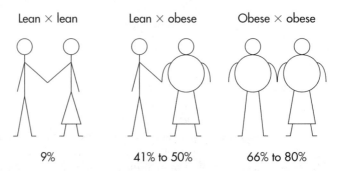

Lean × lean	Lean × obese	Obese × obese
9%	41% to 50%	66% to 80%

Fig. 2-1   Frequency of obesity among offspring of lean and obese parents.

Box 2-1   Neuroendocrine causes of obesity

- Hypothyroidism and hypopituitarism may cause moderate obesity, but the main contributor to excess weight in these conditions is fluid, not adipose tissue.
- Cushing's syndrome rarely causes gross obesity; typically, it has a truncal distribution.
- Castration and ovarian failure predispose to obesity. They are usually accompanied by hot flashes and other symptoms of vasomotor instability plus elevated urinary gonadotropin levels.
- Polycystic ovary (Stein-Leventhal) syndrome may cause a combination of hypothalamic and endocrine obesity. The syndrome is characterized by reduced or absent menses, moderate hirsutism, and weight gain. It usually develops in young women shortly after menarche.
- Insulinoma may predispose to generalized obesity. Typical symptoms of hunger and hypoglycemia indicate the need for further evaluation.
- Hypothalamic lesions resulting from malignancy, trauma, or infection can, in rare instances, cause weight gain by affecting appetite control. Massive obesity may result.
- Prader-Willi, Fröhlich's, and Laurence-Moon-Biedl syndromes are associated with childhood obesity, mental retardation, and failure of sexual development (Fig. 2-2 and Plate 1). Fröhlich's habitus (obesity and apparently delayed genital development) must be distinguished from true Fröhlich's syndrome.

Box 2-2   Main components of energy expenditure

- *Resting energy expenditure (REE).* Normally, REE accounts for more than 60% of total energy expenditure and is related most directly to one's fat-free (lean) mass, which is more metabolically active than fat mass. Since obese persons tend to have increased amounts of fat-free mass (to support the greater fat mass), they have an increase in REE. To date, most studies have shown that REE, adjusted for fat-free mass, is normal in obese persons and in normal-weight persons who are predisposed to obesity.
- *Thermic effect of food (TEF).* The contribution of TEF to total daily energy expenditure is only about 10% of energy intake. Although a number of studies have found TEF to be blunted in obese persons, the potential energy *savings* from an abnormal TEF is probably less than 25 kcal/day, an insufficient amount to explain the development of obesity.
- *Activity-related energy expenditure (AEE).* AEE normally represents 20% to 30% of daily energy expenditure, depending on the amount of one's physical activity. Although obese persons tend to be less physically active than lean persons, their AEE is not necessarily lower because they require more energy to conduct the same amount of activity. It is not known whether the reduced level of physical activity is secondary to their obese state or if it contributed to their weight gain. There is no evidence to date that obesity-prone persons tend to perform identical physical activities more efficiently (using less energy) than normal-weight persons.

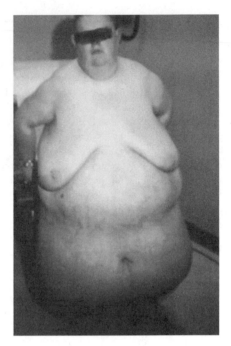

Fig. 2-2   Example of severe obesity in a patient with Prader-Willi syndrome. ▲

Exogenous factors. Exogenous factors that may predispose to obesity include dietary excesses and physical inactivity. One cannot avoid weight gain when calorie intake continually exceeds requirements, nor can one avoid weight loss when calorie intake fails to meet requirements. As noted previously, obese persons must eat more calories to sustain their increased body mass. However, studies of eating behaviors of obese subjects have failed to identify any consistent patterns of calorie intake, eating frequency, or food preferences that account for their obese state. More recently, attention has focused on diet composition. It has been hypothesized that dietary fat intake plays a key role in the long-term regulation of body weight. In this regard, an increase in body fat levels (fat storage) will occur when dietary fat intake exceeds whole body fat utilization (fat oxidation). Dietary fat may have a specific effect because fat oxidation does not increase in direct response to an increased fat intake. By contrast, when carbohydrate is taken in excess, it leads to an increase in carbohydrate oxidation, which reduces the tendency toward positive energy balance.

Large secular-trends surveys appear to indicate that average fat and energy intake in the United States have actually fallen since the late 1970s, even as the prevalence of obesity has risen. The increased availability and use of low-fat and fat-free foods has obviously not produced the desired effect. Data on physical activity are harder to obtain, but it would seem that the average level of physical activity must have declined significantly to account for the divergent patterns of an increase in obesity and a decrease in fat and calorie intake. It is illogical to expect that genetic factors alone are to blame for the increased prevalence of obesity.

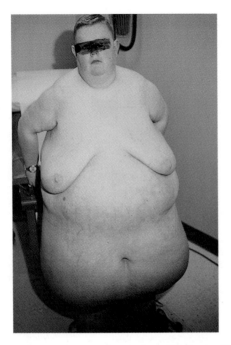

Plate 1　Example of severe obesity in a patient with Prader-Willi syndrome.

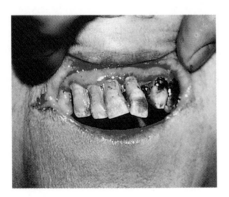

Plate 2　Periodontal disease seen in scurvy.

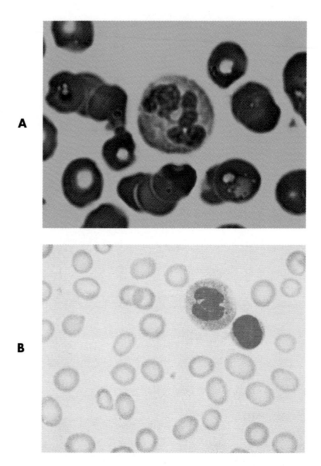

Plate 3 **A,** Blood cells in macrocytic anemia: notice the hypersegmented polymorphonuclear leukocytes. **B,** Blood cells in microcytic anemia.

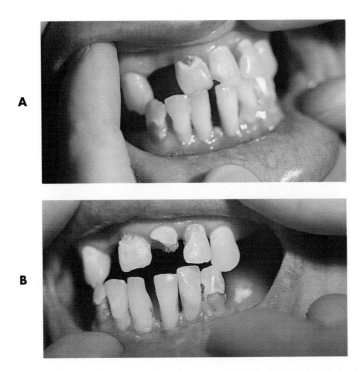

Plate 4   Progression of dental erosion resulting from induced vomiting in a bulimic patient.

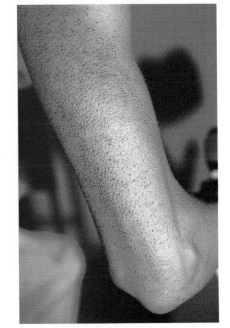

Plate 5   Follicular hyperkeratosis in vitamin A deficiency.

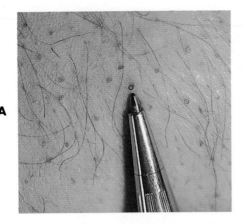 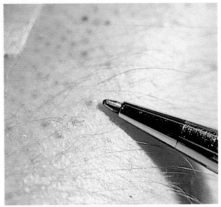

Plate 6 **A,** Corkscrew hairs in scurvy. **B,** Perifollicular petechiae in scurvy.

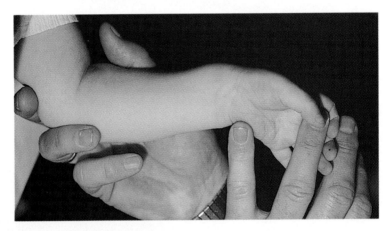

Plate 7 Radial thickening in vitamin D deficiency.

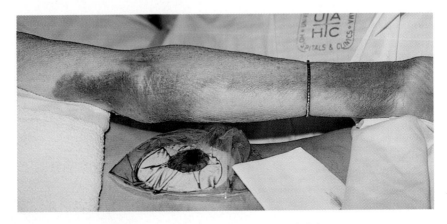

Plate 8 Easy bruisability in vitamin K deficiency.

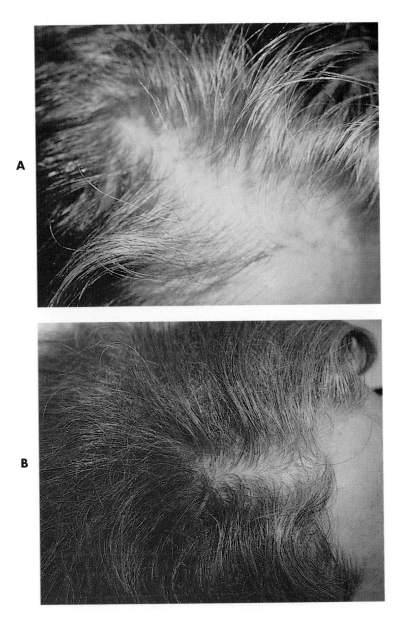

Plate 9 Alopecia before (**A**) and after (**B**) biotin therapy in a patient on long-term total parenteral nutrition without biotin.

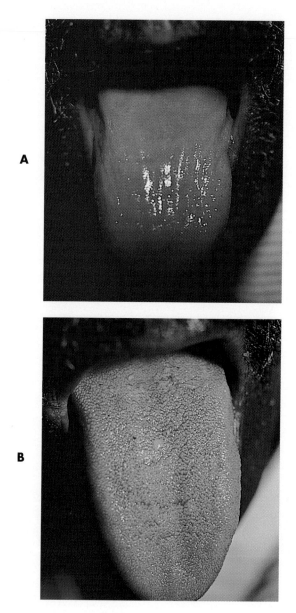

Plate 10 Depapillation of the tongue. Slick tongue before (**A**) and after (**B**) folate replacement in an alcoholic patient.

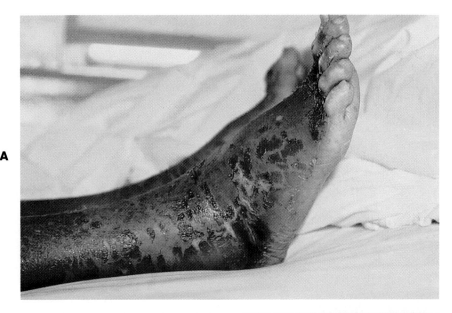

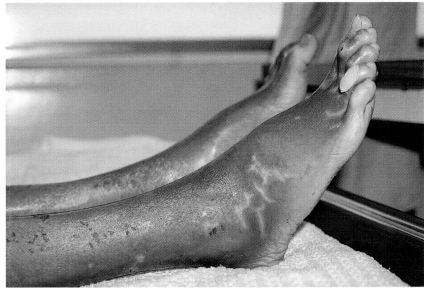

Plate 11 Clinical findings of niacin deficiency before (**A**) and after (**B**) therapy in an alcoholic patient.

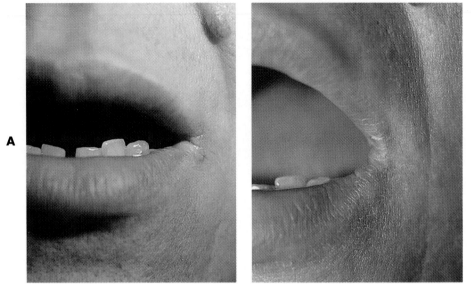

Plate 12 Angular stomatitis of riboflavin deficiency before **(A)** and after **(B)** therapy.

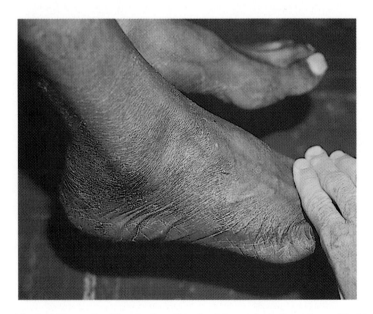

Plate 13 Inability to dorsiflex the foot (footdrop) in an alcoholic patient with thiamin deficiency.

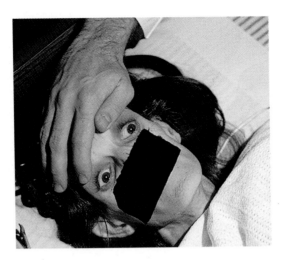

Plate 14 Paralysis of external ocular muscles (ophthalmoplegia) because of thiamin deficiency and phosphorus deficiency.

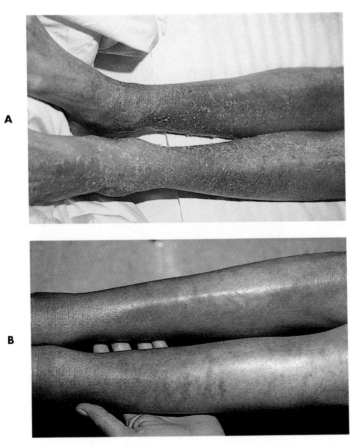

Plate 15 Widespread scaling of the skin before (**A**) and after (**B**) treatment with zinc in a patient with fat malabsorption.

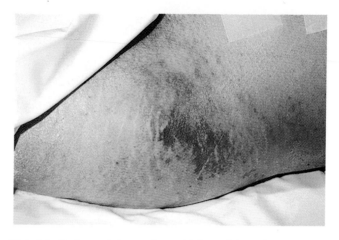

Plate 16   Ecchymosis in a patient with fat malabsorption syndrome.

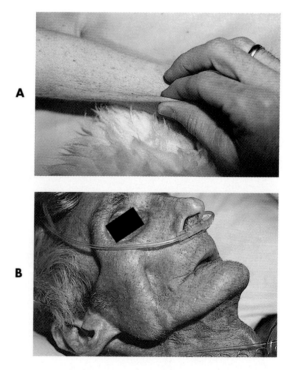

Plate 17   **A** to **B,** Losses of subcutaneous fat reserves and muscle mass in patients with marasmus.

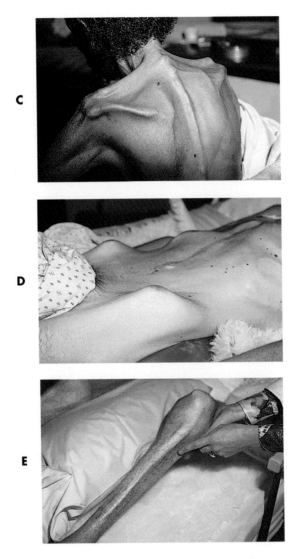

Plate 17, cont'd   C to E, Losses of subcutaneous fat reserves and muscle mass in patients with marasmus.

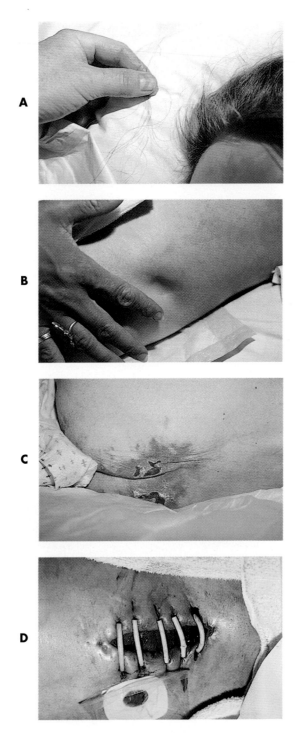

Plate 18 **A** to **D,** Clinical findings in kwashiorkor, including easy, painless hair pluckability, pitting edema, skin breakdown, and delayed wound healing.

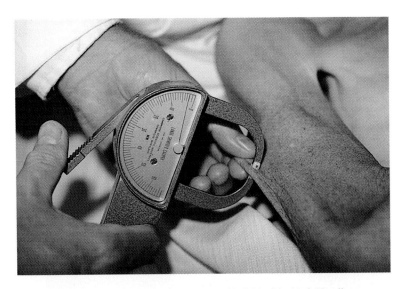

Plate 19   Measurement of the triceps skinfold with skinfold calipers.

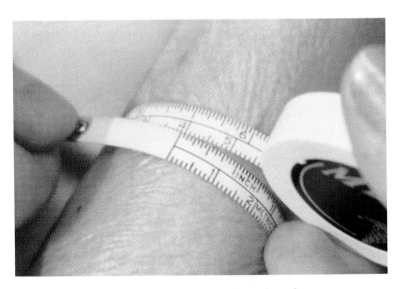

Plate 20   Measurement of the midarm circumference.

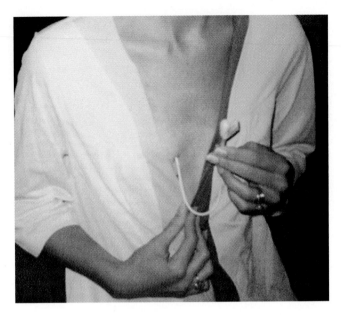

Plate 21   A specialized catheter used for home CVA.

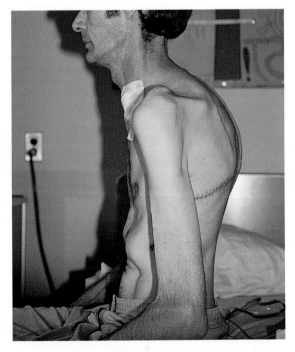

Plate 22   Cachexia in a patient with chronic obstructive pulmonary disease.

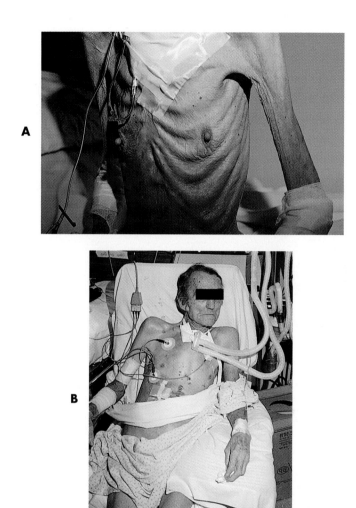

Plate 23 **A,** Patient A: history of weight loss. **B,** Patient B: history of respiratory failure.

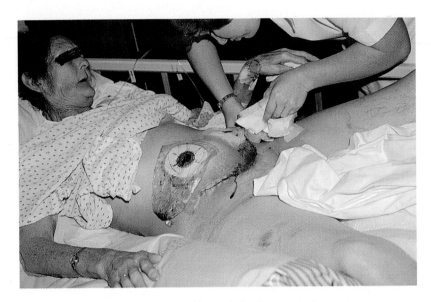

Plate 24 A woman with poorly healing surgical wound.

Clinical assessment of the obese patient

Assessment of degree of obesity. Normative values for defining obesity are not derived from data on optimum health. Nevertheless, it is important to attempt to classify individuals with reference to "desirable" weight. Earlier tables suggested that there was a J-shaped relationship between body weight and mortality; that is, leaner weights were associated with higher death rates. However, more recent studies that controlled for a number of confounding variables (including cigarette smoking, the biologic effects of comorbidities of obesity, and weight loss resulting from subclinical disease) found that lean individuals did not have excess mortality. A variety of data sets have been developed for reference weights, although currently none is considered ideal. Table 2-1 provides a currently used table of height-weight reference values for men and women.

Body mass index (BMI, weight in kg/height in m^2) is generally considered a more reliable index of obesity than the height-weight table. A useful guide for assessing health risk according to BMI is given in Table 2-2.

Measurement of body fat. BMI and ideal body weight present simple and useful clinical indexes of obesity. However, both of these indexes do not take into account the composition of body weight. It is conceivable, for example, that a large-framed individual with a heavy body weight may be classified as obese using the BMI or ideal body weight when in fact they do not have an excess of body fat.

In terms of chemical composition, the body is composed of five compartments: water, bone mineral, fat, protein, and glycogen. The terms *fat mass* and *fat-free mass* are often used to separate body composition into two compartments, fat and nonfat. There is no method to directly measure body fat content, but there are several techniques that indirectly estimate body fat from other measures. Clinically useful techniques include anthropometric measures, such as skinfold thickness, and bioelectrical resistance. Several equations exist for transforming these clinical measures into an estimate of body fat content. Research-based techniques such as underwater weighing and dual energy x-ray absorptiometry may provide more accurate estimates of body fat. For a more lengthy discussion of the various techniques, see the Suggested Readings listed at the end of the chapter.

Distribution of body fat. Body fat distribution is an important predictor of health risk, independent of the degree of obesity. The most convenient measure is the waist/hip ratio, where the waist circumference is taken at its narrowest point and the hip circumference is taken at its widest point. A ratio of greater than 0.80 for women and greater than 0.95 for men reflects an abdominal or android pattern ("apple" shape), which is generally associated with increased visceral fat and greater risk for hypertension, hyperinsulinemia, diabetes, and cardiovascular disease. Studies using computed tomography (CT) or magnetic resonance imaging (MRI) techniques have shown that fat tissue located within the abdominal cavity (visceral fat or intraabdominal adipose tissue) is the compartment of body fat that is most significantly related to the health risks of obesity. Intraabdominal adipose tissue is thought to play a key role in the metabolic risk of obesity, based on its increased metabolic activity together with its anatomic location. It is postulated that increased fat turnover within intraabdominal adipose tissue has marked effects on liver metabolism because of excess hepatic exposure to free fatty acids.

Table 2-1   Healthy weight ranges for men and women

Height	Weight (lb)
4'10"	91-119
4'11"	94-124
5'0"	97-128
5'1"	101-132
5'2"	104-137
5'3"	107-141
5'4"	111-146
5'5"	114-150
5'6"	118-155
5'7"	121-160
5'8"	125-164
5'9"	129-169
5'10"	132-174
5'11"	136-179
6'0"	140-184
6'1"	144-189
6'2"	148-195
6'3"	152-200
6'4"	156-205
6'5"	160-211
6'6"	164-216

From National Research Council, 1989.

Table 2-2   Body mass index

Grade	Height/weight (kg/m²)	Health risk
0	<25	Low or normal
I	25-29.9	Mildly increased
II	30-40	Moderately increased
III	>40	Markedly increased

Diseases associated with obesity

Regarding medical complications of obesity, it is important to keep in mind that not all obese persons have medical complications and the known comorbidities of obesity are not evenly distributed among obese persons. The fact that weight loss improves conditions such as hypertension and hyperlipidemia does not guarantee that the obese state was the primary or sole cause of the condition, since energy restriction or reduction in salt intake may have accounted for the changes. In distinguishing the contribution of obesity per se to overall mortality, a recent prospective study of intentional weight loss and mortality indicated that weight loss for the treatment of obesity reduces mortality when comorbid conditions such as diabetes, hyperlipidemia, or hypertension are present but is less likely to reduce mortality in the absence of comorbid conditions.

Osteoarthritis. Degenerative joint disease or osteoarthritis of the weight-bearing joints is more frequently seen in obese persons. There is also increased likelihood of osteoarthritis in the non–weight-bearing joints, suggesting that the arthritis may not be simply a direct result of mechanical overload. Regardless of whether obesity is the direct cause of the joint disease, it aggravates joint symptoms, exacerbates postural faults, and complicates treatment.

Cancer. Obesity has been associated with increased risk for cancers of the breast, cervix, endometrium, gallbladder, biliary tract, and ovaries in women and of the colon, rectum, and prostate in men. However, only cancers of the breast and endometrium are associated with obesity after statistically accounting for other risk factors. In the case of these two cancers, the mechanism may be related to elevated circulating estrogen levels in obese women resulting from increased conversion in adipose tissue of androgens (androstenedione and testosterone) to estrogens (estrone and estradiol).

Diabetes and hyperinsulinemia. There is a positive association between degree and duration of obesity and risk for diabetes mellitus. The prevalence of diabetes is increased about tenfold with moderate obesity and as much as thirtyfold with severe obesity. Elevated plasma insulin levels are uniformly found in obese individuals in both the fasting and glucose-stimulated states, reflecting insulin resistance. Despite this, not all obese individuals become diabetic. It is likely that obesity only causes diabetes in individuals who are otherwise predisposed.

Hepatobiliary disease. Obesity increases the risk of gallstone formation, probably by increasing fasting and residual gallbladder volumes with resultant bile stasis, and by increasing cholesterol production and bile cholesterol saturation, which enhances cholesterol crystal nucleation. Gradual weight reduction to a normal body weight normalizes risk for gallstones. By contrast, rapid weight loss can increase the chances of stone formation during the period of active dieting by as much as fifteenfold to twenty-fivefold over that of the nondieting obese population. This problem is discussed in Prevention and Treatment of Obesity.

Steatosis (fat accumulation within hepatocytes) is reported to occur to some degree in as many as 88% of obese individuals. Of interest is the fact that the hepatic fat content is not directly related to the degree of obesity, and caloric restriction can reduce the fat accumulation even if the obese state persists.

Hyperlipidemia, hypertension, and coronary artery disease. Most cross-sectional studies have noted a modest positive association between serum triglyceride and cholesterol levels and increasing degrees of obesity: high-density lipoprotein (HDL) cholesterol levels tend to be lower in obese persons. Weight reduction generally improves serum lipid levels during the active period of dieting, but the effect is largely due to energy restriction. On achieving a stable, reduced body weight, lipid levels partially rebound but tend to remain at an improved level as long as the weight loss is maintained.

In population studies, there is a small but statistically significant association between body weight and blood pressure. However, most obese persons are not hypertensive. Weight reduction generally improves blood pressure levels, but as with lipid levels, the most pronounced effect is from energy restriction (and probably an associated decrease in salt intake) rather than from weight loss itself. Maximum and permanent improvement in obesity-associated hypertension requires reduction to and maintenance of a normal body weight.

In general, obese persons are at increased risk for coronary artery disease. However, it is still unclear whether uncomplicated obesity is an independent risk factor for coronary artery disease in the absence of comorbid conditions such as diabetes, hyperlipidemia, and hypertension. Almost three decades of observation of the Framingham cohort suggest that body weight is a significant predictor of heart disease independent of other standard risk factors, although not all studies support this conclusion.

Respiratory problems. The obesity-hypoventilation or Pickwickian syndrome is characterized by marked degrees of obesity, somnolence, periodic apnea (especially during sleep), chronic hypoxemia and hypercapnia (carbon dioxide [CO_2] retention), and secondary polycythemia. The explanations for the inadequate ventilation and reduced functional lung volume are not clear, although there appears to be decreased efficiency of respiratory muscles, reduced respiratory compliance, decreased ventilatory response to CO_2, and increased pulmonary dead space and atelectasis. Complications include pulmonary artery constriction resulting in pulmonary hypertension and right heart failure. Even moderate weight reduction can reverse the hypoventilation syndrome. Periodic apnea can be caused by intermittent upper airway obstruction, distinct from the alveolar hypoventilation syndrome. Such obstruction often responds to surgical therapy.

Prevention and treatment of obesity

Currently, about one fourth of men and one half of women are attempting to lose weight, and they spend $33 billion per year on weight loss products and services. In fact, not all persons desiring to lose weight should do so, and not all treatment programs can be equally endorsed. Box 2-3 offers several criteria to consider in selecting a weight control program. Obesity must be treated like other chronic conditions such as hypertension or diabetes. It cannot be corrected by short-term interventions but requires ongoing effort and long-term support to help the individual establish and maintain control of the disorder. The goals are to establish permanent changes in eating habits and physical activity that become mutually supportive and self-reinforcing.

On the basis of risk for gallstone formation, a safe rate of weight loss has been recommended as an average of less than 1.5 kg/week and no more than 1.5% of body weight each week.

Weight cycling. Weight cycling, or *yo-yo dieting,* refers to repeated bouts of weight loss and regain. Weight cycling causes frustration on the parts of the patient and the therapist. However, with regard to physiologic effects, a recent review by National Institutes of Health (NIH) Obesity Task Force (see Suggested Readings) concluded that there is no convincing evidence that weight cycling has adverse effects on body composition, energy expenditure, risk factors for heart disease, or the effectiveness of future efforts at weight control. Since the average length of time to regain the lost weight is about tenfold longer than that to lose it, it can be argued that the net effect of a weight loss program, even if not permanent, is likely to be positive in terms of temporarily improving health risk. Obese individuals

---

Box 2-3   Criteria for selecting weight control programs

Patient selection

Special attention if:
<20 or >65 years old (younger and older patients may have special nutritional needs)
BMI > 37 kg/m^2
History of other eating disorders (anorexia nervosa, bulimia)
Avoid treatment if:
Pregnant or lactating
BMI < 20 kg/m^2
(NOTE: patients with a BMI < 25, a gynecoid pattern of fat distribution, and no co-morbidities may not be appropriate candidates for weight reduction)

Weight loss claims

Look for:
Prescribed rate of weight loss < 1.5% or 1.5 kg/week
Direct medical supervision for faster rates of weight loss
Outcome data of ≥ 1 year after treatment

Therapeutic approach

Look for:
Team skilled in diet, exercise, behavioral techniques
Diet emphasizing self-selection of foods from conventional food supply for long-term weight maintenance
Program of physical activity geared to individual needs
Behavioral modification, psychosocial support

Medical supervision

Recommended if:
Significant obesity-related comorbidities exist
Diet provides < 800 kcal/day

---

should not allow concerns about weight cycling to deter them from attempting to control their body weight.

Dietary management. The dietary approach must be based on a sound scientific rationale, be safe and nutritionally adequate, and be practical for long-term adherence.

Very–low-calorie diets are designed to provide severe energy restriction (<800 kcal/day) but sufficient protein to minimize loss of lean body mass. Protein losses tend to be less than with fasting but often continue to occur. The main concern about these diets is that they induce rapid weight loss that increases the risk of gallstone formation. They are sometimes useful for patients who are at substantial health risk from severe obesity (e.g., obesity-hypoventilation syndrome), where rapid weight loss is critical. Under these circumstances, direct medical supervision is important.

Moderately–low-calorie, balanced diets are appropriate for most persons desiring weight loss. Although they can have different characteristics, in general they should meet the three criteria outlined above, should provide at least 800 kcal/day (most often 1000 to 1200), and should emphasize low-fat, high–complex-carbohydrate foods. One example is the *EatRight* program used at the University of Alabama at Birmingham and currently published for public use. Using the concept of time-calorie displacement, the dietary approach is based on the spectrum of calorie densities of the various food groups shown in Table 2-3. The low-calorie, low-fat, high-bulk, slow-eating food groups to the right of the chart are emphasized.

Patients are given a list of foods in each category from which to choose according to their preferences. Most female patients who are moderately overweight are instructed to eat the number of servings indicated under each food group in Table 2-3, which provides approximately 1000 kcal/day. Fats are limited to a *maximum* of 3 servings per day, whereas the fruit and vegetable prescription is a *minimum* of 3 and 4 servings per day, respectively—with no upper limit. By encouraging liberal amounts of complex carbohydrates as vegetables, fruits, and unrefined starches, moderate amounts of low-fat meats and dairy products, and only small amounts of fat, satiety and nutritional adequacy are achieved with a low calorie intake and without counting calories. Sweets and snack foods are permitted up to 200 kcal/week as "special occasion" foods. Studies on the *EatRight* program indicate that it is nutritionally adequate, safe, and effective over the long term. It is also ideal for obesity prevention and, with very minor modifications, is appropriate for obese children and for people with diabetes.

Any dietary approach to weight control must emphasize lifelong changes in eating patterns rather than short-term use of a diet. The term *diet* implies temporary intervention, whereas the major challenge in treating obesity is not to lose weight but to modify eating habits to ensure weight loss maintenance.

Physical activity. Physical activity should be included in weight management programs, with the objectives of promoting fat loss while maintaining lean body mass and engendering permanent changes in lifestyle. Repeated studies have demonstrated that a program of routine physical activity is important to long-term

Table 2-3 *EatRight* approach to weight control

	High-calorie, low-bulk, fast-eating				Low-calorie, high-bulk, slow-eating
	Fats/oils	Meats/dairy	Starches	Fruits	Vegetables
kcal/oz	225	75	50	15	10
kcal/serving	45	110	80	60	25
Servings/day (1000 kcal/day)	<3	2½	4	>3	>4

From *EatRight lose weight: 7 simple steps,* Birmingham, Ala, 1997, Oxmoor House, (800) 884-3935.

weight maintenance. As a complement to energy restriction, increased physical activity provides the advantages of improving cardiovascular conditioning and insulin sensitivity and, according to some studies, maintaining muscle mass and bone density while weight is lost. Increased physical activity may best be achieved with a combination of regular exercises several times weekly plus daily "step-losing" activities. Step-losing behaviors such as walking or climbing stairs instead of driving or using the elevator, when routinely established, may be even more effective than programmed exercise in maintaining weight loss.

Behavioral modification and psychosocial support. Behavioral modification and psychosocial support should be included in weight control programs to focus on methods of establishing new behaviors, to incorporate standard therapeutic modalities including self-monitoring and cognitive restructuring, and to provide guidelines for maintaining weight loss. Modification of diet and physical activity patterns frequently requires psychosocial support. Keeping detailed records of dietary intake, exercise, and emotional factors is an important aspect of weight control and appropriately focuses attention on patterns and problems rather than pounds. An important aspect of behavioral support is to help the patient maintain a positive outlook and emphasize even small, positive behavioral changes rather than setbacks. What patients perceive as significant lapses are often no more than exaggerated responses to temporary indiscretions.

Drug therapy. Appetite-suppressant drugs include the serotonergic agonists (e.g., fenfluramine), serotonin reuptake inhibitors (e.g., fluoxetine, sertraline), adrenergic agents (e.g., phentermine, diethylpropion, and phenylpropanolamine), and agents with combined adrenergic and serotonergic effects (e.g., sibutramine). These medications have been found to be more effective than placebo in increasing the rate of weight loss. However, there are two precautions: (1) used singly or in combination, pharmacotherapy generally induces only a modest increase in weight loss over that of placebo, and (2) there are currently too few studies done to determine that available drugs are safe and that they sustain weight loss for periods beyond 1 year. It appears that indefinite use of the medication will be necessary for maintenance of the weight loss. Until more data are available on long-term safety and efficacy, pharmacotherapy is not indicated for the general obese population.

Surgical procedures. Surgery should be limited to individuals who have been severely obese ($\geq$100 lbs or 100% above desirable weight) for at least 3 years, who have serious medical conditions related to their obesity, who have failed repeatedly at attempts to lose weight, and who are judged able to tolerate the operative procedure. The jejunoileal bypass procedure, which was designed to cause weight loss by excluding approximately 90% of the absorptive capacity of the bowel, is no longer approved because of its high rate of complications. The currently used gastric reduction procedures are safer, but they do not necessarily result in patients achieving an ideal body weight. The latter still depends on changes in eating and activity behaviors. Complications of the procedure are primarily postoperative wound infection and postprandial vomiting.

DIABETES MELLITUS

Definition

Diabetes mellitus (DM) is a chronic disorder of metabolism, characterized by hyperglycemia resulting from the inadequate production or effectiveness of insulin. Diabetes mellitus affects approximately 14 million Americans. Each year 500,000 to 700,000 adults and 11,000 to 12,000 children are diagnosed with diabetes.

In 1979 the National Diabetes Data Group (NDDG) established several diagnostic criteria for diabetes. These criteria were revised in 1997. One criterion is a random plasma glucose level of 200 mg/dl (11.1 mmol/L) or greater, with symptoms of hyperglycemia, such as increased thirst (polydipsia), increased urinary frequency and volume of urine (polyuria), fatigue, increased hunger (polyphagia), blurred vision, and weight loss. Another diagnostic criterion is a fasting venous plasma glucose level of 126 mg/dl (7.0 mmol/L) or an oral glucose tolerance test (OGTT) in which the 2-hour plasma glucose level is 200 mg/dl (11.1 mmol/L) or greater. An OGTT is not necessary if the fasting plasma glucose level is 126 mg/dl or greater. A normal blood glucose level ranges from approximately 70 to 120 mg/dl.

Types of diabetes

Type I diabetes mellitus, also called *juvenile diabetes* or *insulin-dependent diabetes mellitus* (IDDM), accounts for 5% to 10% of individuals with diabetes. IDDM is most commonly diagnosed in children and young adults. It is considered an autoimmune disease because the pancreatic beta cells are destroyed by the body's immune system and the pancreas produces little or no insulin. The individual with type I diabetes mellitus is dependent on exogenous insulin to maintain blood glucose control.

Type II diabetes mellitus, also called *non–insulin-dependent diabetes mellitus* (NIDDM) or *adult-onset diabetes,* accounts for 90% to 95% of individuals with diabetes. The onset is typically after 40 years of age. Heredity and obesity appear to be significant factors in its etiology. This type of diabetes is often managed with diet and lifestyle changes, but drug therapies such as oral hypoglycemic agents or insulin may be necessary.

Gestational diabetes exists in women who develop glucose intolerance during pregnancy, usually between the twenty-fourth and twenty-eighth weeks of pregnancy.

Complications

Individuals with diabetes are at high risk for neuropathies and for small vessel and large vessel diseases, such as strokes, retinopathy, and nephropathy. The Diabetes Control and Complications Trial (DCCT) showed that good blood glucose control significantly lowered rates of complications. Although the study included only people with IDDM, researchers believe these findings are applicable to those with NIDDM.

Goals of nutritional therapy

- Maintain blood glucose levels as near normal as possible by balancing food intake and physical activity, using oral hypoglycemic agents or insulin as needed.

- Achieve and maintain optimal serum lipid levels.
- Provide adequate energy to maintain a normal body weight in adults, to enable normal growth in children and adolescents, and to meet the normally increased calorie needs during pregnancy and lactation.
- Provide optimal nutrition.

The diabetic food groups

The development of an individualized nutrition program is not only based on nutritional requirements but also on the individual's learning capabilities. The Exchange Lists for Meal Planning, developed and published by the American Diabetes Association and the American Dietetic Association, are used most often to develop meal plans (Table 2-4). The exchange lists are categories of foods that are nutritionally alike. Each food in the list can be "exchanged" for another food within the same category. In 1995 the exchange lists were reorganized to focus on the major nutrients: carbohydrate, protein, and fat (see Table 2-4). Starch, fruit, and milk lists are now grouped together as part of the Carbohydrate Group. Since a serving of food from any of these three groups contains approximately 12 to 15 g of carbohydrate, foods may be exchanged between the three groups. The vegetable list, in which one serving contains 5 g of carbohydrate, is also listed in the Carbohydrate Group. A new list created in the 1995 revision, Other Carbohydrates, is included in the Carbohydrate Group. Foods that contain added sucrose and fat (e.g., cake, doughnuts, cookies, potato chips) are listed in this group. One serving

Table 2-4   Diabetic exchange groups

Groups/lists	Carbohydrate (g)	Protein (g)	Fat (g)	Calories
CARBOHYDRATE GROUP				
Starch	15	3	1 or less	80
Fruit	15	—	—	60
Milk				
Skim	12	8	0-3	90
Low-fat	12	8	5	120
Whole	12	8	8	150
Other carbohydrates	15	varies	varies	varies
Vegetables	5	2	—	25
MEAT AND MEAT SUBSTITUTE GROUP				
Very lean	—	7	0-1	35
Lean	—	7	3	55
Medium-fat	—	7	5	75
High-fat	—	7	8	100
FAT GROUP	—	—	5	45

Food groups and nutrient composition taken from the American Diabetes Association and American Dietetic Association Exchange Lists for Meal Planning.

from this list has approximately 15 g of carbohydrate and is equivalent in carbohydrate to one starch, one fruit, or one milk. Meats are divided into very lean, lean, medium-fat, and high-fat categories. The Fat Group is divided into three lists (monounsaturated, polyunsaturated, and saturated fats) in an attempt to decrease saturated fat and increase the relative amounts of monounsaturated fats in the meal plan. An example of a 1200-kcal meal plan using the exchange groups is shown in Table 2-5.

Nutritional goals for IDDM

Management of IDDM involves coordinating insulin therapy with dietary intake. Individuals on conventional therapy of one or two injections per day need to eat at times that are synchronized with the time actions of the insulin. Individuals on an intensified insulin regimen of multiple injections or having an insulin pump have more flexibility in the timing of meals and snacks, as well as the amount of food eaten.

Nutritional goals for NIDDM

In overweight individuals, even a moderate weight loss of 10 to 20 pounds has been shown to reduce hyperglycemia and dyslipidemia. This is particularly important for individuals with an android pattern of obesity (increased waist-to-hip ratio), which is more likely to be associated with hyperinsulinemia and insulin resistance. Moderate caloric restriction (i.e., a deficit of 250 to 500 kcal/day) is recommended if weight loss is desired. Other important factors in the treatment of NIDDM are teaching the individual to improve food choices (such as grilled chicken in place of fried chicken or fat-free pretzels in place of potato chips), spreading carbohydrate intake throughout the day, and regular exercise.

Table 2-5   Example of a 1200-kcal diet using the diabetic exchange list based on 50% carbohydrate, 20% protein, and 30% fat

Group	Number of servings	Calories
Starch	4½	360
Fruit	3	180
Milk (skim)	2	180
Other carbohydrates	0	0
Vegetables	3	75
Lean meat	4	220
Fat	5	225
TOTAL CALORIES		1240

Group	Breakfast	Lunch	Supper	Snack
Starch	1	1½	1	1
Fruit	1	1	1	0
Milk (skim)	1	0	0	1
Other carbohydrates	0	0	0	0
Lean meat	0	2	2	0
Fat	2	1	2	0

Calorie and nutrient needs and carbohydrate distribution

Calories should be prescribed to achieve and maintain a reasonable body weight. A reasonable method to estimate caloric needs is a diet history of usual food intake, which is particularly important for children and adolescents. Table 2-6 provides guidelines for estimating calorie requirements based on desirable body weight (DBW).

There are limited scientific data on which to base recommendations for protein intake for individuals with diabetes. The American Diabetes Association recommends 10% to 20% of daily calories as protein. The remaining 80% to 90% of calories are then distributed between dietary fat and carbohydrate. The general recommendations for the U.S. population and individuals with diabetes is to limit total dietary fat to less than 30% of total calories, with less than 10% of calories as saturated fat and up to 10% of calories from polyunsaturated fats, the remainder of fat from monounsaturated fat. Since individuals with diabetes often have hyperlipidemia, the guidelines for the treatment of hyperlipidemia may also need to be followed. Studies have shown that a diet with increased fat in the form of monounsaturated fats and decreased carbohydrates (e.g., 45% to 50% carbohydrate, 30% to 35% fat, 20% protein) can lower plasma triglycerides, glucose, and insulin levels more than a high-carbohydrate, low-fat diet (e.g., 55% to 60% carbohydrate, 20% to 25% fat, 20% protein). However, the lower-fat diet may facilitate reduced calorie intake for patients requiring weight loss.

For many years the most widely held belief about the dietary treatment of diabetes has been that "simple" sugars (i.e., table sugars and syrups) should be avoided and replaced with unrefined and more complex carbohydrates (i.e., whole-grain bread, cereals, and pasta). This belief appears to be based on the assumption that sugars are more rapidly digested and absorbed than starch and thereby increase blood glucose levels to a greater degree. There is little scientific evidence that supports this assumption. More than a dozen studies have substituted sucrose for complex carbohydrates and found no adverse effects on blood glucose levels. Therefore the American Diabetes Association suggests that sucrose and other simple sugars may be substituted for other carbohydrates gram for gram in terms of diabetes control. However, it should be realized that a diet high in simple sugars may be low in fiber and other micronutrients and higher in energy density than a diet based on complex carbohydrates.

Sweeteners such as fructose, honey, corn syrup, molasses, fruit juice or concentrated fruit juice, dextrose, maltose, mannitol, sorbitol, xylitol, and hydrogenated starch hydrolysates have no significant advantage over sucrose. Sorbitol, mannitol, and xylitol are sugar alcohols that cause a lower glycemic response than sucrose and other carbohydrates; however, excessive amounts of these sugar alcohols may cause diarrhea.

Aspartame, acesulfame K, and saccharin are currently approved for use as nonnutritive sweeteners by the FDA. All of these sweeteners may be used in moderation by individuals with diabetes, although data are still lacking to show their usefulness for either the control of diabetes or body weight.

The American Diabetes Association recommends an intake of 20 to 35 g of dietary fiber per day. Soluble fiber (e.g., pectin, oat bran) is capable of delaying glu-

Table 2-6   Estimation of maintenance calories for adult

	Kcal required/lb DBW*	Kcal required/kg DBW
Men and physically active women	~15	~30
Most women, sedentary men, and adults over age 55	~13	~28
Sedentary women, obese adults, and sedentary adults over age 55	~10	~20
PREGNANT WOMEN		
First trimester†	~13-15	~28-32
Second/third trimesters†	~16-17	~36-38
Lactation‡	~15-17	~36-38
GESTATIONAL DIABETES		
Normal weight 120% DBW	~13-14	~28-30
Obese 120% DBW	~11-12	~24-25
CHILDREN		
Age 0-12 months	~55	~120
1-10 years	36-45§	80-100
YOUNG WOMEN		
11-15 years	~17	~35
16 and older (More with increased activity)	~15	~30
YOUNG MEN		
11-15 years	20-36 (mean 30)	50-88 (mean 65)
16-20 years		
Average activity	~18	~40
Very physically active	~22	~50
Sedentary	~15	~30

*DBW, desirable body weight.

May be estimated for women as 100 lb for 5 feet in height and an additional 5 lb for each additional inch over 5 feet in height.

May be estimated for men as 106 lb for 5 feet in height and an additional 6 lb for each additional inch over 5 feet in height.

10% of the total can be added for large frame and 10% subtracted from the total for small frame.

To estimate maintenance calories, multiply DBW in pounds by the calories required.

To lose 1 lb/wk, subtract 500 kcal from daily requirement or increase energy expended through exercise.

To lose 2 lb/wk, decrease calories by 1000/day or increase exercise. To gain weight, do the opposite.

†Follow weight gain on pregnancy weight gain grids to determine actual needs. Calorie level may need to be increased for women who are >40 lb above DBW. Calories based on DBW may not be sufficient to prevent starvation ketosis and for adequate fetal growth. Consultation between physician and dietitian may be needed for women whose estimated calorie needs are <1800 or >2500.

‡Follow weight; actual calorie needs may be less or more.

§Gradual decline in calories per pound as age increases.

cose absorption, but the ultimate effect on blood glucose levels is insignificant. However, the inclusion of soluble fibers especially as unrefined starch, vegetables, and fruit may be beneficial in managing elevated lipid levels and body weight.

Alcohol may be consumed in moderation by individuals with diabetes mellitus. Alcohol cannot be converted to glucose, inhibits gluconeogenesis, and increases the hypoglycemic effects of insulin by interfering with the counterregulatory hormones. Therefore individuals who take exogenous insulin or oral hypoglycemic agents should limit alcohol intake to no more than two drinks per day. One drink is defined as 12 ounces of beer, 5 ounces of wine, or 1½ ounces of distilled alcohol. Food should also be eaten at the time of alcohol consumption to prevent hypoglycemia. Individuals with NIDDM should recognize that alcohol provides significant calories (approximately 100 kcal per drink) and that alcohol can increase triglyceride levels.

Management of low blood glucose

Hypoglycemia, which is usually defined as a blood glucose level less than 70 mg/dl with symptoms of hypoglycemia such as shakiness, light-headedness, or altered sensorium, can be treated with a fast-acting carbohydrate. Causes of hypoglycemia in individuals with diabetes taking insulin or oral hypoglycemic agents include an imbalance of exogenous insulin and food intake, skipped meals or snacks, improper spacing of meals and snacks, alcohol consumption, and exercise. Treatment is initiated with 15 g of fast-acting carbohydrate such as glucose tablets, ½ cup of juice, or ½ cup of a sugar-containing drink. Blood glucose should be rechecked in 15 minutes. If blood glucose is not greater than 70 mg/dl, an additional 15 g of carbohydrate should be consumed. A snack or the scheduled meal should follow. Foods used to treat hypoglycemia are considered to be in addition to the regular meal plan.

Exercise

Exercise has many benefits for the individual with diabetes, including reduced hyperinsulinemia and improved weight control. Exercise-associated hypoglycemia can be a significant problem in individuals who take insulin or oral hypoglycemic agents, whereas those with NIDDM controlled by diet and exercise alone are not at risk of hypoglycemia when exercising. For individuals on insulin or oral hypoglycemic agents, a preexercise snack is recommended if blood glucose is below 100 mg/dl. See Table 2-7 for other recommendations on exercise.

Summary

There is no one "diabetic" diet. The best diet for an individual with diabetes depends on the nutritional assessment and treatment goals. Nutritional therapy for people with diabetes should be individualized, with consideration given to usual eating habits and other lifestyle factors. Monitoring metabolic parameters including blood glucose, glycosylated hemoglobin, lipids, blood pressure, and body weight is crucial to successful outcome.

Table 2-7   Food adjustments for exercise

Type of exercise and examples	If blood sugar is:	Increase food intake by:	Suggested food
EXERCISE OF SHORT DURATION OR OF MODERATE INTENSITY	<100 mg	10-15 g of carbohydrate	1 serving from fruit or bread group
Examples: Walking a half mile or leisurely biking for 1 hour	>100 mg	Not necessary to increase food	
EXERCISE OF MODERATE INTENSITY	<80 mg	25-50 g of carbohydrate before exercise	½ meat sandwich with 1-2 servings milk or fruit group
Examples: Tennis, swimming, jogging, leisure cycling, gardening, cycling, golfing, or vacuuming for 1 hour		Add 10-15 g per hour of exercise if necessary	1 serving fruit or bread group
	80-170 mg	10-15 g of carbohydrate	1 serving fruit or bread group
	180-250 mg	Not necessary to increase food	
	>250 mg	Do not begin exercise until blood sugar is under better control	
STRENUOUS ACTIVITY OR EXERCISE	<100 mg	50 g of carbohydrate *Monitor blood sugar carefully*	1 meat sandwich (2 slices bread) with 1 serving milk or fruit group
Examples: Football, hockey, racquetball, or basketball games; strenuous cycling or swimming; shoveling for 1 hour	100-180 mg	25-50 mg of carbohydrate depending on intensity and duration	½ meat sandwich with 1-2 servings fruit or milk group
	180-250 mg	10-15 g of carbohydrate per hour of exercise	1 serving fruit or bread group
	>250 mg	Do not begin exercise until blood sugar is under better control	

NUTRITION AND CARDIOVASCULAR DISEASE
Risk factors

Cardiovascular disease (CVD) is responsible for 40% of deaths and is the leading cause of deaths in the United States. Coronary heart disease (CHD), responsible for 65% of CVDs, has declined 2% per year since 1968 partially because of changes in diet and smoking. Among preventable causes of all deaths in the United States, smoking is responsible for 19% of deaths, followed closely by diet and activity combined, which is responsible for 14% of deaths. The extensive variation in CHD mortality among countries and the temporal change in the United States rates suggests a prominent role for environmental determinants, particularly cigarette smoking, diet, and activity.

Certain interrelated risk factors predispose to the development of CHD. Those risk factors are dyslipoproteinemia, elevated blood pressure, current cigarette smoking, diabetes mellitus, and increased age. Dyslipoproteinemia includes elevated serum apolipoprotein B (ApoB) lipoproteins, specifically very-low-density lipoproteins (VLDLs) (with elevated triglycerides [TG]), remnant lipoproteins, postprandial lipoproteins, low-density lipoproteins (LDLs) and lipoprotein(a) [LP(a)], and low levels of the ApoA-I–containing HDLs. Other established predictors of CHD include male gender, family history of premature CVD, truncal adiposity or insulin resistance, and physical inactivity. There is a positive curvilinear relationship of CHD deaths with serum total cholesterol (TC) and diastolic blood pressure. This dose-response relationship of TC and CHD shows an increase of 27% in CHD risk for each 10% increase in serum TC. An increment of 1 mg/dl in LDL-C increases CHD risk 1%, whereas a 1 mg/dl decrease in HDL-C increases CHD risk 2% to 3%. At any given serum TC there is a synergy with other CVD risk factors that increases CVD risk by severalfold.

Diagnosis of dyslipoproteinemia. The National Cholesterol Education Program (NCEP) has proposed a clinical strategy of diet or activity modification and medication in the highest quartile of CVD risk and a public health approach for lifestyle changes for the general population. The NCEP categorizes individuals at high risk if TC is greater than or equal to 240 mg/dl (LDL $\geq$ 160 mg/dl), borderline high if TC is 200 to 240 mg/dl (LDL-C 130 to 159 mg/dl), and desirable if serum TC is less than or equal to 200 mg/dl (LDL-C < 130 mg/dl). HDL-C less than 35 mg/dl is considered low and greater than 60 mg/dl is a negative risk factor. A borderline-high LDL-C with two or more CHD risk factors or a high-risk LDL-C requires clinical evaluation, testing for secondary causes of dyslipoproteinemia, initiation of diet therapy, and, potentially, medication. A patient with established CHD whose LDL is greater than or equal to 100 mg/dl should receive maximal diet therapy and be considered for drug therapy. For primary prevention the remainder of the population older than 2 years of age should be provided information on prudent eating patterns, physical activity, and risk factor reduction.

Impact of diet. Several long-term studies documented the direct influence of dietary factors on CHD risk not mediated by serum TC and blood pressure. Adjusted for age, cigarette smoking, and blood pressure, the absolute level of CHD at any given TC level differed threefold in the Mediterranean populations compared with the Northern European populations. Intake of saturated fatty acids and flavonoids explained 90% of the variance in CHD mortality rates. These results indicate that the relationship between diet and serum TC explains only a portion of the relationship between diet and CHD. The Mediterranean diet contained less meat but more fish, fruits, vegetables, and alcohol. This diet, low in saturated fatty acids and rich in monounsaturated fatty acid (MUFA), antioxidants, and phytochemicals, may beneficially affect LDL oxidation and thrombosis independent of effects on lipoprotein concentrations. Other long-term studies indicate that an increase in dietary cholesterol of 200 mg/1000 kcal is associated with a 30% greater risk of CHD, when adjusted for serum TC. The observed association was not mediated by the concentration of serum TC. Thus the mechanisms of these dietary effects on CVD mortality may be by way of fasting or postprandial LP levels, qualitative changes in LP composition or function, or in platelet and thrombotic tendencies. Changes in diet can have a significant effect on CHD mortality and total mortality. If a middle-age man were to modify his diet from 16% of calories from saturated fatty acids and a cholesterol intake of 300 mg/1000 kcal to 7% of calories as saturated fatty acids and cholesterol intake of 100 mg/1000 kcal, decrease his serum TC from 220 mg/dl to 180 mg/dl, decrease his systolic blood pressure by 20 mm Hg, and decrease smoking 10 cigarettes per day, the risk of CHD mortality would decrease by 86% with a decrease in all-cause mortality of 78%. Overall, this would give a man of 55 the same life expectancy of a 41-year-old man.

Pathogenesis

The underlying substrate for a CHD event is thrombosis, stimulated by rupture of an atherosclerotic plaque that has developed over several decades. Atherosclerosis is a dynamic, chronic inflammatory process driven by macrophage recruitment, foam cell formation, and foam cell death. The initial lesion is a fatty streak, a flat intimal lesion composed of subendothelial, cholesterol ester–filled macrophages on top of diffusely thickened intima. The intracellular cholesterol esters are derived from LDL particles with their phospholipid or ApoB modified by oxidation or entrapped by proteoglycans in the subendothelial compartment. LDL is a macromolecular spherical complex of lipids and protein with a core of cholesterol esters and a surface coat of phospholipids, cholesterol, and ApoB. Oxidation appears to be important in producing endothelial dysfunction and macrophage accumulation. Oxidized LDL also activates endothelial cell genes that change its actively anticoagulant, antiinflammatory surface into a procoagulant, proinflammatory surface. The ability of HDL to remove cholesterol from macrophages may be the basis for its protective role and its reputation as a negative risk factor. Some fatty streaks progress to fibrous plaques, lumen narrowing, and raised intimal lesions with a smooth collagen cap. These fibrous plaques increase in volume with proliferation of smooth muscle cells and degeneration of foam cells to produce a lipid core composed of cholesterol crystals. Inflammatory cells, especially T lymphocytes and macrophages at the periphery of the expanding plaque, can disrupt the collagen cap and expose the plaque contents to blood, triggering thrombosis. The clot becomes organized and incorporated into the evolving plaque, or it may cause an ischemic event resulting from lumen narrowing.

The key pathogenic factors are macrophage foam cell accumulation, smooth muscle cell proliferation, and thrombosis. A synergy between these factors stimulates plaque formation or regression. The determinants of these processes appear to be lipoproteins, endothelial dysfunction, platelet activation and aggregation, activation of the coagulation cascade, and inhibition of fibrinolysis. Both genetic and environmental determinants affect risk factors and control these related processes directly and indirectly. With significant lowering of serum LDL, plaques can regress by decreasing the volume of macrophage foam cells while maintaining an intact collagen matrix and cap that stabilizes the lesion. Lowering the concentration of ApoB lipoproteins, limiting their oxidation, and inhibiting thrombosis appear to be complementary strategies for regression and stabilization of lesions.

Effects of specific nutrients (Table 2-8)

Fatty acids. The saponifiable lipids in the diet are predominantly triglycerides that contain various types of fatty acids. Saturated fatty acids containing chain lengths from 8 to 10 carbons are medium-chain fatty acids. Longer-chain saturated fatty acids include lauric ($C_{12:0}$), myristic ($C_{14:0}$), palmitic ($C_{16:0}$), and stearic ($C_{18:0}$) acids. MUFAs include the predominant *cis*-MUFA oleic acid ($C_{18:1}$) and the *trans*-MUFA elaidic acid ($C_{18:1, n = 9 \text{ trans}}$). The polyunsaturated fatty acids (PUFAs) include two families: the ω-6 family, those with the double-bond six carbons from the methyl end of the chain, including linoleic acid ($C_{18:2}$), and the ω-3 family, including linolenic acid ($C_{18:3}$).

In the Seven Countries Study, the Japanese diet, which was very low in fat, and the Mediterranean diet, which was rich in *cis*-MUFA, were associated with the lowest rates of CHD. Saturated fatty acids raise serum TC, LDL-C, HDL-C, and TG. The effects are predominantly due to lauric, myristic, and palmitic acids with little or no effect from stearic acid. The increase in TC is due to an increase in LDL-C with a smaller increase in HDL-C. *Cis*-MUFAs are neutral on serum TC but appear to lower LDL-C while raising HDL-C. PUFAs appear to lower TC and LDL-C while raising HDL-C. *Trans*-FAs are not as well studied but appear to raise LDL-C and to produce a small lowering in HDL-C.

Cholesterol and phytosterol. Dietary cholesterol raises serum TC, with 80% to 90% of the increase in LDL-C and some increase in HDL-C. However, the relationship is curvilinear so that higher dietary intakes have progressively smaller effects on serum TC. Baseline dietary cholesterol is a statistically stronger predic-

Table 2-8 Effect of nutrients on CVD risk*

Nutrient/food	Estimated reduction in CVD risk (%)	Mechanisms
Cholesterol†	30% for 200 mg/1000 kcal/day decreased intake	Decrease postprandial LP
Fish	35% at 30-40 g/day vs. 0 g/day	Antithrombotic
Physical activity	50% if activity is 5-7 times the inactive group	Improve LP Decrease blood pressure
Dietary fiber	19%-26% for every 10-g increase	Decrease LDL
Alcohol	35% at 2-3 drinks/day (J-shaped)	Increase HDL Antithrombotic
Homocysteine†	38% for a 5-μmol decrease in plasma level	Antithrombotic
Folate†	40% for an increase from <6.8 μmol/L to >13.6 μmol/L	Antithrombotic
Vitamin E†	35% with supplement providing 200-400 IU/day vs. dietary intake of 3-6 IU/day	Antioxidant

*Clinical trials demonstrate that nutrients affect CVD risk factors or atherogenic biologic markers (e.g., platelets, clotting factors, homocysteine).

†Independent of effects on serum total cholesterol.

tor of change in serum TC than added dietary cholesterol. When baseline dietary cholesterol is increased, added dietary cholesterol results in diminishing increments of serum TC. This relationship suggests that the addition of 500 mg of dietary cholesterol (approximately two egg yolks) to a diet containing 100 mg of dietary cholesterol at baseline will increase serum TC 16 mg/dl, whereas the same two eggs will increase serum TC only 4 mg/dl if the diet contained 500 mg at baseline. The increase in serum TC is related to increased LDL-C resulting from decreased LDL catabolism by down regulation of hepatic LDL receptors. Only 40% to 60% of dietary cholesterol is absorbed, and a portion of the variable response between individuals relates to differences in absorption. Phytosterols (e.g., β-sitosterol), the sterol fraction in vegetable oils, are poorly absorbed and can block the intestinal absorption of endogenous and exogenous cholesterol on a 1:1 basis.

ω-3 **PUFA, fish oil, and fish.** The oils in fish include the very-long-chain ω-3 PUFA eicosapentaenoic acid ($C_{20:5}$) and docosahexaenoic acid ($C_{22:6}$). These fatty acids have several effects that may be antiatherogenic, including lowering of TG, decreasing platelet aggregation and clotting, and decreasing inflammation. These effects may be mediated by the incorporation of these fatty acids into phospholipids, altering prostaglandin production (particularly thromboxane) while increasing prostacyclin synthesis. Long-term prospective studies have suggested that men consuming 18 to 40 g/day of fish had fewer deaths and a 25% to 65% reduction in CHD after adjusting for usual CHD risk factors. Several prospective studies that have not observed any CVD protection from fish intake either had short-term follow-up or had few men who consumed no fish. In one secondary prevention clinical trial, encouraging 40 g/day of fish was associated with a 29% reduction in mortality but no reduction in reinfarction. Since seafood, unless fried, is generally low in total fat and saturated fatty acids, it is a good replacement for fatty meats and provides ω-3 PUFA in a CVD-healthy diet. However, for specific antithrombotic effects, aspirin or other platelet active compounds are more specific and active and better tolerated than fish oils.

Obesity and physical inactivity. Excess adipose tissue is an important CVD risk factor because of its association with dyslipoproteinemia, elevated blood pressure and blood glucose, and NIDDM. The entire complex of truncal obesity, elevated blood pressure, glucose intolerance, hyperinsulinemia, dyslipoproteinemia, elevated plasminogen activator inhibitor I, and hyperuricemia has been termed *insulin resistance syndrome* or *syndrome X*. These varied features of insulin resistance syndrome are more strongly associated with the amount of intraabdominal (or visceral) adipose tissue than with total adiposity.

The origin of this syndrome appears to be the capacity of energy excess and a certain sex steroid pattern to induce the accumulation of excess visceral adipose tissue. These adipocytes are particularly sensitive to lipolysis and release free fatty acids in the portal circulation of the liver, causing diminished hepatic extraction of insulin and systemic hyperinsulinemia. These free fatty acids promote hepatic TG and ApoB synthesis and VLDL secretion. The overproduction of VLDL causes increased LDL levels. Higher levels of visceral adipose tissue are associated with higher levels of hepatic lipase, which increases the conversion of VLDL to LDL and lowers levels of HDL. These changes are responsible for a dyslipoproteinemia characterized by high VLDL; small, dense, cholesterol-depleted LDL; high ApoB; and low HDL.

Obese adults often have serum TG levels 30 to 100 mg/dl higher and HDL-C 5 to 10 mg/dl lower than normal-weight patients. Even loss of small amounts of adipose tissue can significantly change the metabolic profile to improve glucose tolerance and to reduce serum insulin and dyslipoproteinemia. In general, the higher the TG at baseline, the greater the decrease with weight loss. Men may experience a greater decrease in TG and increase in HDL-C than women, and younger patients (<34 years of age) may have a greater decrease in LDL-C.

Physical inactivity is a significant CV risk factor, conferring a relative risk of 1.9 for individuals with sedentary compared with active occupations. This is comparable with the relative risk of hypercholesterolemia, hypertension, and smoking. Physical activity affects many physiologic and metabolic mechanisms involved in protection against CHD, including increasing glucose tolerance, insulin sensitivity, and HDL-C, while lowering TG, blood pressure, and thrombosis. Low- to moderate-intensity exercise can lower systolic blood pressure by 10 mm Hg and diastolic blood pressure by 8 mm Hg. Unfit men who become fit have a 44% reduction in age-adjusted all-cause mortality and a 52% reduction in age-adjusted CVD mortality. The general recommendation is for 30 minutes of moderate activity, for example, walking 4 miles per hour on most, if not all, days.

Alcohol. There is a J-shaped relationship between total mortality and alcohol intake with the lowest risk among drinkers who consume less than 3 drinks per day. A drink is defined as approximately 12 g of alcohol (e.g., 4 to 5 oz of wine, 12 oz of beer or 1.5 oz of 80-proof liquor). The lower risk is due almost entirely to less CHD. The results are variable between studies but generally cluster at two to three drinks/day providing around 35% protection against CHD and 10% lower total mortality. Approximately 50% of the protection of alcohol against CHD is mediated by increased levels of HDL-C (see Table 2-8). Another portion of the protective effect of alcohol may be an antithrombotic effect by increasing the prostacyclin/thromboxane ratio and decreasing fibrinogen levels and platelet stickiness. Alcohol raises serum TG, particularly among individuals with hypertriglyceridemia where it may increase serum TG 50 to 100 mg/dl. This increase in TG appears to be due to increased secretion of TG in VLDL. There is increased CV and non-CV risk among drinkers of greater than or equal to four drinks per day. Part of the excess mortality is due to hypertension. Alcohol intake is related to an increase of 1 mm Hg per drink per day in both systolic and diastolic blood pressures and may be responsible for 10% of cases of hypertension in the United States. Additionally, at higher intakes of alcohol, other conditions contribute to the higher mortality, including liver cirrhosis, pancreatitis, gastritis, trauma, suicide, certain cancers, cardiomyopathy, cardiac arrhythmias, hemorrhagic stroke, and degenerative nervous system conditions. Since increased health risks predominate in heavy drinkers (at least three drinks per day), they should reduce their intake or abstain. It is important when advising patients on alcohol intake to emphasize their overall risks. For young women without major CHD risk factors the other risks of alcohol should be of more concern. No one should be encouraged to increase alcohol intake. The general recommendation is that if alcohol is consumed, daily intake should not exceed two drinks for men and one drink for women.

Soluble fiber. Water-soluble fiber, that is, fiber that dissolves in water and forms a gel, is a component of many fruits, vegetables, and grains where they comprise 25% to 50% of the total dietary fiber. Beans and oats are particularly good sources, since soluble fiber is approximately 38% and 50%, respectively, of their total fiber content. These water-soluble fibers include pectin, gums, mucilages, algal polysaccharides, some hemicelluloses, and some storage polysaccharides. They are more effective in lowering serum TC than water-insoluble fibers.

The direct mechanism of action of soluble fibers appears to be increasing fecal elimination of bile acids and cholesterol. These actions stimulate hepatic uptake of LDL, thereby lowering serum levels. An indirect action of a diet higher in foods containing soluble fiber is the displacement of fat, particularly saturated fatty acids, from the diet.

The general consensus is that American adults should increase their total dietary fiber from their current mean of approximately 13 g/day to at least 25 g/day. This may have a significant effect on CHD, since a 10-g increase in total dietary fiber, particularly from cereals, is associated with a 19% to 26% reduction in myocardial infarction (MI) risk (see Table 2-8). In children and adolescents up to age 20 years, a reasonable intake is calculated by adding 5 to their age to estimate the number of grams of fiber required each day. These increases could be achieved with the recommended 6 to 11 servings of breads, cereal, rice, and pasta. Similarly, 5 servings of fruits and vegetables may provide an additional 10 to 15 g/day. A single serving of ½ cup of beans provides an additional 4 g of total dietary fiber. Taken together, a daily intake of 1 to 2 servings of beans, 5 fruits and vegetables, and 10 servings of whole-grain products would provide approximately 45 g of total dietary fiber and 15 g of soluble fiber. Overall, since serum TC may decrease 0.5% to 2% per gram of soluble fiber, this may be associated with a lowering of serum TC of 15%.

Soy protein. Soy protein is widely used in Asia at levels of 20 g/day in products like soy milk, tofu, and tempeh. As with soluble fiber, there appears to be a graded response with increased efficacy at higher intakes and with significant hypercholesterolemia. The mechanism of cholesterol reduction may include changes in the amino acid pattern, protein structure, or the content of isoflavones or phytoestrogens. Patients can consume 20 to 30 g/day of soy protein by consuming 2 to 3 servings per day and may lower serum TC 10 mg/dl.

Homocysteine, folate, and vitamins B_6 and B_{12}. There is a high frequency of arterial occlusion and venous thromboembolism in the inherited metabolic disorder homocystinuria. High serum levels of homocysteine have adverse effects on endothelial cells, produce abnormal clotting, and increase platelet adhesiveness and platelet aggregation. In the general population there is an association of high homocysteine and CHD. The commonly accepted range of plasma total homocysteine of 5 to 15 μmol/L includes levels that may predispose to atherosclerosis. The relative risk for CHD for an increase of 5 μmol/L homocysteine is of the same magnitude as an increase of serum TC of 20 mg/dl (see Table 2-8). Hyperhomocysteinemia (serum levels > 15μmol/L) acts independently of other known CHD risk factors but appears to be at least additive or even multiplicative with other risk factors and may be responsible for 4% of CHD deaths in the United States.

→ Folic acid is the most potent of the B vitamins in lowering homocysteine levels. Vitamin B_{12}, a remethylation cofactor rather than cosubstrate, would be expected to have little effect to reduce homocysteine levels. Low dietary intake is the most common cause of compromised folate status, and 88% of American adults consume less than 400 µg/day. Concentrations of homocysteine reach a reduced plateau when folate intakes approach 400 µg/day and serum folate reaches about 15 µmol/L. At these levels of serum folate, that is, the highest quartiles, the risk of CHD is 40% lower than at levels of serum folate less than 6.8 µmol/L in the lowest quartile (see Table 2-8). Fortification of flour is currently mandated for 1998 at a level that will increase intake by approximately 100 µg/day, which would lead to a 1- to 4-µmol/L decline in serum total homocysteine levels. Animal protein is particularly rich in methionine, which is associated with increased homocysteine levels. Reasonable dietary changes would be to reduce meat to reduce methionine intake and to increase vegetables and legumes to increase folic acid intake.

Antioxidants and oxidants. A body of evidence from epidemiologic and basic studies has generated the *oxidation hypothesis*, which states that oxidative modification of LDL and other lipoproteins is important for the development of atherosclerosis and that inhibitors of LDL oxidation will decrease atherosclerosis and its clinical sequelae. This hypothesis is intriguing and promising but not yet proven by well-designed clinical trials. In two large observational studies of male and female health professionals, intakes of vitamin E supplements were associated with a 35% reduction in CHD after adjustment for other CHD risk factors and use of multivitamins, β-carotene, and vitamin C (see Table 2-8). Neither study was able to control for lipoprotein levels, and the only lipid data were self-reported histories of high serum TC. The protective effects of antioxidants are biologically plausible based on the link of oxidation of LDL and foam cell formation. Vitamin C may be synergistic with vitamin E in antioxidant efficacy. Other contributing dietary factors, for example, copper, zinc, manganese, and selenium, are cofactors for cellular antioxidant enzymes including superoxide dismutase and glutathione peroxidase, which may limit cytotoxicity.

The diet also provides another type of phytochemical antioxidant, the flavonoids. Flavonoids are scavengers of free radicals such as superoxide anions and lipid peroxy radicals and will thus interrupt radical chain reactions and reduce oxidation of LDL and its effects.

Iron as a promoter of oxidation has been suggested to play a role in CHD, but the evidence linking iron stores, iron intake, and overall iron nutritional status to the risk of CHD is inconsistent.

Diet therapy

Individual variability. Serum TC levels undergo biologic variation of approximately 10% around the true mean. Lipid measurements also are subject to random day-to-day variation. The clinical significance of these two sources of variations is that the means of at least several measurements on each diet must be used to define individual responsiveness to a diet.

Overall, the range of true responses to diet in individuals is normally distributed so that if the average decrease in serum TC is 22 mg/dl, less than 10% of patients will have less than an 11 mg/dl decrease and 10% of patients will have greater than a 33 mg/dl decrease. Patients who do not improve their lipoprotein profile after dietary therapy should have their compliance to the diet reviewed and weight loss encouraged, if appropriate.

NCEP diets. The NCEP has recommended two therapeutic diets to control elevated levels of LDL-C (Table 2-9). The Step 1 diet has the same dietary goals as for the general population. The Step 2 diet further restricts the intake of saturated fatty acids and cholesterol. The main sources of saturated fatty acids and cholesterol in the U.S. diet are fatty meats, dairy products, snacks and baked goods, and cooking fats. A general therapeutic principle is to use smaller portions or lower saturated fatty acids items or both in each main source for that individual. Examples include low-fat ground beef (<10% fat) in place of regular ground beef, skim or 1% milk in place of whole milk, low-fat cheeses (<5 g/oz) in place of regular cheeses, low-saturated-fatty-acid snacks and baked foods, and low-saturated-fatty-acid oils (<20% saturated fatty acids; e.g., canola oil or corn oil in place of butter). Also, it is appropriate to reduce the intake of hydrogenated oils, since they may have a significant *trans*-FA content. Current *trans*-FA intake is 3% of calories. The fat substitute Olestra is likely to have limited therapeutic efficacy for weight loss or saturated fatty acid replacement unless used in large amounts, in which case it may compromise lipophilic antioxidant status and produce gastrointestinal distress and fecal leakage. Cholesterol is found only in animal products, and its sources are similar to those for saturated fatty acids but also include egg yolks. These can be replaced with egg substitutes or limited to at most four yolks/week (Step 1) and at most 2 yolks/week (Step 2).

Optimal diet. There are nutrient effects that are mediated through serum TC and lipoproteins, truncal adiposity and hypertension, and effects that are likely to be independent of these risk factors. These other effectors may affect oxidation of lipoprotein, homocysteine levels, thrombogenesis, insulin levels, endothelial relaxing factor, arterial inflammation, or other yet-to-be described mechanisms. It

Table 2-9   Dietary recommendations for lowering serum LDL-C (NCEP)

Nutrient	Step 1 diet	Step 2 diet	Average American*
Fat, % energy	≤30	≤30	34-36
SFA, % energy	<10	<7	13-14
MUFA, % energy	<15	<15	14-15
PUFA, % energy	<10	<10	5-6
Cholesterol, mg	≤300	≤200	360 (men)
			220-260 (women)
			200-300 (children)
Carbohydrate, % energy	≥55	≥55	~50
Protein, % energy	~15	~15	14-15

*National Health and Nutrition Examination Survey III (1988-1991).

is helpful for the health care provider to suggest priorities for the patient to modify diet and activity. The foremost priorities are to eliminate cigarette smoking, achieve an ideal body weight, and decrease saturated fatty acids and cholesterol in the diet. For both saturated fatty acids and cholesterol, there are no minimum requirements. Thus it is likely that the lower they are the better, and patients can be encouraged to progressively decrease their intake gradually to levels of saturated fatty acids no more than 4% of calories and cholesterol less than 100 mg/day. The elimination of obesity by decreasing dietary fat to less than 20% of calories and increasing physical activity is a valuable complement to the lowering of saturated fatty acids and cholesterol. The diet should be rich in fruits and vegetables (≥8 servings/day based on energy intake) and whole grain products (10 to 12 servings/day). The protein sources and amounts can shift to a greater dependence on plant sources including soybeans and other beans, since there is no requirement for meat. Starting these dietary changes in childhood is likely to provide the greatest benefit in protection against CVD. The diet should remain nutritionally adequate and support normal growth and development. Daily supplements of folic acid (400 to 1000 μg), vitamin E (400 IU), and vitamin C (1000 mg) have not been proved to be beneficial, but the potential benefit-to-risk ratio appears favorable. Patients should have their lipoprotein level and blood pressure measured every several years starting in childhood. Those individuals who develop these risk factors on a program of diet and activity may require pharmacologic therapy.

NUTRITION AND HYPERTENSION

Approximately 50 million people in the United States have hypertension. The prevalence of hypertension increases with age, and it is more common in African-Americans, in lower socioeconomic groups, and in the southeastern United States. Hypertension is a risk factor for CHD, stroke, renal disease, and overall mortality. The risks associated with hypertension increase independently with increasing systolic and diastolic blood pressures. Much progress has been made over the past 25 years in the detection and treatment of hypertension, which has probably contributed to the decrease in CHD and stroke observed during this same period. However, there still exists a large number of people with undetected and uncontrolled hypertension. Up to one third of people with hypertension are unaware of this condition, and up to one half of hypertensive patients are not on treatment. The classification of hypertension is outlined in Table 2-10. Over 90% of hypertension is essential, or without a known cause. Despite the lack of a specific cause in most cases, dietary modifications can potentially have a substantial effect in the treatment and prevention of hypertension.

Nutritional correlates with hypertension

Increasing body weight increases the risk of hypertension, although not all obese individuals develop hypertension. Individuals with a predominantly upper-body fat distribution (abdominal obesity, "apple" shape) have an increased risk of developing hypertension compared with individuals with a lower-body fat distribution (gluteal obesity, "pear" shape).

Table 2-10 Classification of blood pressure in adults*

Category	Systolic blood pressure	Diastolic blood pressure
Optimal	<120	<80
Normal	<135	<85
High normal	130-139	85-89
Hypertension		
Stage I (mild)	140-159	90-99
Stage II (moderate)	160-179	100-109
Stage III (severe)	180-209	110-119
Stage IV (very severe)	>210	>120

*Adapted from National Institutes of Health: *The Fifth Report of the Joint National Committee on Detection, Evaluation, and Treatment of High Blood Pressure,* NIH Pub No 95-1088, 1995.

In general, epidemiologic and clinical studies support a direct association between dietary sodium intake and blood pressure. This association is seen mainly with sodium chloride and not with other forms of sodium such as sodium bicarbonate or sodium ascorbate. However, most of the sodium consumed is as the chloride salt (i.e., table salt). The obligate dietary requirement for sodium is only about 200 mg/day, yet the average intake in the United States is over 4000 mg/day. Because virtually everyone in the United States has a relatively high intake of sodium, it may be that only susceptible individuals develop hypertension. Similarly, individuals vary in their responsiveness to dietary sodium restriction. Although African-Americans and the elderly may be more sodium sensitive than the general population, sodium sensitivity cannot be predicted in an individual.

In many studies an inverse association has been demonstrated between blood pressure and intake of potassium, calcium, and magnesium. Calcium supplementation may lead to a small decrease in systolic (<2 mm Hg on average) but not in diastolic blood pressure. Similar to sodium restriction, it may be that certain subgroups of people are more likely to respond to supplementation with calcium. However, unless deficiency or decreased intake of a nutrient is present, current evidence does not justify supplementation with isolated nutrients to treat or prevent hypertension in the general population. An increased intake of foods that are good sources of these nutrients may be beneficial for both treatment and prevention. Fruits and vegetables are good sources of potassium; low-fat dairy products, some types of fish (canned with bones), leafy green vegetables, broccoli, and nuts are good sources of calcium; and grains, nuts, and leafy green vegetables are good sources of magnesium.

Compared with saturated fats, polyunsaturated fats may slightly lower blood pressure. ω-3 fatty acids (fish oil) may also lower blood pressure when consumed in large amounts. However, it should be remembered that fats are high in energy density and may contribute to weight gain.

Vegetarians have a lower prevalence of hypertension than the general population. The specific mechanisms responsible for this association are not clear but are probably due to the combined effects of this overall pattern of eating rather than one or two isolated nutrients. Potentially beneficial reasons include a decreased intake of sodium, total calories, and saturated fat and an increased intake of fiber, polyunsaturated fats, and foods high in potassium and magnesium. In addition, vegetarians tend to weigh less than the general population.

It has been suggested that dietary fiber is inversely related to blood pressure, although evidence is inconclusive. Caffeine may exert an acute hypertensive effect, but tolerance develops rapidly in people who consume it regularly.

Treatment and prevention

The assessment of a patient with elevated blood pressure should include a diet and exercise history. If there are reasons from the history or physical examination to suspect a secondary cause, this should be evaluated. Initial treatment should include lifestyle changes and focus on four main areas: weight loss, regular exercise, and dietary restriction of salt and alcohol. Beneficial changes in these areas may prevent the need for medications or decrease the amount of medications required.

Weight loss in obese individuals has the largest potential effect toward lowering blood pressure. Decreased alcohol consumption in people who consume alcohol regularly will also have a large effect in lowering blood pressure. Although some recommendations are for no more than one to two drinks per day as a reasonable goal, the more that alcohol intake is decreased, the lower the blood pressure response will be. Salt restriction may lower blood pressure in hypertensive patients if the individual is salt sensitive. It has been recommended that hypertensive patients should attempt to decrease sodium intake to 2300 mg/day (2300 mg sodium equals 6000 mg sodium chloride, which equals 100 mmol sodium; Table 2-11). The greatest contributors to salt intake in the diet are canned, boxed, or frozen convenience foods (Box 2-4). For this reason, it is important to read labels to help monitor salt intake. After a few months of lower sodium intake, taste preferences change and individuals become more comfortable with a reduced intake, which can help facilitate long-term compliance. Aerobic exercise may help decrease body weight and also has a modest independent effect on lowering blood pressure. Patients should be encouraged to make whatever lifestyle changes they can comfortably make in these areas, keeping in mind that maintaining these changes indefinitely is the primary goal.

The same beneficial lifestyle modifications used to treat hypertension may help prevent it. Population changes in these areas may lead to lower blood pressure values, although it may be impossible to predict which individuals will be favorably affected. Subjects with high normal blood pressure or a family history of hypertension should particularly consider adopting these healthy lifestyle behaviors.

In summary, lifestyle habits that may help prevent high blood pressure include maintaining a healthy body weight; performing regular aerobic exercise; ingesting minimal amounts of alcohol; and consuming a diet high in unprocessed plant products such as fruits, vegetables, legumes, and whole grains, which are low in sodium and high in potassium, magnesium, calcium, and fiber. These lifestyle changes are compatible with other recommendations for disease prevention and therefore may contribute to decreased risk of diseases such as CHD and cancer.

Table 2-11 Modified diets—sodium

Daily sodium (Na) intake*	Food limitations	Practicality
5 to 6 g Na (12.5 to 15 g salt)	Includes table salt, heavily or visibly salted items	Average American diet
4 g Na (10 g salt)	No additional salt on tray or at table	Practical for home use
3 g Na (7.5 g salt)	Food only lightly salted in preparation; restrict heavily or visibly salted items (potato chips, pretzels, crackers, pickles, olives, relishes, sauces, most soups); no salt on tray	Practical for home use
2 g Na (5 g salt)	Above limitations plus no salt in food preparation; avoid most processed foods (canned foods, dry cereals, luncheon meats, bacon, ham, cheese) unless calculated into diet; regular bread, butter, milk in limited amounts	Fairly practical for home use with cooperative patient
1 g Na (2.5 g salt)	Above limitations plus use of only salt-free bread	Practical for home use with only unusually cooperative patient
0.5 g Na (1.25 g salt)	Above limitations plus limitation of meat (4 oz/day), eggs, some vegetables; milk (1 pt/day) and salt-free butter allowed	Not practical for home use

*1 g Na = 43 mEq; 1 mEq Na = 23 mg; 1 g Na = 2.5 g NaCl.

CANCER

The links between diet and cancer have received much attention in both scientific and lay literature in recent years. Although there is evidence that a large number of nutrients modify the development of malignancies, the relative magnitude of the individual and collective effects of nutrients is still unclear. Because cancer is the second leading cause of death in the United States, and because survival rates from the deadliest forms—lung, breast, and colon cancer—are still unsatisfactory, prevention through diet and other means could have a significant impact on the American population.

Cancer develops through a multistage process that usually begins with exposure to a precarcinogen in the environment that must be activated in vivo. Once active, the carcinogen effects tumor initiation by producing a mutation that activates an oncogene or removes a tumor suppressor gene. Fortunately, many mutant cells are probably destroyed before they form a clone. Tumor promotion and progression, which involve additional mutations and the influence of growth factors and often take many years, must occur before a tumor develops that is large enough to produce symptoms. It has become clear that nutrition interacts with each of these stages

---

Box 2-4   Foods to avoid on a sodium-restricted diet

Condiments

Pickles, olives, relishes, salted nuts, meat tenderizers, commercial salad dressings, monosodium glutamate (Accent), steak sauce, ketchup, soy sauce, Worchestershire sauce, horseradish sauce, chili sauce, commercial mustard, onion salt, garlic salt, celery salt, butter salt, seasoned salt

Breads

Salted crackers and breads with salted tops

Meat, fish, poultry, cheese, and substitutes

Cured, smoked, and processed meats such as ham, bacon, corned beef, chipped beef, wieners, luncheon meats, bologna, salt pork, regular canned salmon and tuna; all cheese except low-sodium and cottage cheese; TV dinners, pizza, frozen Italian entrees, imitation sausage and bacon

Beverages

Commercial buttermilk, instant hot cocoa mixes

Soups

Commercial canned and dehydrated soups (except low-sodium soups), bouillon, consommé

Vegetables

Sauerkraut, hominy, pork and beans, canned tomato and vegetable juices

Fats

Gravy, regular peanut butter

Potato or potato substitutes

Potato chips, corn chips, salted popcorn, salted pretzels, frozen potato casseroles, commercially packaged rice and noodle mixes, dehydrated potatoes and potato mixes, bread stuffing

---

of carcinogenesis, making the relationship complex. The following nutrients and dietary habits are thought either to enhance or impede the development of cancer.

Excess intake of energy and dietary fat; obesity

These have been implicated to increase the risk for several cancers, including those of the breast, colon, and uterus. Red meat intake is particularly associated with higher risk for colon cancer, and this may or may not be because of the fat contained in the meat. In fact, much of the association of high dietary fat intake with cancer may be mediated by other constituents that are correlated with fat, such as total energy intake, rather than fat itself. In animal studies, excess energy intake or low energy expenditure (sedentary lifestyle) or both increase the rates of a variety of cancers. Obesity has been linked with increased rates of endometrial and breast cancers, especially when intraabdominal fat is increased. These associations are likely caused by alterations in circulating estrogens in obese women.

Dietary fiber. Certain types of insoluble fiber found in whole-grain foods such as wheat bran appear to have a protective effect against colon cancer. However, some of the apparent effects of fiber noted in epidemiologic studies may be a reflection of other features of populations that have high dietary fiber intakes, such as lower fat or energy intakes.

β-carotene and vitamin A. β-Carotene and related carotenoid and retinoid compounds (such as vitamin A) provide some of the more firmly established diet-cancer links. Data from epidemiologic, animal, in vitro, and clinical studies are largely consistent in showing a protective effect for β-carotene against cancers of the lung, oropharynx, and skin. Epidemiologic studies show that both smokers and nonsmokers who have lower intakes or plasma levels of carotenes or both are at increased risk for lung cancer, possibly through a combination of mechanisms, including the quenching of free radicals, other antioxidant actions, and regulating cell-cell communication through gap junctions.

Human intervention studies are underway to test the cancer-preventive properties of β-carotene or synthetic retinoids. Some of those that have been completed confirm the expected protective effects, but a large trial of β-carotene supplementation in smokers in Finland showed, paradoxically, a small but significant increase in lung cancer. This result may have occurred because carcinogenesis had already progressed in the subjects, who had smoked for an average of 36 years, beyond the point where β-carotene could exert an effect. It may also indicate that other constituents of fruits and vegetables are responsible for some of the protective effects attributed to β-carotene.

Other antioxidants. Vitamin C blocks the transformation in the stomach of dietary nitrates and nitrites into carcinogenic nitrosamines, thus likely inhibiting the development of stomach cancer. The effect of vitamin C on other cancers is difficult to separate from that of other nutrients, such as β-carotene and folic acid, that are in many of the same foods. The ability of vitamin E to protect lipid membranes against oxidation may give it a role in inhibiting the action of carcinogens. Selenium, which is also an antioxidant, may have a protective effect as well. A large trial of supplementation of a high-risk population in China with a combination of antioxidants confirmed a modest protective role for these nutrients.

Folic acid. Red blood cell (RBC) folate levels correlate inversely with cervical dysplasia in women with human papillomavirus infection and with atypical bronchial metaplasia in cigarette smokers—both of which can be premalignant. Higher folate intake is also correlated with lower rates of colon cancer.

Alcohol. Excessive alcohol consumption is the main cause of hepatic cirrhosis in the United States, which in turn is the greatest risk factor for liver cancer. Excess alcohol also interacts with cigarette smoking to increase the risk of oral, pharyngeal, and esophageal cancers. There is evidence that even moderate alcohol intake increases the risk for breast cancer.

Nonnutritive substances. In addition to the known nutrients, nonnutritive substances (phytochemicals) in fruits and vegetables, such as indoles, protease inhibitors, flavonoids, and isoflavones, are probably responsible for some of the benefits of these foods. Because these substances can be obtained only from foods, the use of dietary supplements in lieu of dietary change to prevent cancer is unwise. Although it is not clear precisely which nutrients or substances are most responsible, the benefits of a high intake of fruits and vegetables are beyond dispute.

Dietary recommendations for cancer prevention

The National Cancer Institute, the American Cancer Society, and other groups have issued reasonable dietary guidelines for cancer prevention based on current information. They include the following:

Maintain a desirable weight.

Eat a varied diet.

Include a variety of both vegetables and fruits in the daily diet. (These foods are significant sources of antioxidant nutrients, folic acid, phytochemicals, and fiber, and are low in fat.)

Eat more high-fiber foods, such as whole-grain cereals, legumes, vegetables, and fruits.

Cut down on total fat intake. Major sources of fat include high-fat meats (especially hamburgers), dairy products that are not low-fat, cooking fats such as oils and margarines, processed foods, and sweets and snacks. Low-fat varieties of many of these are available.

Limit consumption of alcoholic beverages, if you drink at all.

Limit consumption of salt-cured, smoked, and nitrite-preserved foods. These foods are strongly implicated in the risk for stomach cancer but are not a major component of the American diet.

ORAL DISEASES
Nutrition and oral health

Oral diseases have a multifactorial etiology that is heavily influenced by health habits, dietary practices, and lifestyle. Pathogenic bacteria in plaque accumulations on dental surfaces and in periodontal tissues are directly responsible for two of the most common diseases: dental caries and periodontal disease. However, the nature of the diet consumed can modulate the virulence and severity of oral disease. There are different ways in which nutrient deficiencies can exert their influence on oral diseases. During tooth formation, malnutrition can give rise to irreversible hypoplastic lesions and discolorations, which may also increase susceptibility to dental caries. A lack of nutrients during critical periods of growth can profoundly affect structure of teeth, time of exfoliation and eruption, and development of salivary glands. The protective role of these salivary glands in the maintenance of oral health can be compromised by nutritional status and drug-induced challenges. Finally, alveolar bone loss can induce tooth mobility, as well as an inability to use prosthetic devices to facilitate masticatory actions in edentulous individuals (those without teeth). Because the mouth is the entry point for nutrients, total-body nutritional status is also influenced by integrity of dental structures, glandular and oral soft tissues, and their supporting bony structures.

Optimal nutrition therefore has two distinct roles in the maintenance of oral health: one is related to the systemic effects exerted by nutrients in the growth and development of all oral tissues and in their maintenance; the other is mediated by local effects of food residues in the oral cavity. The composition of foods and their organoleptic properties, such as taste and texture, will influence the residence time of residues and determine the flow of saliva, thus influencing the implantation, colonization, and metabolic activity of dental plaque bacteria. The interaction between different etiologic factors (Fig. 2-3) will be responsible for the presence and severity of oral disease. Effectiveness in prevention and management of oral diseases will require understanding of their complex etiology and consideration of more than one etiologic factor to ensure success. Thus it will be important to address control of pathogenic bacteria in the mouth; nutritional quality and organoleptic properties of food consumed; amount and composition of saliva bathing oral tissues; and availability of fluoride, oral hygiene, and preventive care to ensure prevention of disease and maintenance of oral health.

Mineralization of teeth and alveolar bone: calcium and fluoride

Teeth are complex structures formed by three distinct calcified tissues: enamel, dentin, and cementum. They are sustained in place by the gingiva and the periodontal membrane, which anchors the teeth within the alveolar socket. The integrity of this bone in terms of thickness of its cortical section and height of the alveolar crest is fundamental to avoid loosening of teeth and eventual loss. Calcium and associated nutrients, such as phosphorus and vitamin D, need to be available in the required optimal quantities during those critical times when they are required for the formation of teeth. There is only one opportunity for optimal structural and morphologic completion. This critical developmental period for tooth mineralization starts about 4 months in utero and continues until 15 to 16 years of age when the second molar of the permanent dentition is completed. Calcium intakes at adequate levels throughout life, but particularly during the formative stages of dental and skeletal development, will result in structures that have decreased susceptibility to osteoporosis and tooth loss.

Fluoride from water and foods also contributes to strengthening of enamel, decreases enamel solubility, stimulates reparative mineralization of enamel surfaces, and exerts an antibacterial effect that increases resistance to caries. The beneficial effect of this element when provided in optimal amounts has been demonstrated in innumerable laboratory and epidemiologic investigations that have shown an inverse relation between dental caries and fluoride concentrations in the drinking water. Fluoride has been found effective in preventing caries when provided in toothpastes, mouthwashes, and topical applications, as well as when administered in drops or tablets or supplemented in salt and milk. Fluoridation of drinking water is implemented at a concentration that ranges from 0.7 to 1.0 ppm fluoride depending on climate and amount of water normally consumed in the locality. Optimal recommendations for dietary fluoride supplementation have been recently published by the American Academy of Pediatric Dentistry (Table 2-12). One should not take more than these recommended doses, particularly during the time of active tooth

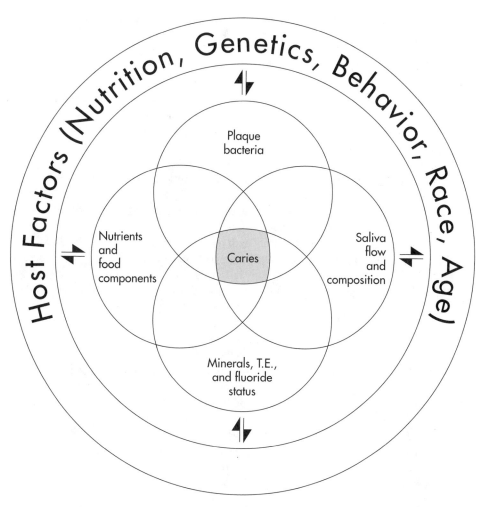

Fig. 2-3 Multifactorial interactions in the etiology of dental caries. *TE,* trace elements. (From Navia JM: Carbohydrates and dental health, *Am J Clin Nutr* 59(suppl) 719S-727S, 1994.)

Table 2-12 Dietary fluoride supplementation schedule

Age	Less than 0.3 ppm F	0.3-0.6 ppm F	More than 0.6 ppm F
Birth-6 months	0	0	0
6 months-3 years	0.25 mg	0	0
3 years-6 years	0.50 mg	0.25 mg	0
6 years-max. 16 years	1 mg	0.50 mg	0

From Dietary fluoride supplementation schedule, position paper on pediatric dentistry, *Journal of the American Academy of Pediatric Dentistry,* 18:24, 1996.

mineralization, when excessive fluoride might produce irreversible dental fluorosis, characterized by discoloration of the enamel and mottling.

Dental diseases: hypoplasia and dental caries

Enamel hypoplasia is a defect of enamel matrix formation that results in a disturbance of mineralization and affects the integrity of the enamel surface because of an insult to the ameloblast cells. Animal and epidemiologic studies have shown that in individuals with chronic malnourished status, enamel calcification will not be complete and the maturation of the enamel surface will be delayed at the time of tooth eruption. The irregularity of hypoplastic enamel provides unique sites for cariogenic bacteria to colonize, and decay of these surfaces is readily seen. Epidemiologic studies done recently in China indicate that children with low birth weight show more hypoplastic teeth and a significantly higher caries incidence than children with normal weight at birth.

Malnutrition not only affects tooth mineralization but also interferes with the caries-protective role of saliva. Protein malnutrition can significantly affect the composition of saliva, as well as its buffering capacity and flow rate. Saliva has a powerful protective role against caries through its capacity to buffer acid production in plaque, formation of a protective pellicle on enamel surfaces, and activation of its antibacterial systems. When proper nutrition is provided, these normal protective mechanisms of saliva minimize the caries challenge. However, when a diet rich in sugars is consumed, these mechanisms can be overcome.

Excessive and frequent exposures to fermentable carbohydrates in the diet of individuals with poor oral hygiene and low levels of fluoride will lead to increased levels of caries. Some foods, such as cheese, have been found to be non–caries-promoting and may even exhibit caries-preventive properties because of their capacity to enhance remineralization. Other foods, such as those rich in fermentable carbohydrates, have a caries-potentiating effect. Food cariogenicity is modified by the length of time a food residue remains in the oral cavity and its composition.

Effect of nutrients on periodontal and soft tissues in oral cavity

Throughout life, maintenance of oral health and integrity of soft tissues is also affected by nutritional deficiencies that may interfere with their healing and repairing mechanisms. The characteristic symptoms of ascorbic acid deficiency (scurvy; Fig. 2-4 and Plate 2) seen in advanced cases (inflammation of the gingiva and increased tooth mobility and tooth loss) represent the clinical consequences of vitamin C–induced defects in oral epithelial basement membrane and collagen. Recent studies have indicated that certain habits, such as smoking, produce a localized deficiency of folate. These compromised nutritional circumstances may lead to impaired healing and even to tumor development. Malnutrition is not the only factor that determines soft tissue lesions, gingivitis, or periodontal diseases, but it is a modulating factor that limits the protective mechanisms necessary to offset the disease stresses on oral tissues exposed to pathogenic bacteria.

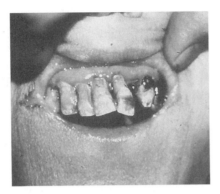

Fig. 2-4   Periodontal disease seen in scurvy. ▲

Dietary modifications for prevention of oral diseases

The rational approach to the prevention of oral diseases is in reality no different from that of any other organ system. The only major difference with other organs is that dental structures have only one opportunity to be formed normally and, consequently, nutritional alterations imposed early in life have irreversible consequences. Adequate intake of nutrients important to biologic mineralization is critical during the early years. Frequent oral hygiene and fluoride exposure are necessary throughout life at optimal levels to reduce the caries challenge and strengthen enamel surfaces. Intake of protein and micronutrients contained in fruits and vegetables are essential to soft tissues and are indispensable for their integrity and maintenance. Foods that increase masticatory actions are beneficial to salivary gland function. This is of special importance for the elderly population, who may have reduced salivary flow because of disease, radiation treatments, or prescribed medications. Finally, an excessive number of sugar exposures during the day should be avoided to prevent stimulation of the resident oral flora and the buildup of pathogenic plaque. Selection of protective foods such as cheese will contribute greatly to the maintenance of the full dentition during all years of life.

OSTEOPOROSIS

Osteoporosis is a metabolic bone disease in which there is an imbalance between bone formation and bone resorption, causing a reduction in bone mass. The end result of low bone mass is the development of traumatic and atraumatic bone fractures. Osteopenia is a decrease in the amount of bone per unit volume relative to that found in normal young adults of the same gender. Osteoporosis refers to osteopenia with normal amounts of matrix and calcified bone. Osteomalacia, on the other hand, is an impaired ability to calcify matrix, resulting in increased matrix and a relative deficiency of calcified bone.

In 1995, it was estimated that approximately 26 million Americans suffered from osteoporosis and of that number, 20 million were women. The estimated annual cost to the U.S. health care system is approximately $10 billion for osteoporosis-related morbidity and mortality.

Osteoporosis is classified in three ways:

1. Primary (no clear cause, idiopathic) or secondary osteoporosis (related to a specific cause such as hyperparathyroidism or malignancy).
2. High- or low-turnover osteoporosis. This classification reflects the activity of osteoblasts (bone formation) and osteoclasts (bone resorption). High-turnover osteoporosis is associated with an increase in both osteoblastic and osteoclastic activity but results in net bone loss resulting from greater osteoclastic activity. Conversely, net bone loss with low activity of osteoblasts and normal activity of osteoclasts is considered low-turnover osteoporosis.
3. Type I, II, or III. Type I osteoporosis occurs in early postmenopausal women and affects mainly trabecular bone (such as the vertebral bodies). Type II osteoporosis is also known as *senile osteoporosis*. It affects both men and women and is related to aging; both cortical and trabecular bone loss occur. Fracture sites are mainly the hip and vertebrae; however, fractures of the humerus, tibia, and pelvis may also occur. Type III osteoporosis is mainly drug-induced, such as corticosteroid-induced osteoporosis. Both trabecular and cortical bone loss can occur.

Pathophysiology

Osteoporosis is the result of uncoupling of the bone remodeling cycle, resulting in low bone mass. Bone remodeling proceeds over several months with an orderly sequence of events at discrete foci called *bone remodeling units*. The process involves the resorption of bone by osteoclasts followed by the recruitment of osteoblasts to fill the resorption cavity. In normal young adults, bone mass is maintained, since bone resorption and formation are tightly coupled. A decrease in bone mass is due to an uncoupling of formation and resorption with a predominance of resorption over formation.

High-turnover osteoporosis occurs in the early postmenopausal period (i.e., within 10 to 15 years after menopause). The activity of both osteoclasts and osteoblasts are increased with the resorptive process predominating. During this period, up to 15% of bone density can be lost, mainly from trabecular bones. High-turnover bone disease is also seen in conditions such as hyperparathyroidism.

Low-turnover osteoporosis occurs in elderly individuals and is characterized by low osteoblastic activity and normal osteoclastic activity, leading to net bone loss. A reduction in osteoblastic activity may be due to age-related decreases in bone-stimulating factors (such as cytokines) or to a decrease in the sensitivity to external factors (e.g., an age-related decrease in vitamin D receptor expression in osteoblasts).

Risk factors

Peak bone mass is generally reached by age 30 (Fig. 2-5). After a period of stabilization, age-related bone loss begins in both female and male adults. The loss of bone mineral density is particularly rapid after menopause, when there is a loss of the trophic effect of estrogen on the bones. Attainment of low peak bone mass can predispose one to osteoporosis. Factors influencing bone mass include genetic

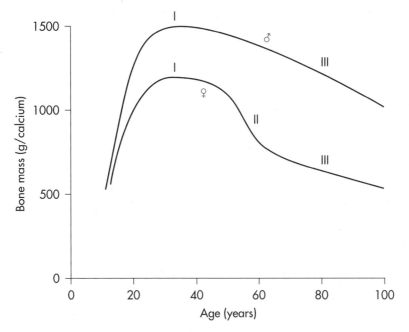

Fig. 2-5   Bone mass as a function of age in women and men. (From Klippel JH: Chapter title. In Riggs BL, Melton LJ III, editors: *Oxford textbook of geriatric medicine,* Oxford, UK, Oxford University Press.) ▲

makeup, nutrition, age, lifestyle, medical disorders, and drug therapies. These factors are outline in Box 2-5.

Genetic factors. Osteoporosis has a genetic component, since individuals with a family history of osteoporosis are more likely to have presenting symptoms of this disorder. Men have greater bone mass than women, even after correcting for body weight. Race is also a risk factor, with osteoporosis being more common in Caucasians and Asians compared with African-Americans. Studies have shown that African-Americans have a 5% to 10% greater bone mass than do age- and gender-matched Caucasians. Obese persons tend to have greater bone mineral density than individuals who have a thin body habitus.

Nutritional factors. Bone mineral density is affected by a number of nutritional factors, including calcium, sodium, protein, and vitamin D intake. Bone mineral density is positively related to calcium intake, especially during the period of peak bone mass development (childhood and adolescence). Calcium intake in several age-groups for both genders in the United States is substantially below the recommended level specified by the NIH Consensus Development Panel (Table 2-13). Individuals who are lactose intolerant may consume less milk products and thus have lower intake of calcium and vitamin D.

Bone mineral density is also related to vitamin D intake. Vitamin D may either be obtained from the diet or from synthesis in the skin after exposure to sunlight. Dietary vitamin D is converted to the active form, 1, 25-dihydroxyvitamin D_3,

---

Box 2-5   Risk factors for osteoporosis

Genetic factors

Family history of osteoporosis
Caucasian or Asian heritage
Asthenic body habitus
Female gender

Nutritional factors

Low calcium intake
Lactose intolerance
Vitamin D deficiency
High sodium intake
High protein intake

Age-related factors

Menopause-reduced estrogen production
Hypogonadism
Reduced serum calcitriol production
Increased serum parathyroid hormone
    (PTH)
Late menarche
Reduced osteoblast function
Reduced calcium absorption

Lifestyle factors

Lack of weight-bearing exercise
Excessive exercise, which produces
    amenorrhea
Lack of exposure to sunlight

Smoking
Excessive alcohol intake
Caffeine

Medical comorbidities

Cardiopulmonary and renal transplants
Cushing's syndrome
Prolactinoma
Diabetes mellitus
Renal failure
Eating disorders
Hyperparathyroidism
Malabsorption
Rheumatoid arthritis
Thyrotoxicosis
Total parenteral nutrition (extended)

Drug therapies

Anticonvulsants
Chronic phosphate-binding antacids
Cyclosporin A
Excessive thyroid replacement therapy
Glucocorticoids
Gonadotropin-releasing hormone ago-
    nist therapy
Heparin
Methotrexate
Tetracycline use extended

---

which is required for the absorption and reabsorption of calcium from the intestine and kidney, respectively. Therefore children with low intake of vitamin D or insufficient exposure to sunlight or both, especially if compounded with low calcium intake, may not attain optimum peak bone mass.

High intakes of sodium increase urinary calcium excretion (hypercalciuria), which may predispose to net bone loss. Whether high protein intake, which can increase urinary calcium excretion, increases bone loss or fracture rate is not known. However, urinary calcium levels return to a normal range after long-term high protein intake.

Age-related factors. Adequate levels of sex hormones are important in the attainment and maintenance of bone mineral density. Late menarche has been correlated with low bone mass. Menopause (surgical or natural), resulting in decreased estrogen level, is associated with losses of 10% to 15% of the appendicular skeleton and 15% to 20% of the vertebrae. In men a decreased testosterone level

Table 2-13   Optimal calcium intake

Age-group	Optimal calcium intake (mg)
INFANTS	
Birth to 6 months	400
6 months to 1 year	600
CHILDREN	
1 to 5 years	800
6 to 10 years	800-1200
ADOLESCENTS/YOUNG ADULTS	
11 to 24 years	1200-1500
MEN	
25 to 65 years	1000
>65 years	1500
WOMEN	
25 to 50 years	1000
>50 years (postmenopausal)	
Taking estrogen replacement	1000
Not taking estrogen replacement	1500
>65 years	1500
Pregnant or nursing	1200-1500

From NIH Consensus Development Panel on Optimal Calcium Intake: Optimal calcium intake, *JAMA* 272:1942, 1994.

(hypogonadism) is a significant risk factor for accelerated bone loss. Hormone replacement in both men and women can slow bone loss.

Studies have shown that around the fourth decade of life the activity of osteoblasts decreases and bone resorption predominates in the bone remodeling units. This imbalance contributes to loss of bone mineral density, which occurs with aging.

In both men and women the efficiency of calcium absorption decreases after the age of 65. During high calcium intake, calcium is absorbed through a passive or vitamin D–independent process, whereas during low calcium intake, absorption of calcium involves the active or vitamin D–dependent process. Studies suggest that low efficiency in calcium absorption is likely due to a decrease in the vitamin D–dependent process resulting from a decline in the intestinal vitamin D receptors. In addition, impaired renal hydroxylation of 25-hydroxyvitamin D_3 to 1α, 25-dihydroxyvitamin D_3 may lead to impaired intestinal calcium absorption and renal calcium reabsorption. In women the decline in estrogen level during menopause is associated with decreased fractional calcium absorption and may also have a direct effect on calcium uptake in the duodenum.

Aging is also associated with increased levels of parathyroid hormone (PTH), with resultant increase in the activity of the bone remodeling unit. Factors causing

PTH elevation include subtle hypocalcemia, parathyroid hyperplasia, altered set-point for calcium-stimulated PTH secretion, altered circadian pattern of PTH secretion, or decreased PTH clearance.

Lifestyle factors. Frequent weight-bearing exercise throughout the life cycle is positively correlated with higher bone mass. Excessive exercise (such as in patients with eating disorders) leading to amenorrhea is detrimental to skeletal health. Long-term smoking and heavy intake of alcohol are both risk factors for decreased bone mass. High intake of caffeine also seems to correlate with low bone mineral density.

Medical disorders and drug therapy. Several medical or surgical conditions have an adverse effect on bone mineral density. These include fat malabsorption, renal failure, hyperparathyroidism, thyrotoxicosis, and eating disorders. Drug therapy can also lead to an accelerated rate of bone loss, such as with long-term use of glucocorticoids, anticonvulsants, and excessive thyroid hormone replacement.

Diagnosis

The diagnosis of osteoporosis is made by combining historical data, results of the clinical examination, laboratory tests, plain radiographs, and specialized radiographic procedures. Diagnostic plans are outlined in Table 2-14.

History and physical examination. The history should emphasize genetic and lifestyle factors, medical conditions, and medications that can affect bone mineral density. Height should be measured using a stadiometer and repeated at each visit. The loss of 1.5 inches is a clue to the presence of osteoporosis and may indicate vertebral compression fractures. Because the clinical manifestations of osteoporosis are often silent, posture, skeletal deformities, and gait are important factors to note. A characteristic change in posture occurs with vertebral fractures: loss of height, a humped back (dowager's hump), loss of waistline contour, and a protuberant abdomen.

Laboratory tests. Laboratory tests are used to rule out secondary causes of osteoporosis and to quantify the rate of bone turnover. A battery of laboratory tests, which should be tailored to the individual patient's situation, is outlined in Table 2-14. Serum osteocalcin is a marker of bone formation when bone resorption and formation are uncoupled, and it is a marker for bone turnover when resorption and formation are coupled.

A measurement of 24-hour urine calcium and creatinine helps detect impaired calcium absorption and hypercalciuria. Urinary hydroxyproline, pyridinoline, deoxypyridinoline, and N-terminal collagen telopepetides can serve as markers of bone resorption. However, urinary hydroxyproline may be increased by dietary collagen intake, which must be minimized before this test.

Radiographs. Plain radiographs are useful in evaluating underlying disorders such as rheumatoid arthritis, the morphology of bones, and the presence of fractures. Because they can only detect losses of greater than 30%, standard radiographs are a relatively insensitive indicator of bone mass. A lateral radiograph of the spine is useful to check for vertebral compression fractures.

A number of more sophisticated tests can be used to assess bone mineral density, such as single-energy x-ray absorptiometry (SXA), dual-energy x-ray absorptiometry (DEXA), quantitative computed tomography (QCT), and radio-

Table 2-14   Diagnosis of osteoporosis

Components of diagnosis	Features	Additional comments
History	Family history of bone disease Lifestyle Medical conditions Medications	See Box 2-5
Physical examination	Height Posture/skeletal deformities Neurologic examination and gait	Compared with age 18 or height on driver's license Dowager's hump, loss of waistline contour, protuberant abdomen
Laboratory tests	Calcium, phosphorus, alkaline phosphatase levels Blood counts Thyroid-stimulating hormone (TSH) Protein electrophoresis Vitamin D levels Hormone levels	Used to rule out secondary causes of osteoporosis, i.e., thyrotoxicosis, metastatic bone disease, hyperparathyroidism, and vitamin D deficiency
	Serum osteocalcin (marker for bone turnover when resorption and formation are coupled, marker for bone formation when resorption and formation are uncoupled) Urinary markers of collagen breakdown largely from bone (pyridinoline, deoxypyridinoline, and N-telopeptide cross-linking of type I collagen)	Bone markers are used to determine the level of bone formation and resorption and to follow response to therapy
Radiographs	Single-energy x-ray absorptiometry (SXA) Dual-energy x-ray absorptiometry (DEXA) Quantitative computed tomography (QCT) Radiographic absorptiometry (RA)	DEXA is the gold standard for measurement of bone density T-score: bone density in standard deviations compared with a "young normal" control population of the same gender Z-score: bone density in standard deviations related to an "age-sex-matched" control
Bone histomorphometry	Bone biopsy Tetracycline labeling	Important test in diagnosis of metabolic bone disease Used as a dynamic assessment of the rate of bone formation

graphic absorptiometry (RA). DEXA is currently the most accurate method. It generates a T-score that relates the bone density to that of a "young normal" control of the same gender and a Z-score that compares it with that of an "age-sex-matched" control. Osteoporosis is defined by DEXA as bone mineral density (BMD) with more than 2.5 standard deviations (SD) below the mean value of peak bone mass in a young normal population. Osteopenia is defined by DEXA as a BMD between -1 SD and -2.5 SD of the mean value of peak bone mass in that same population. Indications for DEXA include parathyroid disease, chronic prednisone therapy, malabsorption, incidental osteopenia noted on plain films, and hypogonadism. It is also useful in the perimenopausal period, when a relatively low bone mineral density makes postmenopausal hormone replacement advisable.

Bone histomorphometry and biopsy. Bone biopsy is another useful test in the diagnosis of metabolic bone disease. Tetracycline labeling (oral dose of demethylchlortetracycline or tetracycline hydrochloride for 2 days, no medication for 10 to 20 days, then repeat the tetracycline for 2 to 4 days) allows the rate of bone formation to be assessed from bone biopsies.

Prevention and treatment

Prevention of osteoporosis is more cost effective than therapy. Prevention should focus on achieving optimum peak bone mass and maintaining it. Children and adolescents should be encouraged to have a balanced diet with an adequate intake of calcium (see Table 2-13). For premenopausal women and men, recommended calcium intakes are similar to those of adolescents (see Table 2-13). Calcium intake may be in the form of food or calcium supplements. Regular weight-bearing exercise is recommended. Alcohol and caffeine should be taken in moderation or not at all, and smoking should be avoided. Elderly individuals over the age of 70 years who have sedentary lifestyles should be encouraged to have sunlight exposure and supplemental intake of vitamin D and calcium. Fall prevention strategies are also important in this age category.

For those diagnosed with osteoporosis, a number of medical therapies are now available. Table 2-15 lists treatments categorized as either antiresorptive or bone formation–promoting therapy. For women, hormone replacement after menopause is considered the gold standard. However, for women who cannot or will not take hormone replacement therapy, a variety of other therapies such as calcitonin and bisphosphonates are now available. Adequate calcium and vitamin D intake are important adjuncts to these therapies. A number of promising agents to improve bone mineral density are currently being tested.

NUTRITIONAL ANEMIAS

Anemia is defined as the diminished oxygen-carrying capacity of the blood resulting from a deficiency of circulating RBCs. Anemia is diagnosed when the hemoglobin is less than 12 g/dl in female adults or less than 14 g/dl in male adults. These hemoglobin levels correspond to hematocrit levels approximately 36% and 42%, respectively. Anemia is considered nutritional in origin when the intake of one or more essential nutrients is implicated in the cause of the anemia. A relative nutrient deficiency may exist in the face of normal dietary intake if metabolic re-

Table 2-15 Prevention and treatment of osteoporosis

		Antiresorptive treatments		
Drugs	**Food/trade name**	**Application**	**Comments**
Estrogen	Conjugated estrogen (Premarin)	Oral	For Type I osteoporosis
	Estropipate (Ogen)		Currently the best option for women
	Ethinyl estradiol		Progesterone should be prescribed in women with an intact uterus to
	Estradiol (Estrace)		prevent uterine cancer; women without a uterus may be treated with
	Prempro	Combinations of	estrogen alone
	Premphase	estrogen and	A slight risk of breast cancer with long-term hormone replacement therapy
		progesterone	(HRT) is possible
	Estradiol transdermal (Estraderm, Climarz)	Dermal patch	
Calcium	Dairy products, salmon,	Oral	For Type I and II osteoporosis
	collard and turnip		For postmenopausal women on HRT
	greens, spinach,		1000 mg of Ca; without HRT 1500 mg of calcium; for women and men
	broccoli, cooked dried		over 65 yrs, 1500 mg of Ca (see Table 2-13)
	beans		Ca supplements are best taken between meals if achlorhydria is not
	Calcium carbonate		present, with no more than 500 mg at a time
	Calcium acetate		Calcium citrate is best for patients with achlorhydria and when iron
	Calcium lactate		supplements are concurrently prescribed
	Calcium citrate		
Vitamin D	Cholecalciferol	Oral	For Type I and II osteoporosis
	Ergocalciferol		Usually 400-800 IU/day as cholecalciferol in multivitamins is sufficient;
	Fortified milk, egg yolks		take with Ca to increase fractional absorption of Ca
	Present in most		For those with low Ca absorption and low urinary Ca (<100 mg/day),
	multivitamins		50,000 IU of vitamin D every 7-10 days may be prescribed
Vitamin D analogs	Calderol (25-hydroxyvitamin D)	Oral	For Type I and II osteoporosis 50 µg of Calderol is equivalent to 50,000
	1,25-dihydroxyvitamin		IU of vitamin D
	D (Rocaltrol)		No more than 0.25 µg/day of Rocaltrol
			Both should be taken with Ca supplement
			Ca levels should be closely monitored

Continued

Table 2-15 Prevention and treatment of osteoporosis—cont'd

Drugs	Food/trade name	Application	Comments
		Antiresorptive treatments	
Calcitonin	Salmon calcitonin (Calcimar)	Parenteral (subcutaneous injection)	For Type I osteoporosis An option for those in whom estrogen is contraindicated; it has analgesic effects. A skin test should be done before prescription.
	Miacalcin	Nasal	Usually taken with Ca supplements Side effects are nausea and flushing; less with nasal form
Bisphosphonates	Etidronate disodium (Didronel)	Oral	For Type I osteoporosis Potent inhibitor of bone resorption Ca supplements should be prescribed An alternative to estrogen treatment Must be used cyclically NOTE: May impair mineralization, leading to long-term effects such as increased incidence of hip fractures
	Fosamax (Alendronate)		Does not need to be prescribed cyclically Ca supplements should be prescribed
PROMOTE BONE FORMATION			
Sodium fluoride	Slow fluoride (slow-release sodium fluoride)	Oral	Pending FDA approval 25 mg twice daily for 4 years resulted in increased spinal and femoral neck bone mass and prevented new vertebral fractures (but not recurrent fractures)
PTH	Growth hormone		More experimental evidence is needed for its potential usefulness
Growth factors	Insulin-like growth factors		More experimental evidence is needed for its potential usefulness

Ca, Calcium.

quirements are high (as for folic acid in hemolysis or pregnancy), if external losses are great (as with loss of iron from chronic gastrointestinal bleeding), or if an antivitamin is being consumed (as for methotrexate, which is a folic acid antagonist). Table 2-16 identifies the causes of nutritional anemias based on cell mean corpuscular volume (MCV). Fig. 2-6 and Plate 3 show examples of microcytic (small; Fig. 2-6, *B*) and macrocytic (large; Fig. 2-6, *A*) RBCs.

Symptoms of anemia include early onset of fatigue with exertion, as well as exercise intolerance. Resting tachycardia with a pulse greater than 100 beats per minute is a helpful diagnostic sign because it demonstrates the body's adaptation to the diminished oxygen-carrying capacity in the blood. Other symptoms of anemia may include palpitations, dizziness, syncope, amenorrhea, and menorrhagia. Pallor of the mucous membranes (i.e., conjunctiva, buccal cavity, tongue) and skin may provide a clue to the presence of anemia, but unfortunately, pallor does not correspond closely with the hematocrit. Other signs of anemia include tachycardia, a wide pulse pressure, systolic ejection murmurs, and venous hum (see Table 2-16).

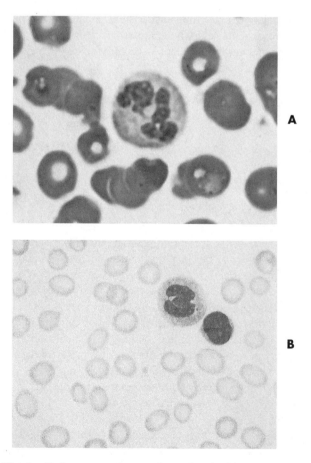

Fig. 2-6 **A,** Blood cells in macrocytic anemia: notice the hypersegmented polymorphonuclear leukocytes. **B,** Blood cells in microcytic anemia. ▲

Table 2-16 Differential diagnosis of nutritional anemias by RBC mean corpuscular volume (MCV)*

Category	Differential diagnosis
Microcytic; MCV < 80	Iron deficiency
	Pyridoxine deficiency
Normocytic; MCV 80-100	Copper deficiency
	Protein-calorie malnutrition
Macrocytic; MCV > 100	Folic acid deficiency
	Vitamin B_{12} deficiency

*Normal values for the MCV will vary in different hospitals; these figures should be considered representative.

Other evaluations that should be considered to determine the cause of an anemia are a complete blood count (CBC) with a white blood cell (WBC) differential and a reticulocyte count. A bone marrow biopsy and aspirate are often useful in providing a definitive diagnosis. The evaluation of the blood smear by the health care professional can provide important clues to the cause of the anemia. The diagnosis of a nutritional anemia is confirmed by the measurement of the suspected nutrient or a metabolite in serum or plasma, blood cells, or urine.

It is important to remember that anemia almost never occurs as an isolated finding; a nutritional deficiency sufficient to limit the production of RBCs usually affects other cells with a high turnover rate such as leukocytes, platelets, and enterocytes. Most cases of megaloblastic anemia are accompanied by reddening and soreness of the tongue along with loss of lingual papillae (called *slick tongue*). These changes may make eating difficult and impose further limitations on food choices and therefore predispose to other vitamin and mineral deficiencies.

Iron deficiency (microcytic) anemia

Anemia resulting from lack of iron is the most common form of nutritional anemia and is perhaps the most common nutritional deficiency in the world. Iron deficiency is due to inadequate intake, inadequate absorption, or excessive losses (i.e., bleeding). Iron deficiency anemia is more likely to occur at major stages of the life cycle: (1) age 6 months to 4 years; (2) early adolescence; (3) during the female reproductive period; and (4) during pregnancy. In men and postmenopausal women, iron equilibrium is accomplished by the absorption of 1 mg/day, on the average, from a diet containing the RDA of 10 mg of iron. This replaces the small amounts of iron lost by both men and women each day from minor injuries and shedding of epithelial cells. During childbearing years, women lose an average of 30 mg of elemental iron during each menstrual period, imposing a demand for an additional 0.5 mg, or a total of 1.5 mg/day, to maintain equilibrium. For premenopausal women, the RDA has been set at 15 mg/day. The RDA for iron during pregnancy is 30 mg/day and during lactation is 15 mg/day.

Food sources provide heme and nonheme iron. From 10% to 15% of dietary iron is heme iron and is found in meats and seafood. About 85% to 90% of dietary iron is nonheme iron and is found in dried beans and peas, kale, bitter chocolate,

Table 2-17   Findings in nutritional anemias

Characteristic	Deficiency states			
	Normal	Iron	Folic acid	Vitamin B$_{12}$
RBC morphology	Normocytic	Hypochromic, microcytic	Macrocytic	Macrocytic
MCV μ^3	80-100	<80	>100	>100
MCHC %	32-26	<32	>32	>32
Hypersegmented neutrophils	Absent	Absent	Present	Present
Bone marrow morphology	Normal	Normoblastic	Megaloblastic	Megaloblastic
Stainable marrow iron	Normal	Absent	Normal/high	Normal/high
Serum iron μg/dl	42-135	<42	Normal/high	Normal/high
TIBC μg/dl	270-400	>400	Normal/high	Normal/high
Ferritin ng/ml	10-300	<10	Normal/high	Normal/high
Serum folate ng/ml	3-10	3-10	Usually <3	Normal/high
RBC folate ng/ml	140-360	140-360	<140	Normal
Serum vitamin B$_{12}$ pg/ml	200-700	200-700	Normal/high	<200
Serum homocysteine level μmol/L	5.4-16.2	Normal	High	High
Serum methylmalonic acid level nmol/L	73-271	Normal	Normal	High

dried fruits, and enriched breads and cereals. Nondietary sources of iron include cooking utensils, water pipes, and therapeutic supplements of iron.

A suspicion of iron deficiency anemia is supported by a low level of serum iron, usually less than 50 mg/dl, and an increase in the total iron-binding capacity (TIBC) greater than 400 mg/dl. Normally the TIBC is approximately one-third saturated; lower values are suggestive of iron deficiency. A low ferritin level can be helpful in the diagnosis of iron deficiency. A serum ferritin level less than 40 μg/L is suggestive of iron deficiency. A ferritin level less than 70 μg/L in the face of inflammation can usually be considered diagnostic of iron deficiency, since ferritin is also an acute phase reactant. Iron deficiency occurs in stages. In the first stage of iron deficiency, the bone marrow iron is depleted. In the next stage of iron deficiency, the serum iron is low and the TIBC becomes elevated. Anemia is a relatively late finding of iron deficiency anemia. Table 2-17 presents some of the characteristic findings in iron deficiency.

It is always important to establish the cause of iron deficiency and to distinguish between inadequate nutritional intake and a correctable cause of blood loss. A 30-day therapeutic trial of an oral iron supplement may be justified in women if the physical examination is normal and if the history provides a likely cause, such as frequent pregnancies or excessive menstrual blood loss. Such a course is almost never justified in men or postmenopausal women. Hypochromic microcytic anemia in those stages of the life cycle is most commonly caused by chronic occult blood loss from the gastrointestinal tract. A microcytic anemia in those age-groups demands careful study of stool specimens for the presence of blood and parasites, as well as complete examination of the upper and lower gastrointestinal tracts with x-rays or endoscopy. In the hospital, excessive blood sampling for laboratory tests may aggravate to iron deficiency anemia. One unit of blood (500 ml) contains 250 mg of iron and may require 2 to 4 months for replacement.

For treatment of iron deficiency anemia, replacement therapy with simple iron salts, such as ferrous sulfate given orally in dosages of 325 mg one to four times daily, is generally quite effective. Adjunctive measures include using iron cookware; taking vitamin C with each meal (a 50-mg vitamin C tablet or a glass of orange juice acts by reducing sugar to increase vitamin C absorption); taking in an adequate amount of high-quality animal protein; and avoiding intake of agents known to inhibit iron absorption, such as phosphates, phytates, tannic aid in tea, and antacids. Therapy is often limited by gastrointestinal intolerance. Parenteral iron is seldom needed but is available in the form of an iron-dextran complex providing 50 mg of elemental iron per milliliter. Its use should be restricted to patients in whom serious attempts at oral therapy have failed or in whom chronic losses exceed the absorptive capacity of the intestine because fatal anaphylactic reactions have been described. Iron can be included in total parenteral nutrition mixtures and is apparently safe at maintenance dosages of 1 to 2 mg/day.

Deficiency of folic acid or vitamin B_{12} (macrocytic anemias)

Folic acid (folate) and vitamin B_{12} deficiencies cause another category of nutritional anemias called *megaloblastic* or *macrocytic,* since there is an accumulation of large immature red cell precursors, known as *megaloblasts,* in the bone marrow. A finding of arrested maturation in bone marrow smears was once the hallmark of diagnosis, but it is gradually being replaced by biochemical assessment of vitamin levels and other metabolic substances in plasma, RBCs, and urine (see Table 2-17).

Vitamin B_{12}. The prototype of vitamin B_{12} deficiency is pernicious anemia, which strictly speaking is not a dietary deficiency because it is caused by intestinal malabsorption. Patients with pernicious anemia lack intrinsic factor (IF), a glycoprotein that is normally secreted by the parietal cells and that binds vitamin B_{12} and allows it to be absorbed in the ileum. Even in the face of adequate intake of dietary sources of vitamin B_{12}, a functional deficiency of vitamin B_{12} occurs because of intestinal malabsorption. Total gastrectomy and ileal resection can also disrupt physiologic mechanisms of absorption, and severe pancreatic disease can also hinder vitamin B_{12} absorption by altering the normal transfer of cobalamins from proteins called *R-binders* to IF. The average time of onset of megaloblastic anemia after total gastrectomy is about 4 to 5 years because of the large residual liver stores in most individuals. Inadequate intake of vitamin B_{12} is a relatively rare cause of megaloblastic anemia, but it should be considered in the differential diagnosis of macrocytic anemia in vegans.

Vitamin B_{12} is found in foods of animal origin. The RDA for vitamin B_{12} is 2.0 μg/day for both men and women. During pregnancy the RDA is 2.2 μg/day, and during lactation it is 2.6 μg/day.

The symptoms and physical findings of vitamin B_{12} deficiency are similar to those of anemia in general, except that vitamin B_{12} deficiency affects the posterior and lateral columns of the spinal cord. Macrocytes (megaloblasts) are found on the peripheral smear. Hypersegmentation of the neutrophils is considered to be present if 5% of the neutrophils have more than 5 lobes. Vitamin B_{12} deficiency is likely when the plasma concentration is less than 150 pg/ml. In vitamin B_{12} deficiency the plasma folate level may be elevated to 15 to 20 ng/ml (normally 3 to 10 ng/ml) because of impaired tissue folate uptake and turnover. Newer tests in the diagnosis of vitamin B_{12} deficiency include elevated serum homocysteine and methylmalonic acid levels (see Table 2-16). Like iron deficiency, vitamin B_{12} deficiency occurs in stages. The first stage of vitamin B_{12} deficiency is negative balance, which is manifest by low levels of the proteins that carry vitamin B_{12}, the transcobalamins. In the next stage of B_{12} depletion the vitamin B_{12} level generally falls to less than 150 pg/ml. In vitamin B_{12}–deficient erythropoiesis, hypersegmentation is seen and the vitamin B_{12} level is generally less than 100 pg/ml. In the final stage of deficiency, the vitamin B_{12} level is less than 100 pg/ml, the MCV is elevated, the hemoglobin level is low, and macrocytes are present.

When vitamin B_{12} deficiency is found, it is important to establish or exclude the diagnosis of pernicious anemia. The Schilling test, which evaluates the absorption of a radioactive dose of vitamin B_{12}, can be used to determine the basis of deficiency. If pernicious anemia is treated with large doses of folic acid alone, degeneration of the posterolateral columns of the spinal cord is aggravated, although the anemia will disappear. Therefore it is generally advisable to assay both B_{12} and folate levels in patients with macrocytosis.

The treatment of vitamin B_{12} deficiency is generally with parenteral B_{12}. An initial injection of 1000 μg/day for several days is advisable. In patients who require continued parenteral therapy, injections of 100 μg every month are generally adequate but should be individually adjusted according to blood B_{12} levels. Oral therapy with 1000 μg/day has also been found to be useful in compliant patients with pernicious anemia.

Folic acid. Folic acid deficiency is seen in individuals who ingest insufficient amounts of folate and in individuals with malabsorption. Folic acid deficiency is common in alcoholics because of poor folate intake and folate malabsorption. Folic acid deficiency has recently been identified as a risk factor for neural tube defects during pregnancy. In contrast to vitamin B_{12} deficiency, dietary deficiency of folic acid is relatively common.

Folic acid is found in yeast, liver and organ meats, leafy vegetables, legumes, fresh fruits, and some enriched bread and cereal products. Orange juice is the highest contributor of folic acid to the American diet. Prolonged cooking and processing of foods can destroy food folate. The RDA for folic acid is 3 μg/kg/day, which translates into approximately 180 μg/day for a woman and 200 μg/day for a man. During pregnancy the RDA is 400 μg/day, and during lactation it is 260 to 280 μg/day.

The characteristics of folic acid deficiency anemia are indistinguishable from vitamin B_{12} deficiency anemia in that macrocytes and hypersegmented neutrophils are found on the peripheral blood smear. Folic acid deficiency is likely if the plasma folate level is less than 3.0 ng/ml. However, RBC folate levels are a more reliable indicator of tissue stores; red cell folate levels less than 140 ng/ml are diagnostic of deficiency. The serum homocysteine level is elevated in folic acid deficiency because of an inability to remethylate homocysteine to form methionine in intermediary metabolism. Folic acid deficiency occurs in stages. The first stage is negative balance, which is manifest by a low serum folate level. In the folate depletion stage, the RBC folate level will generally be less than 140 ng/ml. In folate deficiency erythropoiesis, there is hypersegmentation of neutrophils. In folate deficiency anemia, which is the final stage, the MCV is elevated, the hemoglobin level is low, and macrocytes are present.

Folic acid deficiency is corrected readily in most patients with supplemental oral tablets containing 1 to 5 mg of the vitamin (pteroylglutamic acid–oxidized folate) daily. Oral doses of up to 45 mg/day have been used for periods of several weeks without observed ill effects, but such high dosages are seldom necessary. High levels of folate supplementation may interfere with seizure control in patients receiving anticonvulsant medication. Most multiple vitamins contain 400 μg of folic acid. Vitamins containing more than 1 mg of folic acid are available only by prescription so as not to mask vitamin B_{12} deficiency anemia.

EATING DISORDERS

Although anorexia nervosa and bulimia have been observed for decades, the prevalence of these disorders did not command the attention of the psychiatric, psychologic, and medical communities until the mid-1970s. Previously, anorexia nervosa was considered a disorder of the young, white, affluent girl or woman whose illness was a reflection of disturbed family relationships. However, with changing societal expectations for appearance, clinicians have seen a rapid rise in the number of patients with primary eating disorders. As the number of cases has increased, issues regarding etiology and diagnostic criteria have largely been resolved with greater emphasis on treatment and prevention.

Definition and diagnosis

Anorexia nervosa is self-starvation motivated by excessive concern with weight and an irrational fear of becoming fat. People with anorexia nervosa are characterized by an extremely controlled and restrictive calorie intake and an obsessive, narrowed focus on body fat. The patient will usually deny that any problem exists and will exhibit a loss of perspective with respect to body shape.

Like anorexia nervosa, bulimia nervosa is accompanied by a preoccupation with weight and fear of becoming fat. However, unlike the anorectic person, the bulimic individual does not maintain rigid control of calorie intake. Instead, the bulimic patient will binge eat and then purge by self-induced vomiting, use of laxatives or diuretics or both, excessive exercise, or periods of severe caloric restriction. Similar to bulimia nervosa, binge eating disorder involves episodic consumption of excessive calories in a brief period of time. A sense of helplessness in the face of the impulse to eat is often reported. In contrast to individuals with bulimia, the person with binge eating behavior does not resort to extreme compensatory actions such as vomiting.

Though many of the symptoms associated with eating disorders are also consistent with depression and obsessive-compulsive disorder, the defining symptom of anorexia nervosa and bulimia nervosa is the preoccupation with body weight and fat. Other disorders that must be differentiated from the eating disorders are psychosis involving delusions, gastrointestinal disorders, and substance abuse affecting appetite.

The following problems also may signal the possibility of an eating disorder:
- Amenorrhea for several consecutive months
- Complaints of fatigue, dizziness, diarrhea, headaches, or muscle cramping
- Rigid, arbitrary definitions of "fattening" foods or avoidance of certain food groups (e.g., starches)
- Compulsive, intensive aerobic exercise

Etiology and associated features

Although no specific physical disorder has been implicated in the development of eating disorders, a number of demographic and psychosocial variables are consistently associated with anorectic and bulimic patients:
- Nearly all anorectic and bulimic patients are female.
- Age of onset for anorexia nervosa typically is 14 to 18 years; bulimia is most likely to develop between 18 and 22 years of age.
- Many women patients report a history of obesity.
- A family history of affective illness such as depression or substance abuse is common.
- Families of bulimic patients are likely to be characterized by instability and conflict. In contrast, families of anorectic patients appear closely knit but rigid.
- Because their careers may depend on the ability to maintain a particular body weight, models, gymnasts, dancers, flight attendants, and actresses are at high risk.
- The anorectic patient typically will appear rigid and controlled, whereas the bulimic patient will appear impulsive and out of control.

Medical complications

The medical complications of anorexia nervosa are similar to the metabolic and physiologic adaptations observed in starvation. These may include a slow resting heart rate and low blood pressure. The skin is often cool, and there may be loss of scalp hair and appearance of soft lanugo (fine, soft, blond) hair on the face and trunk. Hypercarotenemia and a yellowish discoloration of the skin may develop, possibly secondary to a decrease in the metabolic conversion of carotene to vitamin A, functional hypothyroidism, or consumption of large amounts of carotene-containing fruits and vegetables.

Virtually all observed endocrine changes of anorexia nervosa are related to abnormalities at the level of the hypothalamus and are reversible with weight gain. The hypothalamic-pituitary-gonadal axis is the most sensitive and earliest endocrine axis to manifest changes related to anorexia. A decrease in production of follicle-stimulating hormone (FSH) and luteinizing hormone (LH), which causes decreased estrogen and progesterone levels, results in amenorrhea. Amenorrhea can occur even before significant weight loss in anorexia nervosa. Gonadotropin-releasing hormone injections can produce ovulation and menstruation, indicating that the hypothalamic-pituitary-gonadal axis is otherwise intact.

The most serious complication of anorexia nervosa relates to the cardiovascular system and the potential for sudden death. As with any other starvation or semistarvation state, there is loss of cardiac mass, which results in loss of physiologic functional capacity. For example, the predicted response of cardiac output and oxygen consumption to exercise is diminished. With this impaired functional capacity, life-threatening irregular heart rhythms may occur, especially when deficiencies of potassium, magnesium, or phosphorus are present. Thus at this advanced stage the patient with anorexia nervosa is at significant risk for sudden death from these cardiac abnormalities.

The medical complications of bulimia, with its binge eating and purging, present a spectrum of anatomic and physiologic changes distinctly different from the adaptive changes related to starvation in the anorectic patient. Binge eating may create marked gastric dilation, and gastric rupture has been reported. Postbinge pancreatitis also may occur. Painless enlargement of the parotid glands may develop several days after a binge; in some cases, it may persist and become disfiguring.

The consequences of repeated self-induced vomiting include severe erosion of the dental enamel (Fig. 2-7 and Plate 4), loss of teeth, esophagitis, hiatal hernia, esophageal tear and rupture, hypochloremic alkalosis and hypokalemia, and even shock. If ipecac is used repeatedly to induce vomiting, myocardial ipecac toxicity may develop and is associated with dysrhythmias and potentially fatal myocarditis. Laxative abuse may result in chronic hypokalemia with renal tubular damage and cathartic dependence to maintain semblance of normal colonic activity.

Treatment

The treatment of an eating disorder depends on several factors: the severity of the problem, physical status, nature of social support, and associated psychopathology. If significant medical complications are present, the patient may require hospitalization, but in the absence of physical distress, other factors determine the prognosis of outpatient treatment.

Initially, symptomatic treatment may begin with weekly follow-up visits. The patient's weight should be monitored for any changes greater than 1 or 2 pounds, which may indicate binge eating, semistarvation, excessive exercise, laxative use, or diuretic use. In addition, the physician should insist that the patient maintain a food diary. Resistance to keeping such a record is a red flag that the patient is defensive about her eating pattern and may be experiencing binge episodes. After several visits the physician will be in a position to evaluate the patient's attitude toward eating, preoccupation with weight loss, and resistance to change.

Whether treating the problem on an inpatient or an outpatient basis, a therapeutic alliance must be established with the patient. This is most easily accomplished by involving the patient in decision making and by setting limited goals to minimize the anxiety that will accompany weight gain. In the inpatient setting, patients should be informed of potential side effects of treatment. For example, edema is often experienced when diuretics or laxatives are no longer available. The subsequent weight gain and discomfort will often be misinterpreted as fat. Reassuring the patient that the swelling will subside may alleviate fears.

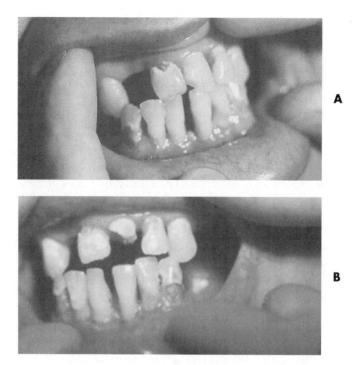

Fig. 2-7 Progression of dental erosion resulting from induced vomiting in a bulimic patient. ▲

If a patient is severely dehydrated or cachectic, intravenous fluids or naso-gastric feeding may be a necessary first step in treatment. The basic rule is to go slowly and to monitor carefully changes in physiologic status to prevent the refeeding syndrome (see Chapter 11). As soon as the patient is stable, reestablishing normal eating patterns is essential. The anorectic patient will initially resist increased oral intake, but setting the expectation of improved calorie intake without requiring immediate weight gain may lessen the resistance. When self-induced vomiting is a focus of treatment, the patient may require observation for 1 to 2 hours after meals to ensure food retention and to discuss developing tolerance to feeling full.

Education is a critical component of the treatment process. For example, the preoccupation with food is often perceived by the patient as evidence of illness. Informing the patient that thoughts about food are as much a physiologic phenomenon as they are psychologic and that eating will relieve them will assist the patient in rethinking and reattributing her behavior. Similarly, food phobias can be addressed by reorienting patients to think that it is not what they eat but how much that affects weight change. An effective psychologic treatment for bulimia involves changing behaviors and attitudes toward food, one's body, and oneself. Cognitive behavior therapy has been well documented in the treatment literature.

The association between affective disorders and eating disorders has led to extensive research evaluating the use of antidepressant medications in the treatment of anorexia nervosa and bulimia. The results have been far more encouraging with bulimic patients than with anorectic patients. Specifically, some patients with bulimia have reduced the frequency of binge eating with high doses of fluoxetine (Prozac) (60 to 80 mg/day). Though not adequately studied, other selective serotonin reuptake inhibitors may also be beneficial. No criteria have been established for determining the usefulness of antidepressant medication in a particular case, but the presence of depressive symptoms in addition to the disrupted eating pattern may justify a trial.

The evaluation and treatment of patients with eating disorders require input from a variety of disciplines—psychiatry, psychology, general medicine, nutrition, and social work. The need for consistent follow-up with families and patients demands the coordination of efforts of the multidisciplinary team.

EFFECTS OF ALCOHOL ON NUTRITIONAL STATUS

Alcohol is toxic; however, small amounts are produced in nondrinkers by the reversal of the reaction catalyzed by alcohol dehydrogenase (ADH). The average intake of alcohol among all Americans is about 4% of total calories and among adult drinkers about 10%. Since ethanol has an energy content of about 7 kcal/g, this is a daily intake of about 15 to 20 g in adult drinkers.

From a nutritional view, the toxic effects of alcohol consumption are detectable once intake exceeds 15% of calories and may be severe at or above 30% of calories. Globally, the toxic effects of alcohol abuse on nutrient status are related to the displacement of nutrients by alcohol-containing beverages, the toxic effect of alcohol on the gastrointestinal tract, the increase in nicotinamide adenine dinucleotide (reduced form) (NADH) levels as a result of the action of ADH on ethanol, and the induction of catabolic pathways for several nutrients.

The effects of alcohol on macronutrients, mineral and vitamin absorption, and metabolism are considered separately.

Macronutrients

Large amounts of ethanol are not used as efficiently as a source of energy as are the major macronutrients. Thus isocaloric substitution of ethanol for carbohydrate results in weight loss, and addition of excess ethanol calories results in lower-than-expected weight gain. In the gastrointestinal tract, ethanol reduces villus height and decreases both lactase and sucrase activity, suggesting that mild malabsorption of carbohydrates may result from ethanol abuse.

The production of excessive amounts of NADH during alcohol abuse provides the metabolic reducing equivalents to biosynthesize and elongate fatty acids. In concert with an increase in NADH, a decrease in nicotinamide adenine dinucleotide (NAD) limits fatty acid oxidation with the well-known consequences of fatty liver, elevated serum VLDL levels and other signs and symptoms related to reduced oxidation and increased production and storage of long-chain triglycerides. It is worth noting, however, that there is a J-shaped curve when death from cardiac disease is plotted versus alcohol intake. Thus 10 to 15 g of alcohol daily is associated with reduced cardiovascular disease, possibly by increasing serum HDL levels. The hyperuricemia of alcohol abuse is also caused by increased NADH levels. Excess lactate, as a result of NADH reduction of pyruvate, interferes with renal clearance of uric acid. It is also possible that excess NADH stimulates purine and uric acid biosynthesis. The net effect is often elevation of serum uric acid levels.

Minerals

Among the major minerals, magnesium, iron, and zinc are most likely to be affected by alcohol abuse. Most alcoholics have low blood magnesium and high urinary magnesium levels. With respect to iron, both deficiency and increased stores are observed. Whereas iron deficiency may result from alcohol-induced gastritis, the etiology of alcohol-induced iron overload (hemochromatosis) is less clear. Red wine contains up to 6 mg of iron per liter and may contribute to increased intake. Transferrin, which is reduced in sialic acid content, occurs with alcohol abuse. This species of transferrin deposits its iron in lysosomes in which there is little recycling of iron, thus increasing iron stores. The potential for hemochromatosis to precipitate liver, kidney, and pancreatic damage may be by iron's prooxidative role. Low blood and liver zinc levels are found in alcoholics, since there is increased zinc loss in the urine. ADH is a zinc-containing enzyme, but the link between these two findings is unclear.

Vitamins

Alcohol abusers are clearly predisposed to deficiencies of thiamin; pyridoxine; folic acid; and vitamins A, D, and E. Displacement of nutritious food by the relatively "empty" calories of alcoholic beverages plays a role. Reduced absorption of thiamin, folic acid, and vitamin A is also important in producing a deficiency of these nutrients. Liver stores of folate, thiamin, and pyridoxine are lower in alcohol abusers, suggesting increased catabolism of these vitamins. Acetaldehyde produced from ADH-catalyzed ethanol oxidation can bind to pyridoxine, possibly displacing it from the active sites of enzymes. Thiamin can also be catabolized by ADH. Alcohol abuse clearly is a risk factor for osteoporosis and low bone density despite apparently normal blood levels of vitamin D. Many fat malabsorption syndromes result in vitamin A, D, and E malabsorption and deficiency; this is especially true of pancreatitis and pancreatic insufficiency resulting from chronic alcoholism. A remarkably high number of alcoholics are deficient in one or more of the above vitamins, suggesting that decreased vitamin intake leads to malabsorption in a pernicious process that eventually depletes the patient.

SUGGESTED READINGS

Factors predisposing to obesity

Bjorntorp P: Visceral obesity: a "civilization syndrome," *Obesity Res* 1:206, 1993.

Bray GA: Fat distribution and body weight, *Obesity Res* 1:203, 1993.

Heyward VH, Stolarczyk LM: *Applied body composition assessment,* Champaign, Ill, 1996, Human Kinetics.

Kuczmarski RJ, Flegal KM, Campbell SM, et al: Increasing prevalence of overweight among US adults, *JAMA* 272:205, 1994.

Lee I-M, Manson JE, Hennekens CH, et al: Body weight and mortality: a 27-year follow-up of middle-aged men, *JAMA* 270:2833, 1993.

Manson JE, Willett WC, Stampfer MJ, et al: Body weight and mortality among women, *N Engl J Med* 333:677, 1995.

Montoye HJ, Kemper HCG, Saris WHM, et al, editors: *Measuring physical activity and energy expenditure,* Champaign, Ill, 1996, Human Kinetics.

NIH National Task Force on the Prevention and Treatment of Obesity: Very low-calorie diets, *JAMA* 270:967, 1993.

NIH National Task Force on the Prevention and Treatment of Obesity: Weight cycling, *JAMA* 272:1196, 1994.

NIH Technology Assessment Conference Panel: Methods for voluntary weight loss and control, *Ann Intern Med* 116:942, 1992.

Roche AF, Heymsfield SB, Lohman TG: *Human body composition,* Champaign, Ill, 1996, Human Kinetics.

Thomas PR, editor: *Weighing the options: criteria for evaluating weight-management programs,* Food and Nutrition Board, Institute of Medicine, Washington, DC, 1995, National Academy Press.

Weinsier R, Wilson N, Morgan S, et al: *EatRight, lose weight—7 simple steps,* Birmingham, Ala, 1997, Oxmoor House.

Williamson DF, Pamuk E, Thun M, et al: Prospective study of intentional weight loss and mortality in never-smoking overweight US women aged 40-64 years, *Am J Epidemiol* 141:1128, 1995.

Diabetes mellitus

American Diabetes Association, American Dietetic Association: *Exchange lists for meal planning,* Alexandria, Va, Chicago, 1995, The Associations.

The Diabetes Control and Complications Trial Research Group: The effect of intensive treatment of diabetes on the development and progression of long-term complications in insulin-dependent diabetes mellitus, *N Engl J Med* 329:977-986, 1993.

The Expert Committee on the Diagnosis and Classification of Diabetes Mellitus: Review: committee report, *Diabetes Care* 20(7):1183-1197, 1997.

Franz MJ, Horton ES, Bantle JP, et al: Nutrition principles for the management of diabetes and related complications, *Diabetes Care* 17:490-518, 1994.

Peragallo-Dittko V, editor: *A core curriculum for diabetes education,* Chicago, 1994, American Association of Diabetes Educators and the AADE Education and Research Foundation.

Tinker LF, Heins JM, Holler HJ: Commentary and translation; 1994 nutrition recommendations for diabetes, *J Am Diet Assoc* 94:507-511, 1994.

Diet, hyperlipidemia, and coronary artery disease

Anderson JW, Johnstone BM, Cook-Newell ME: Meta-analysis of the effects of soy protein intake on serum lipids, *N Engl J Med* 333:276-282, 1995.

Boushey CJ, Beresford SAA, Omenn GS, et al: A quantitative assessment of plasma homocysteine as a risk factor for vascular disease—probable benefits of increasing folic acid intakes, *JAMA* 274:1049-1057, 1995.

Dattilo AM, Kris-Etherton PM: Effects of weight reduction on blood lipids and lipoproteins: a meta-analysis, *Am J Clin Nutr* 56:320-328, 1992.

Gould AL, Rossouw JE, Santanello NC, et al: Cholesterol reduction yields clinical benefit—a new look at old data, *Circulation* 91:2274-2282, 1995.

Hoffman RM, Garewal HS: Antioxidants and the prevention of coronary heart disease, *Arch Intern Med* 155:241-246, 1995.

Hopkins PN: Effects of dietary cholesterol on serum cholesterol: a meta-analysis and review, *Am J Clin Nutr* 55:1060-1070, 1992.

Katan MB: Fish and heart disease, *N Engl J Med* 332:1024-1025, 1995.

Katan MB, Zock PL, Mensink RP: Dietary oils, serum lipoproteins, and coronary heart disease, *Am J Clin Nutr* 61 (suppl):1368S-1373S, 1995.

Klatsky AL: Epidemiology of coronary heart disease—influence of alcohol, *Alcohol Clin Exp Res* 18:88-96, 1994.

Kris-Etherton PM, Emken EA, Allison DB, et al: Trans fatty acids and coronary heart disease risk, *Am J Clin Nutr* 62 (suppl):665S-708S, 1995.

Popkin BM, Siega-Riz AM, Haines PS: A comparison of dietary trends among racial and ethnic subgroups in the United States, *N Engl J Med* 335:716-720, 1996.

Wynder EL, Stellman SD, Zang EA: High fiber intake—indicator of a healthy lifestyle, *JAMA* 275:486-487, 1996.

Hypertension

Beilen LJ: Non-pharmacological management of hypertension: optimal strategies for reducing cardiovascular risk, *J Hypertens* 12 (suppl 10):S71-S81, 1994.

National Institutes of Health: *The Fifth Report of the Joint National Committee on Detection, Evaluation, and Treatment of High Blood Pressure,* NIH Pub No 95-1088, 1995.

Cancer

Block G, Patterson B, Subar A: Fruit, vegetables, and cancer prevention: a review of the epidemiological evidence, *Nutr Cancer* 18:1, 1992.

Hill MJ: Diet and cancer—a review of scientific evidence, *Eur J Cancer Prev* 4(S2):3-42, 1995.

Jacobs MM, editor: Diet and cancer: markers, prevention, and treatment, *Adv Exp Med Biol* 354:1-248, 1994.

Pariza MW: Diet, cancer and food safety. In Shils ME, Olson JA, Shike M, editors: *Modern nutrition in health and disease,* ed 8, Philadelphia, 1994, Lea & Febiger.

Work Study Group on Diet, Nutrition, and Cancer: American Cancer Society guidelines on diet, nutrition, and cancer, *CA Cancer J Clin* 41:334, 1991.

Oral health

American Academy of Pediatric Dentistry: Reference manual 1995-96, *Pediatr Dent* 17:6, 1995.

DePaola DP, Faine MP, Vogel RI: Nutrition in relation to dental medicine. In Shils ME, Olson JA, Shike M, editors: *Modern nutrition in health and disease,* vol 2, ed 8, Philadelphia, 1994, Lea & Febiger.

Enwonwu CO: Interface of malnutrition and peridontal diseases, *Am J Clin Nutr* 61(suppl):430S-436S, 1995.

Johnson DA, Lopez H, Navia JM: Effects of protein deficiency and diet consistency on the parotid gland and parotid saliva of rats, *J Dent Res* 74:1444-1452, 1995.

Li Y, Navia JM, Bian JY: Caries experience in deciduous dentition of rural Chinese children 3-5 years old in relation to the presence or absence of enamel hypoplasia, *Caries Res* 30:8-15, 1996.

Navia JM: Carbohydrates and dental health, *Am J Clin Nutr* 59(suppl):719S-727S, 1994.

Papas AS, Palmer CA, Rounds MC, et al: Longitudinal relationships between nutrition and oral health, *Ann NY Acad Sci* 561:124-142, 1989.

Piyathilake CJ, Hine RJ, Dasayanake AP, et al: Effect of smoking on folate levels in buccal mucosal cells, *Int J Cancer* 52:566-569, 1992.

Pollack RL, Kravitz E: *Nutrition in oral health and disease,* Philadelphia, 1985, Lea & Febiger.

Whitford GM: *The metabolism and toxicity of fluoride, Monographs in oral science vol 16,* ed 2, Farmington, 1996, S Karger.

Osteoporosis

Blumsohn A, Eastell R: Age-related factors. In Riggs BL, Melton III LJ, editors: *Osteoporosis: etiology, diagnosis, and management,* New York, 1995, Lippincott-Raven.

Bunker VW: The role of nutrition in osteoporosis, *Br J Biomed Sci* 51:228-240, 1994.

Chesnut CH, McClung MR, Ensrud KE, et al: Alendronate treatment of the postmenopausal osteoporotic woman: effects of multiple dosages in bone mass and bone remodeling, *Am J Med* 99:144-152, 1995.

Dawson-Hughes B, Dallal GE, Krall EA, et al: A controlled trial of the effect of calcium supplementation on bone density in postmenopausal women, *N Engl J Med* 323:878-883, 1990.

Delmas PD: Biochemical markers for the assessment of bone turnover. In Riggs BL, Melton III LJ, editors: *Osteoporosis: etiology, diagnosis, and management,* New York, 1995, Lippincott-Raven.

Edwards BJ: Age-related osteoporosis, *Clin Geriatr Med* 4:575-588, 1994.

Khosla S, Riggs BL: Treatment options for osteoporosis, *Mayo Clin Proc* 70:978-982, 1995.

Krall EA, Dawon-Hughes B: Walking is related to bone density and rates of bone loss, *Am J Med* 96:20-26, 1994.

Kushida K, Takahashi M, Kawana K, et al: Comparison of markers for bone formation and resorption in premenopausal and postmenopausal subjects, and osteoporosis patients, *J Clin Endocrinol Metab* 80:2447-2450, 1995.

NIH Consensus Development Panel on Optimal Calcium Intake: Optimal calcium intake, *JAMA* 272:1942-1948, 1994.

Pak CY, Sakhaee K, Adams-Huet B, et al: Treatment of postmenopausal osteoporosis with slow-release sodium fluoride, *Ann Intern Med* 123:401-408, 1995.

Reginster JY, Deroisy R, Lecart MP, et al: A double-blind, placebo-controlled, dose-finding trial of intermittent nasal salmon calcitonin for prevention of postmenopausal lumbar spine bone loss, *Am J Med* 98:452-458, 1995.

Reid IR, Ames RW, Evans MC, et al: Long-term effects of calcium supplementation on bone loss and fractures in postmenopausal women: a randomized controlled trial, *Am J Med* 98:331-335, 1995.

Struys A, Snelder AA, Mulder H: Cyclical etidronate reverses bone loss of the spine and proximal femur in patients with established corticosteroid-induced osteoporosis, *Am J Med* 99:235-242, 1995.

Wardlaw GM: Putting osteoporosis in perspective, *J Am Diet Assoc* 93:1000-1006, 1993.

Wimalawansa SJ: Combined therapy with estrogen and etidronate has an additive effect on bone mineral density in the hip and vertebrae: four-year randomized study, *Am J Med* 99:36-42, 1995.

Nutritional anemias

Allen RH, Stabler SP, Savage DG, et al: Diagnosis of cobalamin deficiency I; usefulness of serum methylmalonic acid and total homocysteine concentrations, *Am J Hematol* 34:90-98, 1990.

Beck WS: Diagnosis of megaloblastic anemia, *Ann Rev Med* 42:311-322, 1991.

Colon-Otero G, Menke D, Hood CC: A practical approach to the differential diagnosis and evaluation of the adult patient with macrocytic anemia, *Med Clin North Am* 76:581-597, 1992.

Guyatt GH, Oxman AD, Ali M, et al: Laboratory diagnosis of iron-deficiency anemia. An overview, *J Gen Intern Med* 7:145-153, 1992.

Massey AC: Microcytic anemia. Differential diagnosis and management of iron deficiency anemia, *Med Clin North Am* 76:549-566, 1992.

Eating disorders

Brownell KD, Fairburn CG, editors: *Eating disorders and obesity: a comprehensive handbook,* New York, 1995, Guilford Press.

Fairburn CG: *Overcoming binge eating,* New York, 1995, Guilford Press.

Fairburn CG, Wilson GT, editors: *Binge eating: nature, assessment, and treatment,* New York, 1993, Guilford Press.

Kaplan AS, Garfinkel PE, editors: *Medical issues and eating disorders: the interface,* New York, 1993, Brunner/Mazel.

Alcoholism

Feinman L, Leiber CS: Nutrition and diet in alcoholism. In Shils ME, Olson JA, Shike M, editors: *Modern nutrition in health and disease,* Philadelphia, 1994, Lea & Febiger.

3

Nutrition Throughout the Life Cycle

Nutrition during pregnancy
Breast-feeding
Infancy
Childhood and adolescence
Nutrition and aging

NUTRITION DURING PREGNANCY
Importance of preconceptional nutrition status

The main goals of nutrition-related care are to identify women who are at nutritional risk and to provide appropriate nutritional management. In assessing the woman's history, special attention should be paid to weight status, dietary practices, and use of harmful substances. Excessive use of vitamin and mineral supplements should be avoided, and high levels of vitamin A (>800 retinol equivalents [RE] or 4000 IU/day) should be discontinued in women considering pregnancy. All women of childbearing age who are capable of becoming pregnant should consume at least 0.4 mg of folic acid per day to reduce the risk of having a pregnancy affected with spina bifida or other neural tube defects (NTDs). For those women who have had a child with an NTD, the amount of the folic acid supplement should be 4.0 mg/day. The increased risk of having an NTD appears to outweigh any risk that may occur as the result of the use of large doses of folic acid in these women.

Rapid, substantial weight loss or gain just before conception may influence nutritional status. Preoccupation with weight or widely fluctuating weight, excessive exercise, or excessive dieting may signal a potential eating disorder. Women with poor appetites or who regularly skip meals may be at risk for nutrient deficiencies, particularly if an entire food group is eliminated from the diet. Finally, if the interconceptional period is less than 16 months, iron status may be subnormal.

Physiologic changes of pregnancy affecting nutrition status

Hormone production is influenced by the mother's general health and nutritional status. Progesterone causes a relaxation of the smooth muscles of the uterus so that it can expand as the fetus grows. There is some relaxation of other smooth muscles within the woman's body, including the gastrointestinal tract. This leads to decreased gastrointestinal motility and an increased ability for the body to absorb needed nutrients from the food. Metabolic effects of progesterone include increased fat deposition and increased renal sodium excretion. Estrogen secretion rises sharply near term. Its main role is the growth and maintenance of uterine

73

function. Other effects include an increased affinity of connective tissue for water. This hydroscopic effect, in addition to the sodium loss associated with increased progesterone levels, causes a mixed picture that is often clinically confusing. Patients have presenting symptoms of edema, which may simply be related to estrogen activity but is viewed with alarm because excess fluid retention is one of the symptoms of preeclampsia. When edema is present without the other two symptoms of preeclampsia—proteinuria (protein loss in the urine) and hypertension—there is no increase in perinatal mortality. To the contrary, women with mild edema have slightly larger babies and a lower rate of premature delivery.

Insulin affects blood glucose levels, and its action is critical for a normal pregnancy. The fetus uses only glucose to meet its energy needs. In early pregnancy, women have normal insulin responses to glucose, but later in the pregnancy, it takes more insulin to remove the same amount of glucose from the blood.

Total plasma volume in nonpregnant women averages 2600 ml. By 34 weeks' gestation, it is about 1300 ml higher than at conception. Women with small initial plasma volumes usually have higher increases throughout the pregnancy, as do multigravida women and those with multiple births. In women with relatively small increases in plasma volume, spontaneous abortions, stillbirths, and low-birth-weight deliveries are more likely. The availability of nutrients and the synthesis of normal blood constituents lags behind the increase in plasma volume so that the concentration of various nutrients decreases, although total amount still rises. For example, red cell production is stimulated during pregnancy so that their numbers rise but at a slower rate than the increase in plasma volume. This causes hemodilution and a physiologic drop in hemoglobin levels in the early months of pregnancy.

As the pregnancy progresses, slight cardiac hypertrophy or dilation occurs, which is probably secondary to increased blood volume and cardiac output. Cardiac output increases 30% to 40% by the thirty-second week of gestation. This increased output is largely due to an increased stroke volume in response to increased tissue demands for oxygen.

The elevation of the basal metabolic rate by 15% to 20% at term reflects increased oxygen demands of the uterus, placenta, and fetus, as well as increased cardiac output. Fuel required by the fetus in the third trimester is provided as carbohydrates (70%), amino acids (20%), and fat (10%). The net effect of increased glucose use by the fetus is increased use of fat as a fuel source by the mother. In preparation for the increased need of fuel by the fetus in the third trimester, the mother begins laying down fat stores during the second trimester.

Changes in the gastrointestinal tract occur primarily as a result of the relaxation of smooth muscles. This causes esophageal regurgitation, decreased emptying time of the stomach, and reverse peristalsis, all of which cause heartburn. The decreased smooth muscle tone may also result in increased water absorption from the colon, leading to constipation. Hormonal changes such as a placental rise in human chorionic gonadotropin may contribute to nausea and vomiting. An increased sense of smell is common, and this also often leads to nausea.

Maternal weight gain

Rate of weight gain and total weight gain recommendations. Prepregnancy weight and maternal weight gain during pregnancy influence the birth weight of the infant. Intrauterine growth retardation and low birth weight have been associated with low prepregnancy weight and inadequate weight gain during pregnancy. Accurate and sequential measurements, both preconceptually and during pregnancy, are important components of the nutritional assessment and follow-up of the mother.

According to the Institute of Medicine, National Academy of Sciences recommendations, both the rate of maternal weight gain and total recommended weight gain should be based on prepregnancy BMI, which is defined as the weight in kilograms divided by the height in meters squared (kg/m^2). During the second and third trimesters of pregnancy, the rate of weight gain recommended for women with a low prepregnancy BMI (<19.8) is slightly more than 1 lb/week; for women with a moderate prepregnancy BMI (19.8 to 26.0), the recommendation is about 1 lb/week; and for women with a high prepregnancy BMI (26.1 to 29.0), it is ⅔ lb/week.

A wide range of total body weight gain has been associated with good pregnancy outcomes among women of similar age, weight, height, ethnic background, and socioeconomic status. Therefore the Institute of Medicine, National Academy of Sciences has published ranges for recommended total weight gain. These recommendations for a single-child pregnancy are listed in Table 3-1.

For very obese women (BMI > 29.0), weight loss during pregnancy is not recommended and total weight gain should be decided on an individual basis. Short women (< 62 inches) should strive for gains in the lower end of the recommended range, whereas African-American women and young adolescents should strive for gains in the upper end of the recommended range. The recommended range for a twin pregnancy is 35 to 45 lb (16 to 20 kg).

Fetal weight gain and components of maternal weight gain. Fetal growth follows a sigmoid curve with growth slowing in the final weeks of pregnancy. Fetal growth is most rapid during the second half of pregnancy. The fetus accounts for approximately 25% of the total maternal weight gain. In addition to the fetus, other products of conception contributing to total weight gain include the placenta, contributing about 5% of total weight gain, and amniotic fluid, contributing about 6% of total weight gain.

Table 3-1 Recommended total weight gain for single-child pregnancy

Prepregnancy BMI Weight (kg)/height (m²)	Recommended total weight gain	
	Pounds	Kilograms
Low (BMI < 19.8)	28-40	12.5-18.0
Normal (BMI 19.8-26.0)	25-35	11.5-16.0
High (BMI 26.1-29.0)	15-25	7.0-11.5

Maternal tissue accretion accounts for approximately two thirds of the total weight gain. Contributing factors include increases in weight of uterine and mammary tissues, expansion of maternal blood volume, extracellular fluid, fat stores, and possibly other tissues. The purpose of the additional fat stores is thought to be an energy reserve for pregnancy and lactation.

Specific nutrient needs during pregnancy

Energy and protein needs. Throughout the course of pregnancy, a total of 55,000 kcal are generally required. This translates to 200 to 300 kcal/day above the nonpregnant need. To ensure appropriate weight gain, energy intake above 300 kcal/day may be required during the second and third trimesters and may not be as important during the first trimester.

The RDA for protein is approximately 0.75 grams per kilogram of body weight. The National Research Council recommends an additional 10 to 12 g/day of protein during the last half of the pregnancy to meet the extra demands. Assessment of the adequacy of protein intake is much more important in women whose energy intake is low to avoid the use of protein as an energy source. Additional energy provides a protein-sparing effect that is greater than in the nonpregnant woman.

Minerals and vitamins. Iron is needed for the manufacture of hemoglobin in both maternal and fetal RBCs. The fetus ensures its own production of hemoglobin by drawing iron from maternal sources. Therefore anemia in the mother does not usually result in an infant who is anemic. Iron deficiency anemia in infants is most commonly seen in premature deliveries. Inadequate hemoglobin concentration in the mother means that she must increase her cardiac output to maintain adequate oxygen to the cells. This may fatigue the mother and make her more susceptible to physiologic stress. The National Research Council recommends a general supplementation of 30 mg of iron daily to all pregnant women beginning the twelfth week of gestation. This amount should be adequate in women with normal pregnancies. If a woman develops anemia (defined as a hemoglobin < 11.0 g/dl during the first and third trimesters or < 10.5 g/dl during the second trimester), supplementation with 60 to 120 mg of iron daily is recommended.

Calcium intake during pregnancy should be approximately 1200 to 1500 mg/day. This is the equivalent of four servings of dairy products. If the woman does not regularly consume dairy products or other foods high in calcium, a supplement of calcium of at least 600 mg is recommended.

The RDA for zinc is 15 mg/day. Daily zinc supplementation of 25 mg in women with low plasma zinc levels in early pregnancy is associated with greater infant birth weights and head circumferences, with the effects occurring predominantly in women whose prepregnancy weight is low. Zinc deficiency has been loosely linked to increased likelihood of congenital malformations. It is recommended that a general vitamin and mineral supplement include 15 mg of zinc.

Folic acid is very important before conception and within the first twelve weeks of pregnancy. Adequate intake (400 μg/day) during this time may decrease the risk of NTDs.

Table 3-2 is the suggested approximate composition of prenatal vitamin and mineral supplements for women at increased nutritional risk, including those with a poor-quality diet who are resistant to change and those under the age of 18.

Implementation of nutritional guidelines

Pregnant women should consume a diet that contains a variety of foods, including good sources of calcium, iron, and vitamin C. Health professionals should check to make sure that an entire food group is not being eliminated from the diet. Adequate fluid intake along with regular exercise should also be encouraged as part of a healthy lifestyle during pregnancy.

Sodium. Sodium should not be routinely restricted during pregnancy because water and sodium are required for the expansion of the extracellular and intracellular volumes and to meet the needs of the fetus and amniotic fluid. However, if the woman was restricting sodium before pregnancy for a medical reason, then the restriction should be continued, in consultation with her physician.

Caffeine. Results of studies of the relationship of caffeine intake to pregnancy outcome are ambiguous. One study showed that moderate-to-heavy use of caffeine is associated with an increased incidence of late first trimester and second trimester spontaneous abortion. There is no evidence that caffeine affects embryonic development. A moderate caffeine intake of not more than 2 to 3 servings/day is usually advised.

Alcohol. Alcohol consumption is not recommended during pregnancy because no safe level of alcohol intake has been determined. All alcoholic beverages display a warning from the Surgeon General regarding possible ill effects on the fetus.

Tobacco and drugs. Tobacco and drug use during pregnancy impairs fetal growth. Tobacco and drug use is often accompanied by a decrease in intake of nutrients and/or an increase in nutrient requirements.

Table 3-2   Prenatal vitamin and mineral supplement amounts for women at increased nutritional risk

Nutrient	Daily amount
Iron	30-60 mg
Zinc	15 mg*
Copper	2 mg
Calcium	250 mg
Vitamin B_6	2 mg
Vitamin B_{12}	2 mg
Folate	0.4 mg†
Vitamin C	50 mg
Vitamin D	10 mg (400 IU)

*25 mg of zinc is recommended for women with low concentrations of serum zinc.
†400 μg of folate is the recommendation consistent with the prepregnancy recommendation for all women of childbearing age put forth by the Centers for Disease Control and the U.S. Public Health Service.

Artificial sweeteners. The use of aspartame has been determined to be safe by the FDA, except for individuals who have phenylketonuria (PKU). The use of saccharin is not recommended because studies have been inconclusive about its safety.

Special considerations

Pica. Pica is the persistent compulsive ingestion of substances having little or no nutritional value. Commonly ingested substances include dirt or clay, laundry starch, cornstarch, chalk, baking soda, coffee grounds, and cigarette ashes. Pica can interfere with nutrient intake by replacing nutritious foods or by interfering with the absorption of nutrients such as iron. These substances may contain toxic compounds or quantities of nutrients not tolerated in disease states. Substances such as cornstarch that provide calories can contribute to obesity.

There are several theories about the etiology of pica. Some women ingest these substances as a relief from nausea and vomiting. One hypothesis is that a deficiency of an essential nutrient such as calcium or iron results in the ingestion of nonfood substances that contain these nutrients. Many reasons are based on superstitions, customs, traditions, or practices that are passed from mother to daughter. When evaluating whether a patient may be practicing pica, the health professional should avoid being judgmental. Inquiring about cravings for anything in particular or for any nonfood items would be appropriate when addressing this issue.

Gestational diabetes. Gestational diabetes occurs in women with no prior history of diabetes mellitus and usually resolves after pregnancy. It is associated with perinatal mortality and premature births. Universal screening takes place between 24 and 28 weeks of gestation via a 1-hour, 50-g, nonfasting oral glucose challenge. If the plasma glucose level is greater than 140 mg/dl, a 3-hour, 100-g, OGTT is administered. The diagnostic criteria for gestational diabetes include two or more of the four values during the OGTT being met or exceeded as follows:

Fasting	>105 mg/dl (5.8 mM)
1 hour	>190 mg/dl (10.6 mM)
2 hour	>165 mg/dl (9.1 mM)
3 hour	>145 mg/dl (8.1 mM)

Dietary treatment for gestational diabetes should include all of the recommendations previously discussed plus a diet that provides a caloric distribution of 40% carbohydrate, 20% protein, and 40% fat in several meals and snacks per day. Concentrated sweets should be avoided. The goal of therapy is to achieve normoglycemia, prevent ketosis, and achieve an appropriate weight gain.

Preeclampsia/eclampsia. Preeclampsia is defined as pregnancy-induced hypertension with proteinuria and edema. Eclampsia may result in grand mal seizures and death of the mother. If a patient is diagnosed with preeclampsia, a diet liberal in protein, calories, and fluids with no sodium restriction should be recommended.

Adolescence. Special attention needs to be paid to the pregnant adolescent. Adolescents already have increased needs for specific nutrients such as calcium and iron. Adolescents may also have poor eating habits and/or decreased access to nutritious foods. Adolescence itself is a risk factor for low-birth-weight infants.

Chronic diseases. Pregnant women with a history of diabetes mellitus should have their hemoglobin A_{1c} monitored on a regular basis with a goal level of 5.5% to 6.5%. Blood glucose and urine ketone levels should be monitored. The dietary treatment is similar to that for gestational diabetes.

Maternal PKU is another chronic disease that warrants careful nutrition follow-up. PKU is an inborn error of metabolism in which there is a lack of the enzyme phenylalanine hydroxylase, which metabolizes the amino acid phenylalanine. Before and during pregnancy, patients with PKU are advised to keep their phenylalanine levels very low (2 to 6 mg/dl). This requires the use of low-phenylalanine foods to provide 80% to 90% of daily protein requirements. High phenylalanine levels in the mother have resulted in spontaneous abortion, congenital heart disease, low birth weight, mental retardation, and facial dysmorphology in the infant.

Dietary assessment and nutrition education

The Food Guide Pyramid forms the basis of dietary recommendations for all healthy populations in the United States and can be applied to a healthy diet during pregnancy. In conjunction with the Dietary Guidelines for Americans, a healthful diet during pregnancy can be achieved. Recommendations for the pregnant woman include the following:
- Eat a variety of foods.
- Choose a diet low in fat, particularly saturated fat. Have at least 2 to 3 3-oz servings of meat and 3 to 4 servings of dairy products (at least 4 if under 18 years old), preferably low in fat.
- Choose a diet with plenty of fruits and vegetables, juices, and grain products. Aim for at least 2 servings of fruit, 3 servings of vegetables, and 6 to 11 servings of starchy foods, depending on calorie needs.
- Use sweets, sugars, and soft drinks only moderately.
- Use salt and salty foods as desired unless otherwise directed.

Suggestions for management of common problems of pregnancy

Nausea and vomiting. Take in adequate fluids to avoid dehydration, preferably between meals. Avoid drinking coffee and tea. Try to avoid the smells associated with cooking and food. The odors not commonly associated with food, such as a co-worker's perfume or cigarette smoke, may be particularly offensive because the hormonal changes cause increased sensitivity to smell. Keep a variety of foods around in case cravings occur, and keep fresh lemon to cut and smell. A lemon's freshness has helped in some cases.

Heartburn. Try to decrease emptying time by eating low-fat meals and by eating slowly. Drink fluids mainly between meals. Minimize the use of spices, and avoid lying down for 1 to 2 hours after eating. Wear loose-fitting clothing.

Constipation and hemorrhoids. Drink 2 to 3 quarts of fluids daily, coming from water, milk, juice, or soup. Eat high-fiber cereals and generous amounts of whole grains. It may be helpful to take part in physical activities. Avoid laxatives unless recommended by a physician.

Table 3-3 lists some references for information on governmental food and nutrition programs.

Table 3-3   Food and nutrition resource referrals

Program	Eligibility	Benefits
Women, Infants, and Children (WIC) Program	Pregnant and breast-feeding women, postpartum women, infants, and children < 5 yrs old who are at nutritional risk and at <185% poverty level	Individualized food package provided monthly. Includes foods such as milk, cheese, eggs, cereal, peanut butter, and infant formula. Nutrition education is provided and referral to local agencies facilitated.
Commodity Supplemental Food Program	Pregnant and breast-feeding women, other postpartum women, infants, and children < 6 yrs old at < 185% poverty level	Monthly canned or packaged foods, including fruits, vegetables, meats, and infant formula
Food Stamp Program	U.S. citizens, recognized refugees with visa status, and legal aliens from households with low income and resources. Provided on a sliding scale after formal application process.	Food vouchers to purchase food at area markets
Temporary Emergency Food Assistant Program	Households with < 150% of poverty level	Quarterly distribution of cheese, butter, and rice, and occasionally flour, cornmeal, and dry milk; available monthly
Cooperative Extension Expanded Food and Nutrition Education Program	Households with children < 19 yrs old with income < 125% of the federal poverty level	Education and training on food and nutrition

Summary

Prepregnancy weight, rate of weight gain, and total weight gain during pregnancy are the most important predictors of a successful pregnancy outcome. Women who are at nutritional risk need to be identified and nutrition care plans designed to meet each individual woman's needs. Careful and periodic nutrition follow-up is an essential component of prenatal care.

BREAST-FEEDING

Exclusive breast-feeding is adequate for the first 4 to 6 months of age in almost all infants. One of the U.S. Public Health Service's Healthy People 2000 goals is "to increase to at least 75% the proportion of mothers who breast-feed their babies in the early post-partum period and to at least 50% the proportion who continue breast feeding until their babies are 5 to 6 months old."

Lactation

Lactation is the physiologic completion of the reproductive cycle. All mammalian species produce a milk specific to their own offspring, which is optimal for the ideal growth and development of those offspring. Only the human species has challenged or replaced this stage. Technologic advancement in nutrition has enabled us to manufacture a biochemically acceptable substitute using bovine milk as a base that sustains life and allows growth when the infant's mother does not provide her own milk.

Human milk is not simply a matter of providing macronutrients and micronutrients but the provision of a living dynamic fluid with nutrients, enzymes, epidermal growth modulators, infection protection, and allergy prophylaxis. At the same time, the process provides a hormonal milieu for the mother that promotes psychologic bonding and facilitates the mother's physiologic return to the prepregnancy state while suppressing ovulation and delaying immediate return to fertility.

Adequate release of prolactin and oxytocin is essential for the establishment and maintenance of lactation. Human milk is produced on demand, and involution of the mammary gland is initiated rapidly if milk is not removed from the breast. Prolactin is necessary for the synthesis of milk. Oxytocin is the mediator of the "letdown" or "milk-flow" reflex. Oxytocin release is directly responsible for the contraction of myoepithelial cells that surround the acini of the mammary gland. Oxytocin release usually is stimulated by suckling (tactile stimuli); however, auditory, visual, and olfactory stimuli also may increase its release. Excitement of the sympathetic nervous system appears to inhibit the letdown reflex by directly inhibiting the contraction of myoepithelial cells or by decreasing the blood concentrations of oxytocin that reach the breast. Failure of milk production during highly stressful periods is partially due to these responses.

Maternal dietary requirements

The goals for the postpartum mother include a return to her prepregnant state of health and lactation adequate for successful breast-feeding. A weight loss of up to 20 lb can be expected during the first 3 weeks postpartum. During lactation, an additional 500 to 700 kcal/day and 12 to 15 g/day of protein are required to support the energy and protein requirements of milk production, respectively. Mothers also require additional vitamins and minerals to support lactation. The RDA for lactating mothers is given in Table 1-1.

Nutritional advantages

Human milk is tailored precisely for the growth and development needs of the human infant. The protein content of breast milk is lower than that of other species (1% versus 3% in cow's milk), whose young double their birth weight and wean quickly in days or weeks. The profile of amino acids is ideal for absorption and for utilization, especially by the neonatal brain. The main protein in cow's milk, casein, forms a somewhat indigestible curd and has high levels of phenylalanine, tyrosine, and methionine, for which the infant has little digestive enzyme resources. Cow's milk contains little lactalbumin and cysteine, which the infant can digest readily. Human milk contains taurine, an important nutrient for brain and nerve growth, whereas cow's milk contains none, requiring that taurine be added to most infant formulas.

Breast milk is unique in containing lipases that aid in fat digestion. The fat profile of human milk is predominantly polyunsaturated fats, with a constant amount of cholesterol regardless of the mother's cholesterol intake. Cholesterol is an important constituent of brain and nerve tissue, as well as of many enzymes. Most formulas contain no cholesterol, and the animal fat of cow's milk is replaced with a variety of fats of varying quality. A current concern is that docosa-hexaenonic acid (DHA) and ω-3 oils, while present in human milk and fish oils, are absent in cow's milk and infant formulas. Animal studies suggest a strong relationship between DHA and brain growth. Adding DHA to the diet by using fish oils guarantees neither absorption nor utilization. Human milk is rich in vitamins A, C, and E. The vitamin B content depends on maternal intake and meets calculated standards. Because the primary source of vitamin B_6 and the only source of vitamin B_{12} is animal products, vegetarian mothers, especially strict vegans, may produce milk that is deficient in these vitamins unless they supplement their diets. The vitamin D content of human milk is lower than that of cow's milk, and supplementation is advisable when sun exposure is restricted. All newborns should receive a 0.5- to 1-mg injection or a 2-mg oral dose of vitamin K immediately after birth, regardless of whether breast- or bottle-feeding will be used.

Variations in composition

The composition of milk varies during each feeding and as the child matures. When a feeding is initiated, the mother's milk "lets down," and the first milk or foremilk is released from the ducts as the lacteal cells respond to the surge of prolactin and begin producing milk. The first milk is lower in fat and slightly higher in cells, protein, and lactose. The hind milk is high in fat because the fat globules take more time to form and pass across the cell membrane. Human milk goes through three phases: colostrum, transitional milk, and mature milk. Colostrum, produced at delivery and the first few days postpartum, is high in protein, especially immunoglobulins such as secretory IgA, which provide the infant with initial protection against infection. Colostrum is also high in carotene, which gives it a yellow color. Colostrum provides enzymes that stimulate gut maturation; facilitate digestion, especially of fats by lipase; and stimulate the gut to pass meconium. There is a gradual change from colostrum to transitional milk and then to mature milk over the first 7 to 10 days postpartum. The profile of mature milk persists until about 6 months, when there is a slight decrease in protein content. The immune properties of milk are measurable throughout lactation. At weaning, the milk increases in protein, sodium, and chloride content as the supply diminishes. Mothers who are not fully lactating or are experiencing lactation failure have milk that is higher in sodium and chloride than mature milk.

Immunologic protection

Living cells are present in human milk in concentrations of $4000/mm^3$ in colostrum and $1500/mm^3$ in mature milk. They include macrophages that phagocytize bacteria and viruses in the gut; also included are lymphocytes from the mother's Peyer's patches that also provide immunologic protection in the infant's intestines. The normal flora of the newborn gut include lactobacilli, whose growth is stimulated by the bifidus factor and slightly acidic pH of human milk. The growth of *Escherichia coli* is suppressed by lactoferrin in human milk, which binds the iron that *E. coli* need for survival, whereas growth of *E. coli* is enhanced by iron provided in the diet. Secretory IgA in human milk impedes translocation of organisms across the intestinal wall and mucous membranes from the mouth onward and has been shown in recent studies to reduce respiratory disease, diarrhea, and sepsis. Other humoral factors found in human milk whose precise roles have not all been identified include nucleotides, resistance factor, lysozyme, interferon, complement, and B_{12}-binding protein. All these properties remain unique to human milk, and attempts to fortify infant formulas with some of them, for example, nucleotides, have not been shown to prevent disease.

Fully breast-fed infants experience a lower incidence of and morbidity from bacterial infections, especially of the respiratory tract. Both retrospective and prospective epidemiologic studies also suggest that infants who are fully breast-fed for at least 4 to 6 months may be protected against childhood-onset diabetes, cancers such as lymphoma, celiac disease, and Crohn's disease. The incidence of significant allergic disease (eczema, asthma, and allergic rhinitis) is significantly reduced in the first 2 years of life by breast-feeding, at least in part because of decreased intestinal permeability.

Maintaining lactation

Feeding initiation. Breast-feeding success is enhanced by early initiation. Ideally, the baby should be offered the breast immediately after birth. No test water is necessary when the Apgar scores are good and secretions are modest. Subsequent feedings should be "on demand" but never more than 4 to 5 hours apart in the first week. This is important not only for the infant's nourishment and hydration but also to stimulate the breast to produce milk. Breast-feeding is an infant-driven process. Topping off feedings with water, glucose water, and especially formula is a recipe for lactation failure. Carefully controlled studies have demonstrated clearly that infants who are given water, glucose water, or formula instead of human milk exclusively in the first week lose weight, regain it more slowly, and have higher bilirubin levels and fewer stools.

Feeding frequency. The average infant nurses every 2 hours for 10 to 12 feedings a day during the first few weeks. The gastric emptying time with human milk is no more than 90 minutes, whereas with formulas it is at least 3 hours, and with homogenized milk it is up to 6 hours. Weight gain should be consistent, at least 1 oz/day after 10 to 14 days, when the milk supply is well established. Initial weight loss should not exceed 10% of birth weight and usually averages about 8% when the mother is primiparous. An additional means of monitoring adequate breast milk intake is to count the number of urinary voidings, which should total at least six per day. Stools are an important indication of adequate food in the gut. In the first few weeks, infants produce stool every day, often with every feeding. Signs such as failure to thrive or infrequent stools and voidings deserve evaluation.

Feeding duration. The usual duration of individual feedings is 5 to 20 minutes per breast. Consistent nursing over 25 to 30 minutes per breast may indicate inadequate milk production or inappropriate latch-on. Although most infants extract 80% to 90% of the milk within 5 minutes of nursing, efficiency of sucking varies from infant to infant on the basis of latch-on and suckling vigor. Further, since milk fat is released toward the end of the feeding, arbitrary reduction of feeding times may significantly decrease caloric intake.

Special situations

Working and breast-feeding. Working mothers who wish to continue exclusive breast-feeding may be advised to substitute pumping for some nursings to maintain a total of six or more breast emptyings per day. Increase in nursing frequency on weekends and holidays may be necessary to maintain milk volume. The range of appropriate nursing frequencies is broad when breast-feeding and formula feeding are combined.

Mothers may be advised to begin expressing milk 2 to 3 weeks before returning to work. Initial success is enhanced by pumping the second breast early in the morning, when milk production is at its peak, and immediately after the infant has stimulated oxytocin release by nursing the other breast. Expressed milk may be stored in glass or hard plastic containers, refrigerated immediately, and fed within a day or frozen and fed within 3 months. Some loss of immunologic components will occur if milk is frozen in polyethylene bags. Frozen milk can be thawed quickly by swirling gently under warm running water. This technique prevents the possibility that previously frozen milk will be left at room temperature for long periods during which bacteria may grow and milk fat may break down.

Occluded lactiferous ducts. Occluded lactiferous ducts, characterized by areas of localized breast tenderness, result from milk stasis secondary to infrequent or incomplete breast emptying. If left untreated, occluded ducts may precipitate mastitis. Management includes moist heat and massage and frequent nursing, beginning with the affected breast. Frequent nursing in a variety of nursing positions with concurrent breast massage is the most effective preventive technique.

Mastitis. Mastitis is an inflammation of breast connective tissue or ducts. Symptoms of mastitis include fever, body aches, breast pain, erythematous streaks, and lumps in the breast. *Staphylococcus aureus* is the most common bacterial etiologic agent. *Streptococcus* and *E. coli* are the next most common causes, although other pathogens may cause mastitis. Prompt treatment with an antistaphylococcal antibiotic is indicated for initial bouts of mastitis. Mothers with mastitis can continue to breast-feed. Mothers should be advised to take the full course (7 to 14 days) of oral antibiotics. Recurrent infection is common when mothers discontinue medication after symptoms are alleviated. If mastitis recurs, breast-feeding can be continued during the second course of antibiotic therapy.

Breast abscess. In severe cases of mastitis, usually when antibiotic therapy is either delayed or not completed, breast abscess can occur. Surgical drainage will be required. It is important to counsel the patient to take the full course of prescribed antibiotics, along with application of moist heat to the infected area. Breast abscess is not an indication that breast-feeding should be discontinued. If the surgical incision and drainage tube are away from the areola, bilateral breast-feeding can continue as usual. Otherwise, the infant should nurse from the unaffected breast, with the mother manually expressing milk from the infected breast until the incision heals. It is very important to empty the infected breast at every feeding, using manual expression or a breast pump if nursing is painful. If the breast is not emptied, milk stasis and congestion will become painful and create a potential source for additional infection.

Sore nipples. Sore nipples are normal during the first week of lactation. Pain usually is most noticeable on initial latch-on and subsides after 30 seconds to 1 minute. Sore nipples are associated more with the position of the infant at the breast than with the length of feedings. When mothers complain of sore nipples, the first step is to observe the infant while it is put to the breast, taking particular note of the position: the baby's abdomen should face the mother's abdomen and the infant should directly face the breast. Mothers with persistently sore nipples may be referred to a lactation consultant. Prolonged nipple pain throughout nursing and nipple pain that persists beyond the first 2 weeks may result from incorrect suckling, nipple trauma, or bacterial or fungal infection of the nipple. Virtually all sore nipples benefit from careful attention to rinsing, thorough drying, and 10 to 15 minutes of air exposure after nursing. Suspected bacterial infections may be treated with a topical antibiotic; the breast should be rinsed and dried before nursing. Yeast infections (nipple candidiasis) require simultaneous treatment of mother and infant to prevent reinfection.

Infant refusal to nurse. Refusal to nurse may occur at any time and may last several hours or even days. A variety of conditions have been associated with this unexpected behavior (e.g., thrush, respiratory infections, otitis media, teething, changes in maternal diet, changes in soaps and perfumes, and resumption of menses). Often such episodes are unexplained and resolve spontaneously. When no other symptoms are observed in the infant, reassurance and advice to offer quiet, soothing feeding opportunities may be the most the clinician can suggest. If normal nursing is not resumed in a reasonable time, the child should be examined to rule out underlying illness.

Contraindications

Maternal infections in general do not contraindicate breast-feeding and in most cases even provide additional protection for the infant via the milk. At one time, hepatitis B represented a contraindication to breast-feeding. However, now that all infants born to mothers with hepatitis B are given hepatitis B immune globulin in the first 12 hours of life and then vaccine before hospital discharge, breast-feeding is safe even though the virus might pass into the milk.

Hepatitis C is a nonacute infection that often results in chronic liver disease or cirrhosis, and currently there is no effective treatment. Although the published medical literature contains no evidence of disease transmission through breast milk, the risk of chronic infection is great enough to contraindicate breast-feeding for newborns whose mothers are known to have hepatitis C.

When a mother has active tuberculosis, all mother-infant contact—including breast-feeding—should be suspended until appropriate therapy is initiated and continued for at least 1 week. If maternal disease is discovered before birth and treatment is initiated immediately, breast-feeding should be permitted as long as maternal therapy is continued and infant prophylaxis initiated.

The disease giving most concern presently is acquired immunodeficiency syndrome (AIDS). Not all infants born to human immunodeficiency virus (HIV)-positive mothers are infected with the virus at birth, but those who are infected cannot be identified immediately because passive maternal antibodies are present. In the United States, where the survival of healthy bottle-fed babies is ensured, mothers with HIV should not breast-feed. In developing countries, where infants have a greater than 50% chance of dying in the first year of life if not breast-fed and where the risk of AIDS if breast-fed by an HIV-positive mother is less than 18%, breast-feeding is encouraged. Present data suggest that the virus may pass into the milk, but the milk suppresses the growth of the virus, at least in vitro.

Maternal medications

Although medications pass into milk in varying amounts, depending on the pharmacologic properties of the compound, most medications are safe for mothers to take while nursing. Those that are most effective while delivering the lowest amounts to the infant should be selected. Over-the-counter drugs such as aspirin, acetaminophen, and ibuprofen are usually acceptable in moderate doses for temporary use. Although most antibiotics pass into milk to some degree, those that can be given directly to infants are safe for lactating mothers to take. A short list of drugs contraindicated during lactation is given in Table 3-4. In most cases, acceptable substitutes are available.

Although drugs of abuse represent a risk to nursing infants, in the case of marijuana the risk-to-benefit ratio favors breast-feeding over bottle-feeding. The mother who is bottle-feeding and smokes marijuana in the presence of her infant

Table 3-4 Drugs contraindicated during breast-feeding

Drug	Rationale
Amethopterin, cyclophosphamide, cyclosporine, methotrexate	May suppress the immune system; unknown effect on growth or association with carcinogenesis
Bromocriptine	Suppresses lactation
Cimetidine	Concentrated in breast milk; may suppress gastric acidity in infant, inhibit drug metabolism, and stimulate central nervous system
Clemastine	May cause drowsiness, irritability, refusal to feed, high-pitched cry, neck stiffness
Ergotamine	Doses used in migraine medications cause vomiting, diarrhea, convulsions
Gold salts	Cause rash and inflammation of kidneys and liver
Methimazole	Potentially interferes with thyroid function
Phenindione	Causes hemorrhage
Thiouracil	Decreases thyroid function (does not apply to propylthiouracil)

creates risk without the benefits of breast-feeding. Cigarette smoking has been associated with decreased duration of breast-feeding, but breast-fed infants of smoking mothers have fewer respiratory infections than bottle-fed infants whose mothers smoke. Mothers should be cautioned never to smoke in the presence of the infant and not to smoke within 30 minutes before a feeding to avoid suppressing the letdown reflex and to decrease the possibility of nicotine appearing in the milk.

Radioactive pharmaceuticals used as a single dose for clinical diagnosis require temporary discontinuation of breast-feeding. The breasts should be pumped to maintain lactation, but the milk should be discarded. When radioactive drugs are used in multiple doses for treatment, breast-feeding must be discontinued because no amount of radioactive material is safe for an infant.

Weaning

The introduction of solid foods into the diet of 4- to 6-month-old exclusively breast-fed infants results in reduced milk intake despite attempts to maintain nursing frequency. During the first month, total energy intake also declines slightly. Feeding efficiency increases, and total caloric intake returns to the level achieved during exclusive breast-feeding in the second month after solids are introduced. Single-ingredient foods should be introduced first and new foods offered at intervals of no less than 3 to 5 days to enable the detection of allergies or intolerance to specific foods. Breast-fed infants accept solid foods faster than formula-fed infants.

Weaning may be initiated either by the infant or the mother and is most successful if done gradually. Nursing frequency may be decreased by one nursing every 3 to 7 days. This allows time for breast involution and decreases the possibility of engorgement and mastitis. Solid foods or other liquids may be offered in place of each eliminated feeding.

INFANCY

The first year of life

The first year of life is characterized by rapid growth and changes in body composition and is termed *infancy*. Adequate nutrition is required to promote optimal growth and development, to avoid illness, and to allow the infant to interact with and explore his environment. Infant nutritional requirements are different than those of adults; for example, protein, fat, and energy are important for growth, and iron, zinc, and calcium are required in greater proportions for infants.

Body composition

Knowledge of the body composition of the infant at various stages is of considerable importance. Characterizing changes in body composition is a means for understanding the process of growth and change in function that affect the nutritional needs of a growing infant. The body is composed of fat and fat-free body mass (FFBM), which includes water, protein, carbohydrate, and minerals. The percent of body weight that is fat increases throughout infancy from approximately 14% at birth to 23% by 1 year of age. The accompanying decrease in percent FFBM (86% at birth to 77% by 1 year of age) is due principally to a decrease in water content. The contribution of protein, minerals, and carbohydrate remains relatively constant throughout infancy.

Body composition can be viewed in functional terms such as organ function (brain, heart, liver, kidney), muscle mass, energy reserves (fat mass), extracellular fluid, and the supporting structures (connective tissue, bone). The major organs and muscle mass account for most of the body protein; the fat mass is primarily used for energy when the diet is inadequate; and bone contains a reserve of calcium, phosphorus, and other minerals.

Growth

Growth-related increases in weight, length, and head circumference are extremely rapid before birth and during the first year of life. A normal 1-month-old infant grows approximately 1 cm/week and gains 20 to 30 g/day, which gradually decreases to 0.5 cm/week in length and 10 g/day in weight by 12 months of age. An average newborn weighs 3.5 kg, doubles its weight by 4 months, and triples it by 12 months of age. The energy cost of growth is the cost of depositing fat and protein. Fat deposition requires 10.8 kcal/g, and protein deposition requires 13.4 kcal/g.

During early postnatal development, all organs appear to grow by cell division (hyperplasia) followed by a pattern of increasing cell size (hypertrophy). At birth, 15% of body weight is organ mass, 25% is muscle mass, 14% is fat, and 15% is bone and connective tissue. Throughout infancy, these organ systems continue to grow and mature at a rapid rate. Cell number, measured by increments of deoxyribonucleic acid (DNA), continues to increase rapidly in the brain, heart, kidney, liver, and spleen. The brain doubles in size by 1 year of age. Energy or nutrient deficiencies during this period of rapid cell replication may limit the number of cells formed and possibly cause permanent deficits in the developing brain and nervous system.

Organ maturation

The number of obstacles that the newborn faces in maintaining nutrient balance and their magnitude are inversely related to gestational age. The gastrointestinal tract of the preterm infant and sometimes the term infant may not be ready to perform the vital functions of nutrient intake, processing, assimilation, metabolism, and distribution to other organs. The term infant has mature coordination of sucking and swallowing but poor coordination of esophageal motility; decreased lower esophageal sphincter pressure, which enhances the risk of gastroesophageal reflux; reduced gastric volume and delayed gastric emptying; and variable maturity of several enzymatic and hormonal systems.

The kidneys fine-tune water and electrolyte excretion in relation to intake to maintain a body fluid composition that supports optimal function. The term infant has a full number of nephrons but a low glomerular filtration rate in the first 48 hours; a higher fractional excretion of sodium than in adults; relative difficulty excreting a high acid load; and normal diluting but limited concentrating capabilities.

Premature infant

Special formulas are available for feeding the premature infant with very low birth weight. They are recommended until the infant achieves a body weight of 1.8 kg.

The composition of these formulas differs markedly from that of human milk: in general, they have a higher protein content, contain significant amounts of medium-chain triglycerides, are low in lactose, and contain slightly more sodium.

When the infant with very low birth weight is fed human milk, requirements for normal growth may not be met, although human milk provides immunologic protection needed for the premature infant. Methods are available to fortify human milk for the feeding of the premature infant (Box 3-1).

Infant formulas

When breast-feeding is not feasible, commercially prepared infant formulas are an acceptable alternative. They are stable mixtures of emulsified fats, proteins, carbohydrates, minerals, and vitamins, and they come in ready-to-feed, concentrated liquid, or powdered preparations. Standard infant formulas have an energy density of 20 kcal/oz and an osmolarity of 300 mOsm/L. The American Academy of Pediatrics suggests a caloric distribution of 30% to 55% fat (2.7% of the calories as linoleic acid), 7% to 16% protein, and the remaining 35% to 65% of energy from carbohydrate. The Infant Formula Act of 1980 regulates the composition of infant formulas sold in the United States.

Solid foods

A recommended schedule for introducing solid foods is shown in Box 3-2.

Box 3-1   Guidelines for feeding premature infants

1. Human milk can be fed by continuous nasogastric tube (syringe pumps are recommended), especially if the infant weighs less than 1300 g.
2. When full feeding volume is achieved, fortification of the human milk is instituted. After the infant reaches a weight of 1600 to 1800 g, breast- or bottle-feeding is introduced, and when fed entirely by nipple, fortification can be discontinued.
3. Until the infant's condition is stable, close monitoring of nutritional status is critical, including serum electrolytes, hemoglobin, urea nitrogen, and albumin.

Box 3-2   Schedule for introducing solid foods

Months	Food items
1-4	Breast milk or formula only
4-6	Iron-fortified cereal
6-7	Fruits (strained or mashed); begin introducing a cup
7-8	Vegetables (strained or mashed)
8-9	Finger foods (crackers, banana, etc.) and chopped (junior) baby foods
9	Meats and citrus juice
10	Bite-size cooked foods
12	All table foods

The introduction of solid foods should be based on the individual infant's growth, activity, and neuromuscular development. Infants do not have the oral motor skills to consume solid food or eat from a spoon until 4 to 6 months of age. The potential disadvantages of introducing solid food before this time are shown in Box 3-3.

When adding solid foods to an infant's diet, one new single-ingredient food should be started every 3 to 5 days. This allows the parent to watch for an allergic reaction and gives the infant time to become accustomed to new tastes. Other suggested guidelines for introducing solids are shown in Box 3-4.

The sequence of introducing foods is not critical, although iron-fortified dry baby cereals are usually added first. Rice cereal is commonly the first food because rice is the least allergenic. Eggs and wheat should be avoided during the first 6 to 9 months of age to minimize the possibility of an allergic reaction. Combination foods of strained cereal with fruit, vegetables with meat, high-meat dinners, and other infant or toddler foods may be introduced after single-ingredient foods are well tolerated. Unsweetened fruit juices should be introduced when the

---

Box 3-3   Potential disadvantages of introducing solid foods before 4
to 6 months

- Poor oral motor coordination
- Insufficient energy and nutrient replacement for breast milk or infant formula
- Increased risk of food allergies
- Increased renal solute load and hyperosmolarity
- Disturbance of appetite regulation resulting in overfeeding
- Increased likelihood of infant desiring sugar and salt later in life

---

Box 3-4   Guidelines for introducing solid foods

- Begin with single-ingredient foods, one at a time.
- Give a small amount of each new food, beginning with 1 to 2 tsp and gradually increasing to 3 to 4 tsp/feeding.
- Wait 3 to 5 days before adding another new food; discontinue the last food if allergy is detected.
- Ultimately, offer a wide variety of foods. For older infants, include meats, milk, fruits, vegetables, bread, and cereals for nutritional adequacy and diversity.
- Avoid mixing solids with fluids to allow the infant to learn textures and flavors and to develop facial muscles. *Exception:* for infants with reflux, add rice cereal to thicken feedings.
- Never put a baby to bed with a bottle or allow the baby to suck a bottle continuously during the day. This practice increases the risk of dental caries and may affect tooth eruption.
- Provide solids with textures compatible with the infant's ability to chew and swallow.

infant can drink from a cup. Juices should be given in a cup and not in a bottle, since the latter may predispose the infant to nursing-bottle caries. The protein content of breast milk decreases gradually with the duration of lactation. High-protein baby foods should be encouraged. Sugar and salt should not be added during preparation of homemade baby foods, and frozen or canned foods containing sugar and salt should be avoided.

Between 6 and 12 months of age, infants show increasing interest in self-feeding and develop the ability to grasp and pick up foods. Finger foods should be offered once the ability to chew is acquired. These should be carefully selected to allow for easy manipulation in the mouth and minimize the potential for choking and aspiration (Box 3-5).

Nutritional requirements of infants

The RDAs are the levels of intake of essential nutrients considered to be adequate to meet the known nutritional needs of healthy individuals. These recommendations are based on the average daily amount of nutrients that population groups should consume over time and are not requirements for specific individuals. The RDAs for infants up to 6 months of age are based primarily on the amounts of nutrients known to be provided by breast milk. Those for infants from 6 months to 1 year of age are based on the consumption of formula and increasing amounts of solid food.

Energy

The energy balance of infants may be described simply as: gross energy intake equals energy excreted plus energy expended plus energy stored. The components of energy expenditure are basal metabolic rate (energy needed to maintain body temperature; support the minimal work of the brain, heart, and respiratory muscles; and to supply the minimal energy requirements of tissues at rest), the thermic effect of feeding (energy used for digestion, transport, and conversion of absorbed

---

Box 3-5   Finger foods for infants

Preferred

- Bread, toast, unsalted crackers
- Fruit: fresh or canned (unsweetened), soft, without seeds or peels (banana, apple, peach, apricot)
- Meat, poultry, fish: tender, small cooked pieces or strips without bones (meatballs, meat sticks, hamburger, meat loaf, chicken nuggets, turkey, fish sticks)
- Vegetables: tender, cooked whole pieces or chunks (carrots, green beans, squash, potato)

Avoid

- Popcorn, nuts, seeds, unmashed peas, raisins, potato chips, corn kernels (because of potential for choking and aspiration)

nutrients into their respective storage forms), and physical activity-related expenditure. Energy requirements per kg body weight gradually decline throughout infancy because of decreases in basal metabolic rate per kg and growth rate. It is estimated that the percent of energy intake used for growth decreases from about 27% from birth to 4 months, 11% from 4 to 6 months, and about 5% from 6 to 12 months of age.

Water

Water is required by the infant to replace losses from skin and lungs (evaporative losses) and in feces and urine; a small amount is also needed for growth. Under most conditions, water intake exceeds the requirements for evaporative losses, renal excretion of solutes, and growth, and any excess is excreted in the urine.

Human milk, cow's milk, and infant formulas of conventional energy density (67 kcal/100 ml) provide approximately 89 ml of preformed water in each 100 ml of milk or formula consumed. In addition, foods yield water when oxidized: 0.41 ml, 1.07 ml, and 0.55 ml, respectively, from the complete combustion of 1 g of protein, fat, and carbohydrate. In milks and formulas, preformed water and oxidation water amount to approximately 95% of the volume consumed.

Intestinal solute load. Because the intestine is a semipermeable membrane, rapid introduction of a high-solute (osmolar) load results in a shift of water from the blood stream into the lumen of the bowel, causing osmotic diarrhea. Human milk has an osmolality of 275 mOsm/L. Most of the infant formulas have a solute load of 300 mOsm/L and are tolerated well.

Renal solute load. Certain elements of the diet require excretion by the kidneys, either because they are metabolic waste products or because they are ingested in quantities greater than are required by the body. Water is required to excrete these materials, which include urea, sodium, potassium, chloride, and to a lesser extent sulfates and phosphates. For each gram of protein ingested, close to 4 mOsm of solute are produced in the form of urea. Because our bodies tend to stay in balance with regard to sodium, potassium, and chloride, for each milliequivalent of these substances ingested, a milliosmol of solute must be excreted (Table 3-5).

Because of immaturity, the infant's kidneys can only concentrate urine to an osmolality of about 600 mOsm/L. If an infant is fed 1 L of whole cow's milk, which contains a potential renal solute load of 308 mOsm/L, more than half of the water ingested in the milk will be required to excrete the solute. The actual volume of water required is calculated as follows:

$$308 \text{ mOsm}/600 \text{ mOsm} \times 1000 \text{ ml} = 513 \text{ ml}$$

Carbohydrates

Carbohydrates should comprise 35% to 65% of the total energy intake of the term infant, usually in the form of disaccharides or glucose polymers. Glucose is the principal nutrient that the neonatal brain uses, and inadequate carbohydrate intake can lead to hypoglycemia, ketosis, and excessive protein catabolism. Most milk-based formulas contain lactose as the principal carbohydrate in amounts similar to

Table 3-5   Potential renal solute load of human milk formulas and cow's milk

| | Potential renal solute load (mOsm/L) | | |
| | Components | | |
Food	Urea	Na + Cl + K + P	Total
Human milk	57	36	93
Milk-based formula	86	49	135
Soy protein–based formula	103	62	165
Evaporated milk formula	158	102	260
Whole cow's milk	188	120	308

that of human milk (6 to 7 g/100 ml). Several hypoallergenic formulas contain sucrose, maltose, fructose, dextrins, and glucose polymers as their carbohydrate sources. Since they are lactose free, they are also useful in managing disorders such as galactosemia and primary lactase deficiency and in recovering from secondary lactose intolerance.

Fat

Dietary fat serves as a concentrated source of energy, carries fat-soluble vitamins, and provides essential fatty acids (EFAs). EFAs are precursors for the synthesis of prostaglandins and serve other essential functions. The American Academy of Pediatrics recommends that 30% to 55% of total energy intake be from fat and that 2.7% be from linoleic acid.

The fat content of infant formulas is derived from a variety of long-chain vegetable triglycerides such as soy, corn, and safflower oil and from medium-chain triglycerides (MCT). Linoleic acid is found only in the long-chain vegetable oils in various concentrations. Breast milk contains 8% to 10% of total calories as linoleic acid, and most infant formulas have at least 10%. Some special formulas contain MCT, fatty acids from 6 to 12 carbons in length compared with long-chain triglycerides, which are greater than 16 carbons long. MCT is partially soluble in water and is not dependent on bile acids for solubilization, so it can be absorbed by patients with malabsorption and hepatobiliary disease. Because of its solubility, MCT can appose the mucosal surface and be hydrolyzed by mucosal lipases. This obviates the need for pancreatic lipase. A large percentage of absorbed MCT is transported directly into the portal circulation, bypassing the lymphatic channels necessary to transport long-chain triglycerides. For this reason, MCT oil is useful in managing diseases such as intestinal lymphangiectasia. The disadvantages of MCT oil are that it is not very palatable, it has a cathartic effect when given in large amounts, it is expensive, and it does not contain EFAs.

Protein

Protein provides nitrogen and amino acids for the synthesis of body tissues and enzymes, hormones, and antibodies that regulate and perform physiologic and metabolic functions. Excess dietary proteins are metabolized for energy, increasing the renal solute load and water requirements. The American Academy of Pediatrics recommends that 7% to 16% of total energy be from protein, or 1.6 to 2.2 g/kg/day. Healthy term infants may grow well with a protein intake (from breast milk) slightly below 1.6 g/kg/day.

The protein in commercial formulas was originally from cow's milk, which has a whey:casein ratio of 20:80. Several recent infant formulas contain whey:casein ratios of 60:40, which is closer to the 65:35 or 70:30 ratio and amino acid composition of human milk. The curd formed from whey in the acidic stomach is small, soft, and easily digestible and is emptied quickly.

Other protein sources used in infant formulas include soy protein isolates and protein hydrolysates. Infant formulas containing soy protein are well received by vegetarian families who may wish to avoid cow's milk and animal products. Soy proteins contain trypsin inhibitors that may interfere with absorption. These inhibitors are largely inactivated by heat treatment of the protein isolate. Soy also produces tightly bound protein-phytate mineral complexes that may reduce the bioavailability of some minerals. For these reasons, soy formulas are not recommended for routine infant feeding.

Between 20% and 80% of infants who are allergic to casein are also allergic to soy, so hydrolyzed casein is the protein of choice for these infants. The enzymatic hydrolysis process results in a mixture of amino acids and peptides of various chain lengths and destroys its allergenicity, making it ideal for treating protein hypersensitivity.

Vitamins

Many of the vitamins play important roles as cofactors and catalysts for cell function and replication. The content of most commercial infant formulas is also adequate to meet the requirements of most healthy infants when they consume approximately 750 ml (26 oz) of formula each day. Vitamin supplementation may be necessary for infants whose intake is less than this, when steatorrhea is present (hepatobiliary disease, pancreatic insufficiency, or small intestinal disease causing malabsorption), or when prescribed medications affect vitamin absorption or utilization. Table 3-6 provides guidelines for using vitamin and mineral supplements in healthy infants and children.

Minerals

The American Academy of Pediatrics recommends a dietary calcium:phosphorus ratio between 1:1 and 1:2 for optimal calcium absorption. The ratio declines during infancy with the introduction of solid foods. There are also minimum and maximum levels for sodium, potassium, and chloride in formulas, which will meet growth needs and leave little residue to be excreted in the urine. The ratio of sodium to potassium should not exceed 1, and the ratio of sodium plus potassium to chloride should be at least 1.5.

Iron deficiency is the most common cause of anemia in infants and children. In the healthy term infant, there is no need for exogenous iron between birth and 4 months of age. The usually abundant neonatal iron stores gradually decline during this period to provide for the synthesis of hemoglobin, myoglobin, and en-

Table 3-6 Guidelines for the supplementation of vitamin and mineral supplements in healthy infants and children*,†

Group	Multivitamins	Individual vitamins			Minerals	
		D	E	Folate	Iron	Fluoride
Preterm infants						
Breast-fed‡	+	+	±	±	+	−
Formula-fed	+	+	±	±	+	−
Term infants (0-6 months)						
Breast-fed	−	+	−	−	−	−
Formula-fed	−	−	−	−	−	−
Infants > 6 months§	−	+	−	−	±‖	±‖
Children > 1 year	−	−	−	−	−	±
Pregnant women	±	−	−	±	+	−
Lactating women	±	−	−	−	±	−

+, Needs supplement; −, does not need supplement; ±, prescription of supplement depends on the clinical situation.
*Vitamin K is not shown but should be given to all newborn infants.
†Extra calcium for pregnant and lactating women is not shown.
‡The sodium content of human milk is marginal for preterm infants.
§If high-risk (poor intake, steatorrhea, or medication use that affects vitamin absorption or utilization), multivitamins and multiminerals (including iron) are preferred.
‖See discussion in text.

zymes, but iron deficiency is rare in the first several months unless there has been substantial loss of iron through perinatal or subsequent blood loss.

There are two broad categories of iron in food, heme iron and nonheme iron. Since infant diets contain little meat, the vast preponderance of iron is in the nonheme form. The absorption of nonheme iron depends on how soluble it becomes in the duodenum, and this in turn is determined by the composition of foods consumed in a given meal. The most important enhancers of nonheme iron absorption are ascorbic acid and meat, fish, and poultry. Major inhibitors are bran (whole-grain cereals), oxalates (spinach), polyphenols (tannates in tea), and phosphates (cow's milk, egg yolk). Absorption of the small amount of iron in breast milk is uniquely high, 50% on average, in contrast to 10% from unfortified cow's milk formula and 4% from iron-fortified cow's milk formulas and dry infant cereals.

Box 3-6 suggests ways to optimize iron status in infants.

Trace Minerals

Breast-feeding and commercial formulas provide adequate amounts of trace minerals for full-term infants. The fluoride concentration of breast milk ranges from 3 to 10 μg/L. Fluoride is poorly transported from plasma to milk, and concentrations in milk remain low even if the mother consumes fluoridated water. There is no convincing evidence that orally ingested fluoride is important in preventing dental caries (i.e., by altering the composition of the dental enamel). However, there is clear evidence that oral consumption may contribute to fluorosis of the

---

Box 3-6 Optimizing iron status in infants

Unfortified foods

- Maintain breast-feeding for at least 4 months.
- Do not give fresh cow's milk until after about 9 months.
- Use vitamin C–rich foods and fruit juice or meat with meals of solid food after about 6 months.

Iron- and vitamin C–fortified foods

- If cow's milk formula is used, choose one fortified with iron and vitamin C.
- Use infant cereal or milk-cereal products fortified with iron and vitamin C.
- Use vitamin C–fortified fruit juice with meals of solid foods.

Iron supplementation (ferrous sulfate or similarly bioavailable compounds)

- Supplement low-birth-weight infants with the following amounts of iron from formula or drops, beginning no later than 2 months of age and continuing through the sixth month:

Birth weight	Supplemental iron dose
1500-2500 g	2 mg/kg/day
1000-1500 g	3 mg/kg/day
<1000 g	4 mg/kg/day

- For established iron deficiency: 3 mg/kg/day

---

permanent dentition. No fluoride supplements are therefore recommended for infants. After teeth have erupted, it is recommended that, when feasible, fluoridated water be offered several times daily to infants fed by breast or cow's milk or formulas prepared with water that contains no more than 0.3 mg/L.

CHILDHOOD AND ADOLESCENCE

The childhood years (ages 1 to 10) and the adolescent years (ages 11 to 18) are characterized by changes in growth rates, body composition, and nutrient requirements. Between infancy and adolescence, body fat decreases and FFBM increases. Growth proceeds at a slower rate as energy and protein requirements decrease.

Normal growth rates

Growth is predictable in a normal child. The rate of growth varies with age and can be quantitated using standard height velocity charts for males and females. The child's stature should be measured in the supine position until he or she is 24 to 36 months of age. Two people are required to make an accurate measurement, with one holding the child in the proper position while the other measures. Children from 2 to 18 years are measured standing.

The birth weight triples by 12 months of age and quadruples by 2 years. Thereafter, the weight gain slows to a relatively steady yearly increase of 2 to 3 kg (4.5 to 6.5 lb) until the onset of the adolescent growth spurt. The linear growth velocity after the first year of life decreases more slowly than weight gain. Between

3 and 10 years of age the height gained by girls and boys remains consistently between 5 and 8 cm/year. A normal 2 year old has reached 50% of adult height, and a normal 10 year old has reached about 80% of height potential. The head circumference of a newborn in the United States is about 34 cm. The brain normally doubles in size during the first year of life. By 3 years of age the head circumference has increased to approximately 50 cm. Thereafter, head circumference does not change markedly.

Distance curve. Fig. 3-1, *A,* shows the height growth curve for a typical boy and girl from birth to 19 years. It is the most commonly used description and the most closely associated with the pattern of growth observed in everyday life.

Velocity curve. Fig. 3-1, *B,* shows the growth velocity curve, which is calculated by dividing the difference between two height measurements as near to 1 year apart as possible by the exact time elapsed between them. It is plotted at the midpoint of the time interval. There are three epochs of growth: early, rather fast growth before the age of 2; a relatively unchanging pattern of growth during preschool and primary school years; and then the adolescent growth spurt. There is little difference between boys and girls before 10 years of age. The typical girl starts her adolescent growth spurt earlier and for a few years is taller than a boy of the same age. Some 2 years later the boy starts his spurt and by the age of 14 is the taller. The difference in mature height between men and women in the United States is 12.5 cm.

Nutrient requirements

An adequate intake of energy, protein, and all other essential nutrients is required for the rapid rate of growth and development characteristic of the young child. Mean weights and heights and the RDAs for energy and protein are given in Table 1-1. This illustrates the decreased protein and energy required as growth decelerates. For example, for toddlers, preschoolers, and preadolescents the energy and protein requirements are 102 kcal and 1.2 g/kg body weight, 90 kcal and 1.1 g, and 70 kcal and 1.0 g/kg body weight, respectively. The wide range of the recommendations for energy intake reflect the variation in individual growth and physical activity of children. It is estimated that children from 1 to 2 years of age use approximately 3% of energy intake for growth, and after 3 years of age, most children use less than 2% of energy intake for growth. Protein requirements are those adequate for 95% of the population, whereas energy requirements are expressed as the population mean. Insufficient dietary carbohydrate and fat will result in the utilization of dietary protein and lean body mass to provide individual energy needs. Minerals, such as calcium, iron, and zinc, are also essential for normal growth and development.

Toddlers (1 to 3 years). A child's developmental stages, behavioral characteristics, and food selection choices must be considered when providing food for toddlers ages 1 to 3. Between 1 and 3 years of age, weight gain per year decreases from 6.5 kg to 2.5 kg and height gain per year declines from 25 cm to 7 cm. Growth in head circumference also slows down to an increase of 0.5 to 1.2 cm/year by 3 years of age. There is a concurrent decrease in energy and protein needs to approximately 100 kcal/kg of energy and 1.2 g/kg of protein.

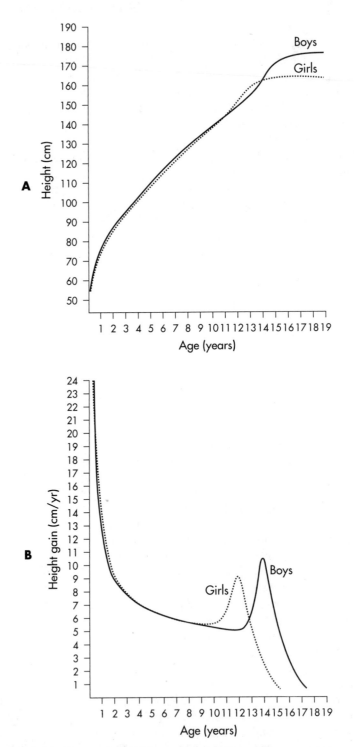

Fig. 3-1 Height distance curve (**A**) and velocity curve (**B**) of a typical boy *(solid line)* and girl *(broken line)*. (Modified from Tanner JM, Whitehouse RH, Takaishi M: Standards from birth to maturity for height, weight, height velocity, and weight velocity: British children 1965, *Arch Dis Child* 41:454-613, 1966.)

Feeding behavior develops progressively during the toddler years, as can be seen in Box 3-7.

Oral and neuromuscular development improves the ability to eat. Increased refinement of hand and finger movement occurs, and the subsequent appearance of most of the primary teeth leads toddlers to self-feeding. As children gain proficiency in coordinating arm, wrist, and hand movements, they demand increased responsibility in feeding themselves and reject any offers of assistance. Finger foods, spoons, and cups should be encouraged to help continue development of manual dexterity and coordination.

Three meals and two snacks should be offered each day, but food intake will vary. Avoid foods likely to be aspirated, such as hot dogs, nuts, grapes, round candies, popcorn, and raw carrots. Set limits so that demands for food and drink do not become attention-getting devices that might lead to inappropriate intake if not recognized.

The eating patterns of most toddlers are characterized by decreased food intake relative to body size. This change in food consumption after infancy, often worrisome to parents, is normal and related to the dramatic reduction in growth rate. Major conflicts are often created because of the discrepancy between the child's appetite and food intake and the parents' expectation of what the child should eat. Box 3-8 lists some suggestions to facilitate the feeding of toddlers.

Toddlers should be offered a variety of foods from each of the sections of the Food Guide Pyramid at regular intervals. Toddlers may also exhibit erratic food preferences. Food readily accepted one day may be totally rejected the next day. Milk consumption usually decreases as solid food intake increases. To foster sound

---

Box 3-7 Toddler feeding behaviors

Age	Feeding behavior
12 months	Chews solid food
	Begins to use spoon but turns it before reaching mouth
	May hold cup; likely to tilt cup, causing spilling
18 months	Uses spoon well with frequent spilling
	Turns spoon in mouth
	Holds glass with both hands
24 months	Feeds self without inverting spoon
	Uses spoon well with moderate spilling
	Holds glass with one hand
	Plays with food
	Distinguishes between food and inedible materials
36 months	Self-feeding complete with occasional spilling
	Can manage knife and fork with some help on difficult foods
	Obtains drink of water from faucet
	Pours from pitcher

Modified from Grand RA, Sutphen JL, Dietz WH, Jr, editors. *Pediatric nutrition: theory and practice,* Stoneham, Mass, 1987, Butterworth.

Box 3-8   Suggestions to facilitate the feeding of toddlers

1. Try to relax; feeding, eating, and meal times should be pleasant for everyone.
2. Avoid battles over eating. Encourage your child, but avoid forced feeding or punitive approaches.
3. You are responsible for deciding when, where, and what food your child is offered (with consideration for your child's preferences); your child decides how much to eat.
4. Use positive reinforcement (e.g., praise for eating well).
5. Withholding food is not an appropriate form of punishment.
6. Accept your child's wish to feed himself or herself. Accept that there will be a mess and be prepared (e.g., newspaper on the floor).
7. Try to eat together as a family. Good eating behavior can be modeled, and young children like to mimic older siblings and parents.
8. Allow about 1 hour without food or drink (except water) before a meal to stimulate the appetite.
9. Consumption of excessive fluids reduces the intake of solid foods; offer solids first and limit juices to 4 to 8 oz/day.
10. Establish a routine of meals and snacks at set times, with some flexibility; however, avoid snacks right after an unfinished meal.
11. Recognize your child's cues indicating hunger, satiety, and food preferences.
12. Limit possible distractions (e.g., television) during meals.

eating habits, the child's environment should be pleasant and enjoyable during mealtime. The child should be allowed to eat with other family members when possible and should not be punished for spilling milk or making a mess with food. Quiet surroundings (television turned off) decrease distractions and thus enhance food intake.

Preschool age (4 to 6 years). In this age-group the child poses fewer nutritional problems. Mealtime is more pleasant for all family members. The preschool child is developmentally able to self-feed without assistance, has more coordinated gross motor skills, and has changing and varied interests. The appetite tends to be sporadic and parallels weight gain. Food becomes a secondary interest. More time is spent away from home at day care centers, baby-sitters, or friends' homes, and food consumption between meals increases. To promote sound nutritional habits and prevent nutritional deficiencies (or excesses), parents should be informed of the basic principles of nutrition and meal planning and serve as role models for the preschool child. The quality of foods from the Food Guide Pyramid should be emphasized. Snacks or desserts high in concentrated sweets or of low nutritional value should be discouraged to prevent obesity and dental caries and promote sound nutritional habits. Skim or low-fat milk may be substituted for whole milk, especially if the child is overweight.

Preadolescent (7 to 10 years). This age-group is characterized by a moderate growth rate, about 2 to 4 kg/year and 5 to 6 cm/year. Nutrient and energy intakes are important because preadolescents are laying down reserves in preparation for the adolescent growth spurt. However, excessive weight gain in anticipation of this growth spurt may result in childhood obesity. The eating habits of preadolescents are often influenced more by peer pressure than by parents' actions. The adaptation to school may present nutritional problems for this age-group. Breakfast may be eaten alone or skipped altogether, and snacks after school are often unsupervised. These adaptations may be less of a problem if sound eating habits are established early in life.

Nutrition education should be integrated into the school curriculum. This should encourage children to learn the principles of basic nutrition related to their physiologic needs and to incorporate these into their daily lives. This training will allow children to accept more responsibility for their health and optimize nutritional intake in adulthood.

Adolescence (11 to 18 years). Nutrient requirements increase markedly during adolescence because of the rapid growth and virtual doubling of body mass. The current recommendations of dietary energy intake are based on estimation of energy expenditure or surveys of energy intake related to average body weights. Adolescents often show marked variation in energy expenditure, and recommendations represent average rather than individual requirements. Dietary proteins are essential to provide amino acids for growth, but they also supply energy needs. Protein will only be made available for growth if total energy needs are met in the diet. The value of dietary protein will also be affected by the amino acid composition. The calcium requirement depends on vitamin D, phosphorus, and dairy product intake. The skeleton contains 99% of the body calcium, and 45% of the skeletal mass is formed during adolescence. The greatest demand of calcium will occur during the adolescent growth spurt, and increased intake should allow for the normal variation in the timing of this event. The adolescent requirement for iron is related to increases in blood volume, hemoglobin, and myoglobin synthesis, and in girls, increased losses with menstruation. The timing of this increased need for iron will be subject to the enormous variation in the pace of puberty. Iron losses before menarche are considered to be the same as in adults, approximately 0.5 to 1.0 mg/day, and recommendations are based on the assumption that only 10% of the intake will be absorbed.

The food habits of the adolescent differ from those of any other age-group. They are characterized by an increasing tendency toward skipping meals, snacking, inappropriate consumption of fast foods, dieting, and fad diets. This behavior can be explained by the teen's newly found independence, difficulty in accepting existing values, poor body image, search for self-identity, peer acceptance, and conformity of lifestyle. Understanding these factors is necessary to counsel a teenager properly regarding diet. Particular care needs to be taken to provide adequate intake of calcium, iron, and zinc, which are frequently marginal in the adolescent's diet. The vegetarian teenager who does not eat eggs or cheese or drink milk may develop deficiencies of vitamins D and B_{12}, calcium, iron, zinc, and perhaps other trace elements. Dental caries, obesity, bulimia, and anorexia nervosa are common in the adolescent and are best handled with professional advice. (For more information on eating disorders, see Chapter 2.)

NUTRITION AND AGING

Older adults comprise a rapidly expanding segment of the U.S. population. Those over the age of 85 constitute the fastest-growing group. Whereas in 1991 there were 3.2 million persons 85 and older, by 2040, over 12 million people are projected to be over the age of 85. Those over 85 tend to be more frail, afflicted by a variety of chronic diseases, and at highest nutritional risk.

A broad spectrum of nutritional problems exists among older adults, particularly among the frail elderly. The prevalence of protein-energy malnutrition ranges from 5% to 10% among community-dwelling older adults to 30% to 50% among hospitalized or institutionalized older adults. Obesity and dyslipidemia affect up to 40% of noninstitutionalized adults over 60. The prevalence of vitamin deficiencies varies broadly in this population but is most pronounced among individuals with lower incomes.

Risk factors for undernutrition in older adults

Risk factors for poor nutritional status include inappropriate food intake, poverty, social isolation, disability, multiple medical problems, chronic medication use, and advanced age. Irregular dietary patterns and restrictive dietary modifications can both contribute to inadequate food intake in older adults, and low income often affects the quantity and quality of food available. Individuals on a fixed income with large expenditures for medications may forego buying groceries to pay bills. The result is that low income is highly associated with inadequate nutrient intake. Losses of friends and family often accompany aging and may lead to social isolation and poor dietary intake. Functional impairment resulting from arthritis, stroke, or other chronic illness may affect an older person's ability to obtain, prepare, and consume a nutritionally adequate diet. Medical problems that may have an impact on nutritional status include dementia, depression, alcohol abuse, oral health problems, swallowing difficulties, underlying malignancies (especially gastrointestinal and lung), chronic obstructive pulmonary disease, severe congestive heart failure, and sensory impairment. Common drugs prescribed to older individuals include antibiotics, diuretics, nonsteroidal antiinflammatory agents, digoxin, antihypertensives, and prednisone. Each of these drugs has the potential to affect nutritional status through drug-nutrient interactions, anorexia or nausea, changes in fluid or electrolyte status, and abnormalities of lipid and carbohydrate metabolism. Advanced age in and of itself is not equivalent to poor nutrition; however, because dependency and chronic illness increase in prevalence with advancing age, the oldest elderly are most prone to nutritional problems.

Changes in body composition

With aging there is a decrease in lean body muscle mass and a relative increase in total body fat. For the average population between the ages of 25 and 75, total body fat doubles as a proportion of the body's composition. Exercise programs may prevent or reverse some of the decrease in lean body mass. The implications of this change in body composition are severalfold. As muscle mass decreases, energy requirements decline. Decreased muscle mass also means decreased protein reserves during periods of stress. The increased proportion of fat mass also results in a relative increase in the volume of distribution of fat-soluble drugs.

Changing nutritional requirements with aging

Calories. Energy requirements decrease over the life span, largely due to the decline in physical activity and metabolically active lean body mass. This decline in lean body mass causes a decrease in basal metabolic rate of about 1% to 2% per decade from age 20 to 75 years. Recommended caloric intake based on the 1989 RDA is 2300 kcal for men and 1900 kcal for women age 51 and over. Generalized estimates, however, should be used cautiously because they do not take into account individual activity levels or concurrent diseases.

Protein. Protein needs do not decline with age. One g/kg/day (14% to 16% of daily caloric intake) is recommended as a safe level for most healthy older persons. Frail, chronically ill older adults may require 1.0 to 1.25 g/kg/day of protein to maintain adequate nitrogen balance. During periods of stress resulting from infection or trauma, protein intake should be increased to 1.2 to 1.5 g/kg to provide a cushion against progressive protein depletion.

Fiber. There is no RDA for fiber, and it is unclear how much fiber should be recommended in the diet of older persons. The National Cancer Institute recommends daily intakes of 25 to 35 g/day. This amount is achievable with five servings of fruit or vegetables plus the use of whole-grain breads and cereals. Encouraging adequate fluid intake is essential on a high-fiber diet to prevent dehydration and constipation. Abdominal discomfort or flatulence is common during adaptation to increased fiber intake; therefore fiber content of the diet should be increased gradually over several weeks.

Water. Because of the changes in thirst mechanisms, decreased ability to concentrate urine, and the decrease in total body water that occurs with aging, older adults are at high risk for dehydration. Prescriptions for fluid intake should be written for at-risk patients, particularly those who are institutionalized, with a goal of at least 1500 to 2000 ml per day (or 1 ml/kcal ingested or 30 ml/kg body weight). Another approach is to provide enough fluids to keep urine osmolality below 800 mOsm/L.

Vitamins. In general, vitamin requirements are the same in older adults as for younger adults. Exceptions include vitamins D, B_6, and B_{12}, in certain groups of elderly people for which higher intake may be indicated. Lack of sunlight exposure, impaired skin synthesis of previtamin D, and decreased hydroxylation of vitamin D in the kidney with advancing age contribute to marginal vitamin D status in many older adults. In all older adults, increased consumption of dietary sources of vitamin D should be encouraged. In elderly people who are not exposed to sunlight, administration of a low-dose vitamin supplement (400 IU/day) may be warranted.

Vitamin B_6 contributes to the maintenance of normal cognitive function in older adults. It also plays a role in immunocompetence. Many older adults appear to be vitamin B_6 deficient based on biochemical studies. This may be in part due to poor intake and in part due to less bioavailability of vitamin B_6 once ingested. Intake of 2.0 mg to 2.2 mg/day is recommended.

The prevalence of vitamin B_{12} deficiency in older adults ranges between 5% and 20%. In the past most vitamin B_{12} deficiency was thought to be due to impairment of intrinsic factor secretion. It is now known that many older adults poorly absorb protein-bound B_{12}. This is due to maldigestion of the food protein–vitamin B_{12} complex in the stomach and uptake of vitamin B_{12} by greater numbers of bacteria in the stomach, particularly among individuals with atrophic gastritis. In many cases, these patients can be treated with oral B_{12} rather than B_{12} injections and may benefit from an increase in the dietary intake of food vitamin B_{12}. Given the potentially significant effects of vitamin B_{12} deficiency on the nervous system, it seems prudent to advocate a daily intake of 3.0 μg or more daily of vitamin B_{12}.

In addition to vitamin deficiency, hypervitaminosis is seen in older adults resulting from consumption of megadoses of fat-soluble vitamins. Malaise, liver dysfunction, headache, hypercalcemia, and leukopenia (low WBC count) may be seen with ingestion of large quantities of vitamin A. Overingestion of water-soluble vitamins may result in toxicities. Diarrhea, causing a false negative on fecal occult testing, and renal stones may occur with vitamin C megadoses. In addition, large doses of vitamin C are contraindicated in individuals with declining creatinine clearance. Peripheral neuropathy may be an adverse consequence of vitamin B_6 excess.

Minerals and trace elements. Aging probably does not substantially alter requirements of minerals and trace elements. Exceptions to this generalization are for iron and calcium. The RDA for *iron* declines from 15 mg to 10 mg in women who are no longer menstruating. Dietary iron deficiency is fairly uncommon among older adults. When it does occur, it is usually the result of loss of blood from the gastrointestinal tract.

Although the recommended *calcium* intake is between 1000 and 1500 mg/day for older women and between 800 and 1000 mg/day for men, most older persons consume far less than 1000 mg/day. Supplementation with calcium carbonate or calcium citrate may be of value for individuals who consume inadequate amounts of calcium-containing foods. Calcium citrate supplementation is useful in individuals with achlorhydria and in those consuming iron supplements.

Marginal *zinc* status is common in older adults and may result in impairments in wound healing, immunity, taste, and smell. Institutionalized and hospitalized adults are at particularly high risk for zinc deficiency, although zinc supplementation has not been shown to accelerate healing except in zinc-deficient patients. Recommended intake is at least 10 mg/day. Individuals with infection, trauma, or surgery may require higher intakes. Excessive intake of zinc has been shown to impair immune response and interfere with copper absorption.

Nutritional assessment for the older adult

Because of the increased prevalence of undernutrition, routine nutritional assessment is especially important to overall health maintenance in older adults. Adequate and cost-effective health care must include not only disease diagnosis and treatment but also disease prevention and health promotion, an integral part of which is optimizing nutritional status. Evaluation of nutritional status is described in Chapter 10. Specific assessment for the older adult is outlined in Box 3-9.

Box 3-9   Nutritional assessment of the older adult

History
  Current illnesses
  Chronic illnesses and disabilities
    Ability to perform ADLs and
    IADLs
  Medications, including
  nonprescription
  Psychosocial
    Adequate income
    Transportation
    Mental status evaluation
    Depression screen
  Alcohol and tobacco use
  Advanced directives
  Dietary intake
    Recent changes

24-hour recall
  Food frequency questionnaire—
    global or targeted
  Targeted review of systems—recent
    weight loss
Physical examination
  Height and weight
  Mobility
  Oral examination
  Skin integrity
  Edema
Laboratory
  Complete blood count
  Blood urea nitrogen and creatinine
  Albumin

ADLs, activities of daily living; *IADLs,* instrumental activities of daily living.

History. The nutritional history for the older person is based on historical factors that place the older adult at increased risk of malnutrition. Recent involuntary weight loss (more than 10 lb in 6 months or 5% of body weight in 1 month) should stand out as an indicator of high risk for nutritional compromise, as well as increased morbidity and mortality. The health care provider should keep in mind that some older adults are reluctant to disclose information that they believe could result in recommendation for placement in a nursing home. Poverty, social isolation, lack of access to transportation for shopping, illness, or disabilities that preclude adequate meal preparation may be concealed by an older adult proudly trying to maintain independence in the community. Dementia and depression may prevent adequate self-assessment and preclude an adequate history. The Folstein Mini-Mental State Exam and the Geriatric Depression Scale are easily administered screening tools for detection of dementia and depression, respectively, and should be used on a routine basis. Family members and caregivers can complement information given by the patient. Functional status is integrally related to nutritional status and can be assessed by asking about activities of daily living (e.g., bathing, dressing, feeding, continence, toileting, and transferring) and instrumental activities of daily living (e.g., shopping, food preparation, using the telephone, housekeeping, laundry, transportation, medications, and finances). The medication history is facilitated by the "brown bag" approach, in which the patient brings in all medications, both prescription and over-the-counter. Alcohol and tobacco use should also be included in the history, since they often have a negative impact on nutritional status. Finally, inquiries about advanced directives, with specific reference to wishes regarding aggressive nutritional interventions such as total parenteral nutrition, are also important considerations in this population.

A thorough nutrition history is important, looking for risk factors that predispose to poor nutrient intake, increased nutrient needs, or nutrient losses. A 24-hour dietary recall is easily performed, provides useful information, and has proven validity in the older population. Food diaries are more burdensome and no more reliable. Food frequency questionnaires may be helpful, particularly if targeted to specific nutrients such as vitamin D and calcium. A targeted review of systems can provide information that may be helpful in formulating interventions and should contain questions to elicit the presence of anorexia, poor dental health, dysphagia, early satiety, nausea, vomiting, dyspepsia, dehydration, constipation, diarrhea, weakness, fatigue, and sensory impairment including alterations in taste and smell.

Physical examination. Actual measurement of weight is very important and can be facilitated by a scale with an attached rail for postural stability, a platform scale for wheelchairs, or a bed scale. Obtaining an accurate height can be problematic in older individuals because of narrowing of the intervertebral disc spaces, kyphosis, scoliosis, and osteoporotic vertebral fractures. This reduction in height gives a false-high value for a common measure of obesity—the BMI (weight in kg/height in m²). Examination of previous height such as on the patient's driver's license or measurement of knee height or arm span to calculate height can be helpful. Other anthropometric measures are less reliable in older adults because of loss of skin elasticity and a smaller proportion of total body fat in subcutaneous tissues. Observing the patient move from a chair to the examining table can provide valuable information about mobility. Dehydration and fluid retention may be readily apparent on examination of the skin and mucous membranes. Muscular wasting is associated with chronic protein calorie undernutrition. An oral examination is essential to uncover signs of vitamin deficiencies (see Chapter 2) and untreated dental problems common in older adults.

Laboratory studies. Serum albumin is the best studied indicator of visceral protein stores, but since it is influenced by nonnutritional factors such as concurrent illness and fluid status, it is not a specific for malnutrition. However, hypoalbuminemia (less than 3.5 g/dl) is very suggestive of protein malnutrition in older persons and has been associated with subsequent morbidity and mortality in older populations. Cholesterol determination is also helpful. A cholesterol less than 160 may be an indicator of malnutrition, and in the nursing home population, it has been associated with subsequent mortality. More evidence is accumulating that lowering of a high cholesterol level can decrease subsequent cardiovascular mortality in the older adult with multiple cardiac risk factors or a history of coronary artery disease. A CBC is useful not only in screening for nutritionally related anemias but also for total lymphocyte count. A total lymphocyte count (the percentage of lymphocytes in the differential multiplied by the total WBC count) less than 1500 is suggestive of protein malnutrition.

Thyroid dysfunction is extremely common in older women and should be included in the evaluation of any older woman with a suspected nutritional problem, including women taking a thyroid supplement who may not be on the optimal replacement dose. Hyperthyroidism can result in a hypermetabolic state and predispose to osteoporosis, and hypothyroidism can depress mood and alter mental status, interfering with appetite and food intake. Lastly, if vitamin, mineral, or trace mineral deficiencies are suspected based on history or physical examination, blood levels should be measured.

Treatment of undernutrition

For older persons with poor dental health, prompt intervention can improve appetite, increase ability to chew, and result in increased nutritional intake. Chronic medical conditions such as diabetes or congestive heart failure should also be optimally treated. Many health problems in the elderly cannot be cured but can be significantly improved or palliated, such as nasal oxygen during frequent small meals for the person with emphysema who is having difficulty eating because of dyspnea. Overly restrictive diet prescriptions should be reconsidered. In a patient who is losing weight on a low-fat, low-salt diet, changing to a diet of choice may reverse the weight loss without compromising medical status. Physical and occupational therapy can help optimize functional status and assist the older person to overcome obstacles to meal preparation with therapy, special devices, equipment, and even modifications to the house. Social supports may be necessary for many older persons, and services such as transportation, housekeeping, visitation for the lonely homebound, home-delivered meals, or enrollment in community nutrition centers can assist older persons to improve or maintain their nutritional status. Alternate living situations, such as group-living facilities, may be the solution for some older persons such as a lonely widower who cannot cook.

Older persons who are institutionalized have special nutritional needs. Depression is common at the time of institutionalization and should be recognized and treated, since it can result in decreased appetite. Many persons are admitted from the hospital and have had preexisting nutritional deficiencies that only became clinically significant during the illness. Others experience further nutritional deterioration during their hospitalization. Persons used to a certain ethnic diet may have difficulty eating generic institutional food. Preferences should be noted and accommodated as much as possible.

If dietary modifications are insufficient to maintain nutritional intake, supplements may be helpful. Powdered protein and calorie supplements can be added to foods to increase nutrient density without changing the flavor, texture, or color. Commercially available liquid diet supplements can help meet 100% of a patient's needs. Since many patients substitute calories from their regular diets for calories from the liquid supplement, adding an exercise regimen appears to have a more positive impact than dietary supplementation alone. Milk-based products may be problematic in the elderly, who frequently have lactose intolerance.

When patients can no longer meet their nutritional requirements orally, the issue of enteral and parenteral feeding arises. This decision must be made with thoughtful consideration of the overall goals of care, which should be based on the patient's wishes. Gastrostomy tube feeding should be considered early for any patient requiring enteral feeding. If enteral or parenteral feeding is indicated, the methodology is well described in Chapter 11.

SUGGESTED READINGS

Nutrition during pregnancy

American College of Obstetricians and Gynecologists: Nutrition during pregnancy, *ACOG Technical Bulletin 179,* Washington, DC, 1993, The College, pp. 1-7.

Copper RL, DuBard MB, Goldenberg RL, et al: The relationship of maternal attitude toward weight gain to weight gain during pregnancy and low birth weight, *Obstet Gynecol* 85:590-595, 1995.

Erick M: *No more morning sickness,* New York, 1995, Plume Books.

Goldenberg RL, Tamura T, Neggers Y, et al: The effect of zinc supplementation on pregnancy outcome, *JAMA* 274:463-468, 1995.

Institute of Medicine: *Nutrition during pregnancy: weight gain, nutrient supplements,* Washington, DC, 1990, National Academy Press.

Institute of Medicine: *Nutrition during pregnancy and lactation: an implementation guide,* Washington, DC, 1992, National Academy Press.

US Public Health Service: *Recommendation on folic acid,* Washington, DC, 1992.

Worthington-Roberts BS, Williams SR: *Nutrition in pregnancy and lactation,* ed 5, St Louis, 1993, Mosby.

Breast-feeding

Committee on Drugs, American Academy of Pediatrics: Transfer of drugs and other chemicals into human milk, *Pediatrics* 84:924, 1989.

Lawrence RA, editor: *Breastfeeding: a guide for the medical profession,* ed 4, St Louis, 1994, Mosby.

National Research Council, Food and Nutrition Board: *Recommended Dietary Allowances,* ed 10, Washington, DC, 1989, National Academy Press.

US Department of Health and Human Services: *Healthy People 2000: national health promotion and disease prevention objectives,* Washington, DC, 1990, US Government Printing Office.

Infancy

Fomon SJ, editor: *Infant nutrition,* St Louis, 1993, Mosby.

Grand RA, Sutphen JL, Dietz WH, Jr, editors: *Pediatric nutrition: theory and practice,* Stoneham, Mass, 1978, Butterworth.

National Research Council, Food and Nutrition Board: *Recommended Dietary Allowances,* ed 10, Washington, DC, 1989, National Academy Press.

Tsang RC, Nichols BL, editors: *Nutrition during infancy,* St Louis, 1988, Mosby.

Childhood and adolescence

Fomon SJ, editor: *Infant nutrition,* St Louis, 1993, Mosby.

Grand RA, Sutphen JL, Dietz WH, Jr, editors: *Pediatric nutrition: theory and practice,* Stoneham, Mass, 1987, Butterworth.

National Research Council: *Recommended Dietary Allowances,* ed 10, Washington, DC, 1989, National Academy Press.

Suskind RM, Lewinter-Suskind L, editors: *Textbook of pediatric nutrition,* ed 2, New York, 1993, Raven Press.

Nutrition and aging

Barrocas A, Belcher D, Champagne C, et al: Nutritional assessment—practical approaches, *Clin Geriatr Med* 11:675-708, 1995.

Folstein MF, Folstein SE, McHugh PR: Mini-Mental State: a practical guide for grading the cognitive state of patients for the clinician, *J Psychiatr Res* 12:189-198, 1975.

Russell RM, Suter PM: Vitamin requirements of elderly people: an update, *Am J Clin Nutr* 58:4-14, 1993.

White JV: Risk factors for poor nutritional status in older Americans, *Am Fam Physician* 44:2087-2097, 1991.

Yesavage JA, Brink TL, Rose TL, et al: Development and validation of a geriatric depression screening scale: a preliminary report, *J Psychiatr Res* 17:37-49, 1983.

4

Case Studies

Obesity

A 36-year-old woman is about 120 lb (56 kg) over her ideal weight. Her only child, who is 14 years old, her sister, and both of her parents are overweight. She has struggled with her weight problem since childhood and feels strongly that her energy requirements are low relative to others.

Before embarking on yet another weight-loss program, she saw a physician whose examination revealed that she had a BMI of 41 and a waist:hip ratio of 0.90. Laboratory testing showed that her blood triglyceride level was elevated at 260 mg/dl and that her HDL-C level was low at 35 mg/dl.

TRUE or FALSE   It is reasonable to assume that in this particular case:
1. Her obesity is primarily the result of her genetic predisposition, in contrast to exogenous factors (e.g., diet, physical activity).
2. Her resting energy expenditure is most likely to be lower than that of normal-weight women of her same height and age.
3. Recognizing the degree of her obesity and her pattern of fat distribution, further medical evaluation is likely to reveal the presence of a neuroendocrine abnormality such as hypothyroidism or Cushing's syndrome.
4. Her pattern of fat distribution may be described as android or "apple," which puts her at greater risk for medical complications than persons with a gynecoid or "pear" shape.
5. This pattern of dyslipidemia is not atypical of persons with obesity and raises the likelihood that weight loss alone will ameliorate the pattern.

Hyperlipidemia and CHD

A 49-year-old businessman was seen by his physician for angina-type chest pains that followed bouts of exertion. He had never maintained a regular pattern of exercise, and his usual diet consisted of the following:

Breakfast: Fried eggs, biscuit with margarine and jelly, coffee
Lunch: Hamburger with fries and soda
Supper: Steak or pork chops, potato, rolls with margarine, tea; ice cream for dessert

He drank no alcohol and did not smoke. There was no family history of premature cardiac disease. He stated that he takes no medications.

Physical examination. He was of normal weight but had poor muscle tone. His blood pressure was normal.

Laboratory data. On a fasting blood sample, his serum total cholesterol was 240 mg/dl, triglycerides 200 mg/dl, and HDL-C 33 mg/dl. An exercise tolerance test revealed no evidence of heart disease.

TRUE or FALSE   Appropriate considerations at this time include the following:

1. It is reasonable to conclude that his LDL-C level is within the normal range.
2. He should have a repeat lipid profile, including lipoprotein fractionation.
3. He should undergo further evaluation to rule out the possibility that his dyslipidemia is due to another disorder such as diabetes or liver disease.
4. Based on this diet pattern, it is very likely that his serum homocysteine level would be increased, in turn increasing his risk for CHD.

Reasonable considerations regarding his treatment at this time include which of the following? (Respond TRUE or FALSE to each statement.)

5. In modifying his diet to improve his lipid levels, he should aim to replace, almost gram for gram, the saturated fat (such as from the meats and ice cream) with polyunsaturated fat (such as from margarines, corn oil, fish, nuts, and seeds).
6. Increasing his physical activity level should be recommended on the basis that, among other advantages, it should increase his serum HDL-C level.
7. Alcohol intake, in moderation, should be encouraged to increase his HDL-C concentration.

See Appendix A for answers and discussion.

Part

2

NUTRIENTS AND THE METABOLIC PROCESS

This section presents the macronutrients and micronutrients, including vitamins, minerals, water, protein, carbohydrate, fat, and energy. Sections outlining their physiology and biochemical pathways, absorption, metabolism and excretion, RDA, food sources, signs of deficiency, and effects of large doses are included for easy reference. (See Tables 1-1 and 1-2.)

Nutrient deficiencies and excesses

Nutrient deficiencies occur by mechanisms of:
- Low nutrient intake
- Inadequate absorption
- Inadequate utilization
- Increased requirements
- Increased excretion
- Increased distribution

Although nutrient deficiencies are commonly thought to be prevalent only in underdeveloped countries, certain groups in developed countries also are at high risk.

Conditions of nutrient excess may occur unknowingly through food ingestion (e.g., vitamin A toxicity from excess liver consumption) or knowingly through the ingestion of supplements.

Megadose vitamin therapy is mandated in certain vitamin-dependent genetic diseases, in diseases associated with defective vitamin transport across cell membranes, and as an antidote to antivitamin drugs. Megadose vitamin therapy for the treatment of other medical problems (e.g., the common cold) merits further scientific scrutiny and research because megadoses of certain vitamins are associated with a low benefit-to-risk ratio and with toxicity.

5

Macronutrients

Energy
Proteins and amino acids
Fats
Carbohydrates and fiber
Water and electrolytes

ENERGY

Energy is needed for metabolic processes that support physical activity, growth, pregnancy, and lactation. Energy allowances are expressed in terms of the physiologically available or metabolizable energy provision of foods actually eaten. Energy allowances, or energy content of foods, are expressed in terms of kilocalories or the international unit of energy, the joule; 1 kcal is equal to 4.184 kJ. The Atwater energy conversion factors for food components are used to establish the energy content of diets. For carbohydrates and protein a value of 4 kcal/g is used for each. For fats a value of 9 kcal/g is used, whereas for ethanol (alcohol) a value of 7 kcal/g (5.6 kcal/ml) is used.

Basal energy expenditure (BEE) required for metabolic processes at rest can be estimated from the following Harris-Benedict equations (where W = weight in kg, H = height in cm, and A = age in years).

For men:

$$BEE \text{ (kcal/day)} = 66.47 + 13.75 \text{ (W)} + 5.00 \text{ (H)} - 6.76 \text{ (A)}$$

For women:

$$BEE \text{ (kcal/day)} = 655.10 + 9.46 \text{ (W)} + 1.86 \text{ (H)} - 4.68 \text{ (A)}$$

BEE is estimated to increase by 20% for routine activity and by an additional 10% to 30% for patients with multiple fractures, 20% to 50% for patients with sepsis, and 90% to 100% for patients with burn injury. See Chapter 11 for further discussion.

Energy allowances are made in general terms at a level considered to be in agreement with good health of the average person. This requires consideration of differences in energy needs associated with age, activity, gender, body size, climate, pregnancy, and lactation. Precise measurement of energy balance is not always feasible. Consequently, energy requirements in RDAs are expressed as average needs for categories of individuals, recognizing that maintenance of desirable body weight throughout adult life depends on energy balance. Recommended levels of intake are given in Table 1-1.

113

PROTEINS AND AMINO ACIDS

The body is in a dynamic state, with proteins and other nitrogenous compounds being degraded and resynthesized continuously. With no special storage form of protein, the body requires a continuous intake of protein to replace the amino acids lost. Dietary protein serves as the source of the 20 amino acids commonly found in tissues. Nine of these amino acids (tryptophan, histidine, lysine, leucine, isoleucine, valine, threonine, phenylalanine, and methionine) are essential for humans and cannot be synthesized in the body. Histidine is required during periods of growth. Adults may be able to biosynthesize enough histidine to supply needs. Cystine can be synthesized from methionine, and tyrosine can be synthesized from phenylalanine. The remaining amino acids can be readily formed by the body and are considered nonessential amino acids.

Except for the branched-chain amino acids, the liver is the main site for the metabolism of amino acids. The branched-chain amino acids (valine, leucine, and isoleucine) are degraded mainly in peripheral tissues, particularly the skeletal muscle, but also by the kidneys and adipose tissue. In muscle and adipose tissue the metabolism of the branched-chain amino acids is coupled to the release of glutamine and alanine. These amino acids function as carriers of ammonia groups (NH_2) to the liver, where the nitrogen may be converted into urea. In starvation or fasting, the release of alanine and glutamine provides for gluconeogenesis to assist in the maintenance of blood-sugar concentrations. In addition to alanine, other glycogenic amino acids are glycine, valine, cystine, serine, aspartic acid, asparagine, threonine, methionine, glutamine, glutamic acid, proline, arginine, and histidine. Tryptophan, tyrosine, phenylalanine, and isoleucine are partially glycogenic. Leucine and lysine are ketogenic amino acids because they directly produce acetyl coenzyme A (CoA) or acetoacetate. Tyrosine, phenylalanine, and isoleucine are partially ketogenic because only a portion of their carbon atoms contribute to ketogenesis.

The aromatic amino acids serve also as precursors of hormones. Tryptophan is converted to serotonin, and tyrosine is a precursor of thyroxine and the catecholamines epinephrine and norepinephrine.

The dietary allowance for proteins is 0.8 g/kg of body weight per day. Additional adjustments, as shown in Table 1-1, are made for children and pregnant and lactating women.

FATS

About 35% of the calories in the average U.S. diet are derived from fat, which has a caloric value of 9 kcal/g. Dietary fat occurs as a heterogeneous mixture of lipids, which consist mostly of triglycerides. Food fats also contain small amounts of phospholipids, cholesterol, sphingolipids, glycolipids, and phytosterols. Fat in the average diet is composed of approximately 35% saturated fatty acids, 40% monounsaturated fatty acids, and 15% polyunsaturated fatty acids. In addition to providing a substantial proportion of energy in the diet, fats furnish essential fatty acids, serve as a carrier for fat-soluble vitamins and for food flavors, and give food desirable texture. Most fats, of either vegetable or animal origin, are readily digested and absorbed by the normal person. Less than 5% are unabsorbed and excreted in the feces. Long-chain triglycerides require the action of pancreatic lipase and bile salts for absorption, whereas short-chain triglycerides can be absorbed directly.

The essential fatty acids are linoleic acid, linolenic acid, and arachidonic acid. These fatty acids or their metabolites serve as precursors for prostaglandins, thromboxanes, prostacyclins, and leukotrienes.

The requirement for essential fatty acids has not been fully defined. For populations consuming relatively low-fat diets (fat less than 25% of calories), a minimum of 3% of energy should be provided from linoleic acid. Health organizations have recommended that the total fat intake in the U.S. diet not exceed 30% of total calories. Of this, approximately one fourth to one third should be polyunsaturated fatty acids. Vegetable oils are usually a rich source of polyunsaturated fatty acids.

A dietary deficiency of essential fatty acids is rare in the adult human, but it has been observed with the use of prolonged fat-free parenteral nutrition. A deficiency can be diagnosed by analysis of the fatty acids present in plasma or red cell membranes.

The transport of lipids and recommendations regarding lipid intake in circulation are discussed in Chapter 2.

CARBOHYDRATES AND FIBER

Although carbohydrates are not essential in the same sense as the essential amino acids and fatty acids, they are our most important source of dietary energy. Each gram of carbohydrate provides approximately 4 kcal. A variety of fuels can serve as energy for most tissues, but the brain, RBCs, and the renal medulla are normally dependent on carbohydrates, although with extended starvation, the brain resorts to use of ketone bodies that are formed from fatty acids. Absorbable carbohydrates can be easily converted into glucose, but gluconeogenesis from fats or proteins is limited to the glycerol parts of fats and the glycogenic amino acids. Carbohydrates exist in the diet in two types: (1) available carbohydrates that are digested, absorbed, and used in the body (monosaccharides such as glucose and fructose; disaccharides such as sucrose, lactose, and maltose; polysaccharides such as starches, dextrins, and glycogen) and (2) unavailable carbohydrates (such as dietary fiber).

Lactose is present exclusively in milk, and its utilization depends on lactase action in the intestine for hydrolysis to glucose and galactose. In some populations, such as Orientals and African-Americans, many adults have a lactase deficiency and are lactose intolerant. Although there is no specific dietary requirement for carbohydrate, it is suggested that about 50% to 60% of the caloric intake should be derived from available carbohydrates. Restriction of carbohydrate in the diet to less than 60 g/day is likely to lead to ketosis, excessive breakdown of tissue proteins, loss of cations (especially sodium), and dehydration.

The unavailable carbohydrates, primarily fiber, provide bulk in the diet and aid in elimination. Fibers represent a diverse variety of polysaccharides, mainly structural components of plant cells, which include cellulose, hemicellulose, pectins, and lignins. Although dietary fiber has no demonstrated metabolic requirement, it appears that the incidence of certain diseases, such as cardiovascular disease, diverticulosis, colon cancer, and diabetes, is inversely related to dietary fiber consumption.

Different types of plant fibers have different effects. Wheat bran, for example, has an effect on stool weight but no effect on serum cholesterol. Pectin and oat bran have little effect on stool weight, but serum cholesterol may be lowered. The fiber intake in U.S. diets averages about 10 to 20 g/day, although it is recommended that the intake be closer to 20 to 35 g/day.

WATER AND ELECTROLYTES
Salt and water

Total body water constitutes about 60% of body weight, two thirds of which is distributed in intracellular fluid and one third in extracellular fluid. Of the extracellular fluid, three fourths is found in the interstitial fluid and one fourth in plasma. Abnormalities of extracellular fluid volume are generally caused by net gains or losses of sodium and an accompanying gain or loss of water. Volume depletion may result from unreplaced losses such as with prolonged sweating, vomiting, diarrhea, or burn injury. Fluid volume excess tends to result from diseases that prevent normal excretion of sodium and water, such as kidney or heart failure. However, no laboratory tests accurately predict the degree of the volume deficit or excess, and serum sodium concentration is not a guide to volume status because it reflects only the relationship between total body water and sodium. That is, changes in sodium concentration tend to be corrected even at the expense of temporary distortion in volume.

Although a multitude of factors determine water requirements, under ordinary circumstances a reasonable allowance is 1 ml/kcal for adults and 1.5 ml/kcal for infants. (Sodium requirements are described in Chapter 2.)

Potassium

Sodium and potassium have inverse relationships in terms of their distribution. Potassium is the primary intracellular cation with only 2% found in the extracellular fluid. Over 90% of ingested potassium is absorbed. The kidney is primarily responsible for maintaining potassium balance, and wide variations in intake are not reflected in changes in plasma concentration if there is normal renal function. Low serum levels usually reflect total body potassium deficits of over 200 mEq.

Potassium is widely distributed in foods. Good sources include meat, milk, and fruits. Usual adult intake ranges from 2 to 6 g/day (50 to 150 mEq). The higher level of intake appears beneficial in terms of blood pressure control (see Hypertension in Chapter 2). In healthy individuals, toxicity can result from rapid intakes of over 12 g/m^2 of surface area per day (about 18 g for an adult).

6

Vitamins

Vitamin A
Vitamin B$_6$
Vitamin B$_{12}$
Vitamin C (ascorbic acid)
Vitamin D
Vitamin E
Vitamin K
Biotin
Folic acid, folate
Vitamin B$_3$ (niacin)
Pantothenic acid
Vitamin B$_2$ (riboflavin)
Vitamin B$_1$ (thiamin)

VITAMIN A

Physiology and biochemical pathways

Vitamin A deficiency, expressed commonly as night blindness and keratomalacia (softening of the cornea), remains a major problem in many areas of the world, particularly in Southeast Asia. Young children are most likely to be affected. Both the retinol and carotenoids in the diet must be considered when determining the adequacy of vitamin A intake. In individuals consuming primarily plant foods, β-carotene and other vitamin A precursors, on conversion to retinol, represent the main source of vitamin A in the diet. Vitamin A functions in vision in the form of retinol, is necessary for growth and differentiation of epithelial tissue, and is required for reproduction, embryonic development, and bone growth.

Absorption

Most of the β-carotene and other provitamin A precursors in the diet are normally cleaved within the mucosal cells of the duodenum and jejunum. The retinaldehyde formed from the cleavage is reduced to form retinol, is esterified, and is then transported via the lymph to the liver. Retinol is either stored in the liver or transported by plasma retinol–binding protein to active tissue sites. Protein-calorie malnutrition and zinc deficiency may impair the absorption, transport, and metabolism of vitamin A. The absorption of retinol and β-carotene is reduced in diseases that cause fat malabsorption, such as celiac disease. Retinol storage and transport are impaired in liver disease.

117

Metabolism and excretion

Retinaldehyde and retinol are reversibly interconverted during intermediary metabolism. Retinaldehyde is converted to retinoic acid, which has biologic activity in growth and in cell differentiation but not in reproduction or vision. Most of the vitamin A in the body is stored in the liver. Vitamin A in the body is destroyed at a fairly steady rate, and the metabolites are excreted in the urine. Oxidized products of the vitamin are largely excreted in the bile, partly as β-glucuronides. Part of the biliary retinol β-glucuronide is reabsorbed and transported back to the liver.

Recommended dietary allowance and nutrient interactions

Because of the ability of β-carotene and certain other carotenoids to serve as precursors of vitamin A, requirements are expressed in terms of retinol equivalents (RE), where 1 RE equals 1 μg of retinol. For this purpose, 6 μg of β-carotene and 12 μg of other provitamin A carotenoids are equivalent to 1 μg of retinol. 1 RE equals 3.33 IU of vitamin A activity from retinol and 10 IU of vitamin A activity from β-carotene. Because carotenoid and preformed vitamin A make up approximately 25% and 75% of the diet, respectively, an average value is 1 RE equals 5 IU. The recommended allowance for vitamin A as retinol equivalents is given in Table 1-1.

Food sources

Vitamin A is found in liver, butter, cheese, egg yolk, margarine, dried milk, cream, kidneys, and fortified milk, with less present in fish and seafoods. Carrots, spinach and other greens, mangoes, apricots, peaches, nectarines, sweet potatoes, tomatoes, pumpkin, squash, lettuce, and most other vegetables and fruits serve as sources of β-carotene and other provitamin A carotenoids.

Evaluation of nutritional status

The most common procedure to evaluate vitamin A status is to measure the retinol level in plasma or serum. The normal range of vitamin A content for a child is 20 to 90 μg/dl; for an adult, the normal range is 30 to 90 μg/dl. Lower values are indicators of deficiency or depleted body stores. Serum values greater than 100 μg/dl are indicative of toxic levels of vitamin A. Retinol esters may also be observed in fasting blood with the intake of toxic quantities of the vitamin.

Dark adaptation tests and electroretinogram measurements are also useful but difficult to perform on young children. Measurements of plasma retinol–binding protein levels can also serve as an indication of vitamin A nutritional status because they correlate with plasma retinol levels.

Signs, symptoms, and treatment of deficiency state

Skin lesions such as follicular hyperkeratosis (Fig. 6-1 and Plate 5) and night blindness are among the earliest signs of vitamin A deficiency. Severe depletion may result in conjunctival xerosis (drying) and progress to corneal ulceration, perforation, and finally destruction of the eye (keratomalacia). These changes are usually seen in children. Rapidly proliferating tissues are sensitive to vitamin A deficiency and

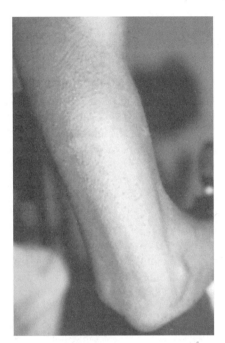

Fig. 6-1   Follicular hyperkeratosis in vitamin A deficiency. ▲

may revert to an undifferentiated state. The bronchorespiratory tract, skin, genitourinary system, gastrointestinal tract, and sweat glands are adversely affected.

In cases of severe vitamin A deficiency in children, a single intramuscular injection of 30 mg of retinol (as palmitate) has been used. The World Health Organization treatment protocol for vitamin A deficiency in children older than 1 year is the use of 110 mg of retinol palmitate orally or 55 mg intramuscularly, plus another 110 mg orally the following day and again before discharge.

Use and effects of large doses

An intake of retinoids greatly in excess of requirements results in a toxic condition known as *hypervitaminosis A*. It may occur in children and adults because of overzealous prophylactic vitamin therapy, extended self-medication, food fads, or use of high doses for the therapy of acne or other skin lesions. A daily intake of more than 7.5 mg (about 37,000 IU) of retinol is not advised, and chronic use of amounts over 20 mg (100,000 IU) can result in dry and itching skin, desquamation, erythematous dermatitis, hair loss, joint pain, chapped lips, hyperostosis (bony deposits), headaches, anorexia, edema, and fatigue. Derivatives of vitamin A have been helpful in the treatment of certain skin diseases. For example, retinoids such as tretinoin (for acne) and isotretinoin (for recalcitrant cystic acne) are useful and have largely replaced the use of retinol for these conditions.

VITAMIN B$_6$

Physiology and biochemical pathways

Vitamin B$_6$ comprises the compounds pyridoxine, pyridoxal, and pyridoxamine. The three forms can interconvert in the body. Vitamin B$_6$ in the phosphorylated coenzyme form takes part in numerous reactions associated with protein metabolism. The reactions include transanimation, deamination, and decarboxylation. The functions of vitamin B$_6$ are diverse and include glycine and serine interconversion, homocysteine conversion to cystathionine, niacin and serotonin formation from tryptophan, and formation of δ-aminolevulinic acid for heme synthesis. The vitamin is present in phosphorylase, the enzyme that converts glycogen to glucose-1-phosphate.

Absorption

Most of the phosphorylated forms of vitamin B$_6$ are hydrolyzed by intestinal phosphatases before absorption. Vitamin B$_6$ is absorbed by a nonsaturable process. Vitamin B$_6$ from some plant products may be present in bound forms (β-glucoside conjugates) that are not biologically available for the human.

Metabolism and excretion

The liver plays a significant role in the conversion of pyridoxine to pyridoxal and pyridoxal phosphate for use by other tissues. In patients with cirrhosis, the hepatic levels of vitamin B$_6$ are considerably reduced and the ability to convert pyridoxine to pyridoxal phosphate is impaired. Pyridoxal phosphate is the main form of vitamin B$_6$ in plasma. The phosphorylated forms of vitamin B$_6$ are tightly bound to albumin and unavailable to tissues. Free pyridoxal is readily taken up by tissues. Small amounts of vitamin B$_6$ are excreted into the urine. The majority of ingested vitamin B$_6$ is converted to 4-pyridoxic acid and excreted. Stores of vitamin B$_6$ in the body are small (20 to 30 mg) and can be depleted within 30 days with the ingestion of vitamin B$_6$–deficient diets.

Recommended dietary allowance and nutrient interactions

The requirement for vitamin B$_6$ increases with the amount of protein in the diet. With an average intake of 100 g of protein per day, 2.2 mg of pyridoxine per day is required by adults. Lower intakes of protein may reduce the need for vitamin B$_6$ to 1.5 mg/day. Some women using oral contraceptives may have an increased requirement for vitamin B$_6$. In general, this effect is of minor clinical concern. Prolonged use of drugs such as isoniazid, penicillamine, cycloserine, and hydralazine may require vitamin B$_6$ supplements to reduce the neurologic side effects. Vitamin B$_6$ supplements in patients receiving levodopa for the treatment of Parkinson's disease should be avoided because B$_6$ may interfere with the metabolism of levodopa.

Food sources

Most of the vitamin B$_6$ in food is in the form of pyridoxine, pyridoxal phosphate, and pyridoxamine phosphate. Vitamin B$_6$ losses are often high in the processing and canning of meats and vegetables and in the milling of wheat. Fish, poultry, and other meats are good sources of the vitamin, as are vegetables such as carrots, cabbage, peas, potatoes, tomatoes, brussels sprouts, and cauliflower.

Evaluation of nutritional status

Vitamin B_6 status may be evaluated with the use of several laboratory procedures. Blood transaminase activities and xanthurenic acid excretion after a tryptophan load are commonly used for assessment. Plasma levels of pyridoxal and pyridoxal phosphate or the urinary excretion of 4-pyridoxic acid are also useful indexes.

Signs, symptoms, and treatment of deficiency state

Vitamin B_6 deficiency is rarely encountered, and the clinical signs and symptoms associated with deficiency are not well established. The most common clinical manifestations are central nervous system changes and abnormal electroen-cephalograms. Hyperirritability and convulsive seizures may occur in infants. In adults, one is more likely to see eczema and seborrheic dermatitis in the regions of the ears, nose, and mouth; chapped lips; glossitis; and angular stomatitis. Occasionally, hypochromic, microcytic anemia may be observed. Increased excretion of xanthurenic acid occurs because of impaired metabolism of tryptophan with vitamin B_6 deficiency. Since a deficiency of vitamin B_6 would probably be associated with deficiencies of one or more other B vitamins, treatment with a B-complex multivitamin preparation is appropriate. In the United States, symptoms of B_6 deficiency are most likely to be seen in the form of neuritis resulting from isoniazid treatment.

Use and effects of large doses

Vitamin B_6–dependent syndromes will require treatment with high doses of the vitamin. Pyridoxine has low toxicity. However, daily supplements of 200 mg of pyridoxine over several months may result in a dependency when the supplement is discontinued. A toxic sensory neuropathy has been reported in people consuming more than 500 mg daily for an extended period. Isoniazid combines with pyridoxal or pyridoxal phosphate to inactivate the vitamin. Supplements of pyridoxine may be necessary to compensate for this inactivation. Vitamin B_6 reduces the beneficial effects of levodopa in the treatment of Parkinson's disease.

VITAMIN B_{12}
Physiology and biochemical pathways

Vitamin B_{12} is a generic term for cobalamins that are active in humans. Structurally, vitamin B_{12} contains cobalt and a corrin moiety. Two cobalamins, 5'-deoxyadenosylcobalamin and methylcobalamin, function as vitamin B_{12} coenzymes in humans. Vitamin B_{12} is also commonly called *cyanocobalamin.* Deoxyadenosylcobalamin is a cofactor of the mitochondrial mutase enzyme that catalyzes the isomerization of methylmalonyl coenzyme A to succinyl coenzyme A, an essential reaction in lipid and carbohydrate metabolism. Methylcobalamin is essential in folate metabolism because of its participation in the methionine synthetase reaction. The interaction of the two vitamins is essential for the conversion of homocysteine to methionine, for protein biosynthesis, for synthesis of purines and pyrimidines, for methylation reactions, and for the maintenance of intracellular levels of folates.

Absorption

Impaired absorption of vitamin B_{12} is most commonly associated with pernicious anemia, wherein the patient usually has a deficiency in the production of gastric intrinsic factor essential for the absorption of the vitamin (see Chapter 2). Intrinsic factor is a highly specific binding glycoprotein secreted by parietal cells of the stomach. In the normal person, vitamin B_{12} is absorbed through receptor sites in the distal ileum. Transcobalamin II, present in the plasma, transports vitamin B_{12} to the tissues that require it.

Metabolism and excretion

Various diseases can result in decreased absorption of vitamin B_{12}. Included are gastric achlorhydria and decreased secretion of intrinsic factor secondary to gastric atrophy (such as with aging and pernicious anemia) or total gastrectomy, impaired pancreatic function accompanied by reduced production of enzymes necessary for the release of vitamin B_{12} from binding proteins, production of antibodies to intrinsic factor, and disease of ileal mucosal cells or surgical removal of the distal ileum. In vitamin B_{12} deficiency, folate becomes trapped as methyltetrahydrofolate to produce a deficiency in the functional form of folate essential for hematopoiesis and other reactions. Vitamin B_{12} is stored in the hepatic parenchymal cells, where 1 to 10 mg may be present, representing up to 90% of the body's store of the vitamin. About 3 μg of vitamin B_{12} are secreted into the bile each day but are normally reabsorbed in the ileum. Little of the vitamin appears in the urine.

Recommended dietary allowance and nutrient interactions

Studies involving body stores and turnover rates of vitamin B_{12} indicate that 0.1% to 0.2% of the vitamin is lost from the body daily. Based on these investigations, the RDA for vitamin B_{12} for adults is 2 μg/day, which allows for incomplete absorption and provides for a substantial body reserve. For the infant an intake of 0.5 μg/day is recommended. During pregnancy and lactation an additional intake of 2.2 μg/day is recommended (see Table 1-1).

Food sources

Microorganisms are the sole source of vitamin B_{12} in nature. All plants are devoid of vitamin B_{12}. Consequently, strict vegetarian diets are free of vitamin B_{12}. Animal products, including meats and meat products (especially liver, kidney, and heart), fish, poultry, shellfish, eggs, milk, and dairy products, are the usual dietary sources. Vitamin B_{12} is rather stable to heat and usual cooking practices.

Evaluation of nutritional status

Measurement of serum vitamin B_{12} levels is commonly used to evaluate vitamin B_{12} status. Radioassays or microbiologic assays are available for the determination of B_{12} status. Serum levels below 200 pg/ml indicate low body stores of vitamin B_{12}. Levels below 100 pg/ml are generally diagnostic of vitamin B_{12} deficiency.

Red-cell vitamin B_{12} levels are less reliable than serum levels for evaluating vitamin B_{12} status.

Methylmalonate excretion is increased with vitamin B_{12} deficiency but is seldom measured as an index of vitamin B_{12} status. The deoxyuridine suppression test is useful in the assessment of vitamin B_{12} nutriture, but the test is not simple to perform. Methylmalonate may also be assayed in the plasma.

Signs, symptoms, and treatment of deficiency state

Deficiency of vitamin B_{12} will result in a sore tongue, paresthesias of the extremities (numbness and tingling), weakness, and other neurologic changes. Vitamin B_{12} deficiency can also cause megaloblastic anemia. Prolonged deficiency can result in irreversible damage to the nervous system. A deficiency of either vitamin B_{12} or folate will result in a morphologically identical macrocytic anemia, megaloblastic bone marrow changes, and hypersegmented polymorphonuclear neutrophils (see Fig. 2-6, *A*). The similar clinical findings in folate and B_{12} deficiency make it necessary to determine levels of both vitamins before starting therapy. When a dietary deficiency of vitamin B_{12} occurs (as with vegans), an oral supplement of 1 μg/day is adequate. When the deficiency is due to inadequate absorption, monthly injections of 100 μg are appropriate therapy, although oral therapy of 1000 μg/day may suffice in some cases. Such patients should have their serum vitamin B_{12} levels monitored every 6 to 12 months.

Use and effects of large doses

Vitamin B_{12} has very low toxicity. However, the use of megadoses of the vitamin has application in the treatment of B_{12} deficiency and in the treatment of the rare situation in which there is a congenital defect in vitamin B_{12} metabolism (e.g., vitamin B_{12}–responsive methylmalonic acidemia).

VITAMIN C (ASCORBIC ACID)
Physiology and biochemical pathways

Vitamin C exists in two forms, ascorbic acid and dehydroascorbic acid, although most of the vitamin exists as ascorbic acid. Specific biochemical functions of vitamin C are incompletely defined, but it appears to participate in a number of reactions, mostly involving oxidation. As such, vitamin C participates in the hydroxylation of proline to hydroxyproline and lysine to hydroxylysine. Consequently, impairment of collagen synthesis occurs in vitamin C deficiency. Vitamin C also participates in the synthesis of carnitine, tyrosine, adrenal hormones, and vasoactive amines and in microsomal drug metabolism, leukocyte functions, folate metabolism, and wound healing.

Absorption

Absorption of vitamin C appears to occur in the distal region of the small intestine by means of a sodium-dependent active transport system. Some ascorbic acid may also be absorbed at a slow rate by simple diffusion. Normally 80% to 90% of dietary intake of vitamin C (up to 100 mg/day) is absorbed. At higher intakes, vitamin C is less well absorbed.

Metabolism and excretion

Absorbed vitamin C readily equilibrates throughout the body pool. The average adult has a body pool of between 1.2 and 2 g that is used at a rate of 3% to 4% per day. Highest concentrations of the vitamin are found in the adrenal and pituitary glands, with lesser amounts in the brain, liver, pancreas, and spleen. Daily intake of 60 mg of vitamin C will provide a body pool of approximately 1.5 g of the vitamin. Excess vitamin C is readily excreted in the urine as metabolites or as unchanged ascorbic acid. The renal threshold for ascorbic acid is about 1.5 mg/dl of plasma.

Recommended dietary allowance and nutrient interactions

An interaction appears to exist between vitamin C, iron, and copper that influences normal heme function through the oxidation-reduction of iron or by regulating iron absorption and availability at the intestinal level or both. The absorption of nonheme iron in the diet can be enhanced fourfold or more by the simultaneous ingestion of 25 to 75 mg of vitamin C. The RDA for vitamin C is given in Table 1-1. The vitamin C requirement of cigarette smokers is higher than that of nonsmokers by as much as 50%. The use of oral contraceptives lowers the plasma concentrations of ascorbic acid; however, the significance of this observation is not known. Studies suggest that the elderly may have an increased requirement for vitamin C. Working in a hot environment increases urinary excretion and also may increase the requirement for the vitamin.

Food sources

Vitamin C is highly water soluble but is labile in solution and readily destroyed by heat, oxidation, and alkali. Relatively large amounts of the vitamin are present in most fruits, including strawberries, citrus fruits, and tomatoes, and in various vegetables, including green peppers, broccoli, cauliflower, cabbage, and greens.

Evaluation of nutritional status

The measurement of serum or plasma levels of ascorbic acid is the most commonly used and practical procedure for evaluating vitamin C status. Serum vitamin C levels of 0.2 to 0.3 mg/dl indicate low or inadequate intake of the vitamin. Levels below 0.2 mg/dl indicate deficiency. Leukocyte vitamin C levels can provide information concerning body stores of the vitamin, but the analytic measurement is somewhat tedious.

Signs, symptoms, and treatment of deficiency state

A deficiency of vitamin C can lead to scurvy. Scurvy is associated with a defect in collagen synthesis that is demonstrated by impacted hair follicles, corkscrew hairs, failure of wounds to heal, defects in tooth formation, and rupture of capillaries that leads to perifollicular petechiae (pinpoint hemorrhages around hair follicles) and ecchymoses (large areas of dermal hemorrhage) (Fig. 6-2 and Plate 6). Scurvy may be associated with loosening of the teeth (see Fig. 2-4), gingivitis, and anemia. The oral signs of scurvy do not occur in edentulous individuals. Adults with scurvy should be given 1 g of ascorbic acid by mouth daily.

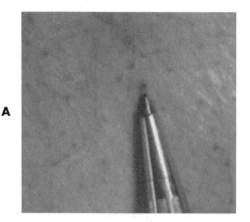
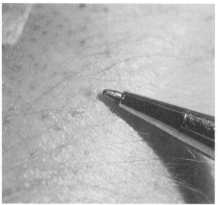

Fig. 6-2   **A,** Corkscrew hairs in scurvy. **B,** Perifollicular petechiae in scurvy. ▲

Use and effects of large doses

In the absence of scurvy, the administration of ascorbic acid in large amounts produces few demonstrable effects. Although megadoses of vitamin C have been reported to have beneficial effects on the common cold and to increase resistance to various diseases, these claims have not been well documented or accepted. For most individuals, ascorbic acid has low toxicity and excessive intake is tolerated. Adverse effects include diarrhea, increased uric acid excretion, hemolysis in patients with erythrocyte glucose-6-phosphate dehydrogenase deficiency, and oxalosis in patients with chronic renal failure. Large doses may interfere with tests for glucose in the urine (false-negative with the glucose-oxidase method, false-positive with copper reagents), may give a false-negative result in tests for occult blood in the stool, and may interfere with anticoagulant (heparin and warfarin) therapy. Large doses of vitamin C should be avoided in individuals with hemochromatosis or other iron storage diseases. Vitamin C will increase absorption and mobilization of iron and facilitate oxidation-reduction (redox) cycling of iron, resulting in the generation of damaging free radicals.

VITAMIN D
Physiology and biochemical pathways

The intestinal absorption of calcium and phosphorus is stimulated by the active metabolite of vitamin D, 1,25-dihydroxycholecalciferol ($1,25\text{-}(OH_2)D_3$), and as such, vitamin D serves as a regulator of calcium and phosphorus homeostasis. Vitamin D occurs in two forms: vitamin D_2 (ergocalciferol) and vitamin D_3 (cholecalciferol). Vitamin D_3 is the naturally occurring form and is produced by the action of sunlight on the 7-dehydrocholesterol in the skin. Vitamin D_2 is formed by ultraviolet irradiation of the plant sterol ergosterol. Vitamin D_2 and vitamin D_3 appear to be equally active in humans. Vitamin D is required for maintenance of skeletal integrity and proper utilization of calcium and phosphorus. Infants and children have the greatest need for vitamin D. When intake is inadequate, rickets may develop. In adults, osteomalacia may occur as a result of vitamin D deficiency.

Absorption

Dietary vitamin D is absorbed from the duodenum and jejunum in association with fat and is incorporated primarily into chylomicrons that are taken up by the liver. Fat malabsorption impairs the absorption of vitamin D.

Metabolism and excretion

Cholecalciferol is hydroxylated in the liver to produce 25-OH-D$_3$. The most potent metabolite of vitamin D, 1,25-(OH)$_2$D$_3$, is produced in the kidneys and is controlled according to requirements for growth, pregnancy, and lactation. Its formation is stimulated by parathyroid hormone, low serum phosphate, estrogen, prolactin, and growth hormone, and it appears to decrease with aging. Vitamin D is degraded by hepatic hydroxylases and excreted in the bile. Only 2% is excreted in the urine.

Recommended dietary allowance and nutrient interactions

Vitamin D requirements are expressed in terms of micrograms of cholecalciferol or in international units; 1 μg of cholecalciferol is equal to 40 IU. The RDA for vitamin D is shown in Table 1-1.

Food sources

The need for vitamin D is normally met by the action of sunlight on 7-dehydrocholesterol in the skin to produce vitamin D$_3$. In areas where sunlight is limited seasonally, the formation of vitamin D may be inadequate to meet needs. The sources of dietary vitamin D are limited primarily to liver, eggs, butter, fortified milk, and fatty fish.

Evaluation of nutritional status

Vitamin D status may be evaluated through the measurement of serum levels of 25-OH-D$_3$ and of 1,25-(OH)$_2$D$_3$. Serum measurements of 25-OH-D$_3$ provide a reliable index of vitamin D stores. Levels of 1,25-(OH)$_2$D$_3$ are less reliable for this purpose. For adults, an acceptable level of serum 25-OH-D$_3$ is 10 to 55 ng/ml and serum 1,25-(OH)$_2$D$_3$ is 10 to 50 pg/ml. Vitamin D deficiency may be accompanied by a decrease in serum phosphate and calcium and an increase in serum alkaline phosphatase, urinary hydroxyproline, and parathyroid hormone levels. Roentgenogram findings may assist in the evaluation of rickets and osteomalacia.

Signs, symptoms, and treatment of deficiency state

Rickets and osteomalacia are not commonly seen in the United States. Rickets in children is characterized by disorders of cartilage cell growth, enlargement of the epiphyseal growth plates, and accumulation of unmineralized bone matrix (Fig. 6-3 and Plate 7). In adults, vitamin D deficiency causes osteomalacia. Patients receiving anticonvulsant agents (e.g., phenobarbital or phenytoin) for prolonged periods may develop rickets or osteomalacia.

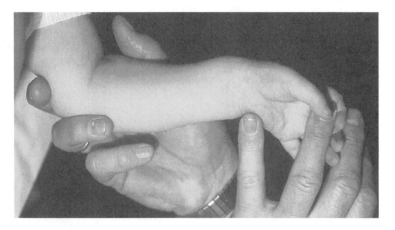

Fig. 6-3   Radial thickening in vitamin D deficiency. ▲

Breast-fed infants or those fed unfortified formula should receive 400 units of vitamin D daily as a supplement. Fully developed rickets is usually treated with 1000 units of vitamin D daily. The major therapeutic uses of vitamin D are for prevention and cure of nutritional rickets, treatment of metabolic rickets and osteomalacia, and treatment of hypoparathyroidism. Chronic renal failure is characterized by a decreased ability of the kidneys to convert 25-OH-D$_3$ to 1,25-(OH)$_2$D$_3$.

Use and effects of large doses

Toxicity caused by excess vitamin D administration is associated with plasma 25-OH-D$_3$ concentrations of more than 400 ng/ml. The initial signs and symptoms of vitamin D toxicity are weakness, fatigue, headache, nausea, vomiting, hypercalcemia, and impaired renal function. Hypercalcemia may arrest growth in children. Large doses of vitamin D cause bone decalcification. Because of the potential for toxicity, vitamin D should not be administered in excess of the RDA in Table 1-1.

VITAMIN E
Physiology and biochemical pathways

Vitamin E is the name given to the family of tocopherols with a substituted chromanol ring and a saturated or unsaturated side chain. The biologic activity of these vitamins is proportional to their proficiency as antioxidants, with α-tocopherol having the highest activity.

Vitamin E is lipid soluble and is found in all cell membranes. The greatest amount is found in adipose tissue, where the concentration is approximately 1 mg/g of lipid. The biologic function of vitamin E is not specific in the sense that it participates as a coenzyme for enzyme-catalyzed reactions. The role of vitamin E as a free radical scavenger appears to be its primary biologic function. In this capacity, it scavenges free radicals generated by oxidases (e.g., xanthine oxidase and cytochrome P-450–dependent oxidases) and generated by the breakdown of hydrogen peroxide. In this process the chromanol ring is converted to the relatively stable free radical tocopheroxyl, which may react with oxygen to form quinone. In the absence of the vitamin, free radicals peroxidize and oxidize polyunsaturated fatty acids, resulting in membrane dysfunction, altered lipoprotein metabolism, and the deposition of lipofuscin or ceroid pigment (granules composed of oxidized lipid and protein).

Absorption

Vitamin E is absorbed in the proximal small intestine through a process that requires bile and pancreatic enzymes. Absorption is impaired in chronic cholestasis and pancreatic insufficiency. Transport from the intestine is via chylomicrons and is similar to that of dietary triglycerides. Thus abetalipoproteinemia impairs transport.

Metabolism and excretion

Tocopherols protect polyunsaturated fatty acids in cellular and intracellular membranes from peroxidative damage. Thus the function of tocopherol is complementary to the function of glutathione peroxidase (a selenoenzyme), which catalyzes the reduction (i.e., detoxification) of peroxides in the cytoplasm.

Oxidation of tocopherol to quinone destroys the biologic activity of the vitamin. Quinone and other oxidized metabolites are found in urine and feces. Ascorbic acid may reduce the tocopheroxyl radical or tocopherones (another oxidation product) back to tocopherol and may recycle the vitamin.

Recommended dietary allowance and nutrient interactions

One international unit has been defined as 1 mg of dl-tocopheryl acetate, a synthetic form of the vitamin. Synthetic dl-tocopherol has a potency of 1.1 IU/mg. One international unit is equivalent to 0.67 mg of dietary α-tocopherol, although various forms of vitamin E have differing activities. The RDA for vitamin E varies with age, gender, pregnancy, and lactation. Recommended amounts are listed in Table 1-1. Requirements may be increased by the intake of foods high in polyunsaturated fatty acids and low in the vitamin (e.g., fish oil). Large doses of vitamin E interfere with vitamin K metabolism and should be avoided during anticoagulant therapy. Doses of 400 mg/day of α-tocopherol also interfere with arachidonic acid metabolism. Vitamin E absorption by infants is poor, and there is some evidence that low-birth-weight and premature infants need at least 8 mg of tocopherol per day. Oxidation of polyunsaturated fatty acids (as measured by breath pentane) in smokers has been reduced by supplements of 800 mg/day.

Food sources

As a rule, tocopherols are present in vegetable oils in proportion to the linoleic acid content of the triglyceride. Therefore good sources of the vitamin include cottonseed, corn, soybean, and safflower oils. Other moderately good sources include yellow-green vegetables, eggs, and whole-grain food products.

Evaluation of nutritional status

There are high-performance liquid chromatography (HPLC) and colorimetric assays for serum and plasma vitamin E. Normal values are 0.5 to 1.2 mg/dl. Greater than 10% hemolysis by the peroxide-induced erythrocyte hemolysis test is also an indication of deficiency because this value corresponds to a vitamin E concentration of approximately 0.4 mg/dl. Vitamin E mobilized from liver is bound to VLDLs; therefore hypolipidemic patients will have lower serum levels. There is some evidence that a ratio of serum tocopherol to total lipid is a better indicator of vitamin E nutriture. A value below 0.8 mg tocopherol per 1 g of total serum lipid is considered deficient in adults and children.

Signs, symptoms, and treatment of deficiency state

The cell membranes of a variety of organs may be altered by vitamin E deficiency; therefore signs and symptoms may be nonspecific. Signs and symptoms include hemolytic anemia, myopathy with creatinuria, weakness, ataxia, impaired reflexes, ophthalmoplegia, retinopathy, and bronchopulmonary dysplasia (if on a respirator). In severe deficiency, permanent damage to nervous tissue has been demonstrated, whereas psychomotor dysfunction has been demonstrated in some vitamin E–deficient patients. However, pure dietary deficiency is rare. Premature and low-birth-weight infants and patients with cholestasis and other fat malabsorption syndromes are predisposed to vitamin E deficiency. Deficiency states may be corrected with oral intake of 0.2 to 2 g. In the case of severe malabsorption, the parenteral route may be required.

Use and effects of large doses

Large doses of vitamin E have been used prophylactically in premature infants to protect against hemolytic anemia, retinopathy, and bronchopulmonary dysplasia. Large doses are also indicated in chronic cholestasis, pancreatic insufficiency, uncontrolled celiac disease, and other fat malabsorption syndromes. In addition, certain rare inborn errors of metabolism that result in hemolytic anemia also respond. These include glucose-6-phosphate dehydrogenase deficiency, thalassemia major, glutathione peroxidase deficiency, and glutathione synthesis deficiency. Vitamin E appears to stabilize the RBC membrane in patients with sickle cell anemia. Vitamin E, unlike other fat-soluble vitamins, is remarkably nontoxic. High doses may interfere with vitamin K metabolism, resulting in an increase in clotting time, and may interfere with arachidonic acid and prostaglandin metabolism. Impaired immune function, sepsis, and impaired wound healing have been reported in infants treated with high doses. On the other hand, ingestion of up to 500 mg/day for 3 years failed to produce evidence of toxicity.

Recent studies have demonstrated that doses of 200 to 500 mg/day will protect the LDL particle from oxidative damage. It is known that oxidized LDL is not recognized by the liver receptor and will accumulate in plasma and contribute to the formation of the atherosclerotic lesion. Thus vitamin E may have a protective effect with respect to cardiovascular disease.

VITAMIN K

Physiology and biochemical pathways

A vitamin K–dependent process in the liver is responsible for the synthesis of prothrombin (factor II), the zymogen of the blood coagulation enzyme thrombin. In the absence of vitamin K or in the presence of vitamin K antagonists such as warfarin sodium, vitamin K–dependent posttranslational glutamyl carboxylase is inhibited and abnormal forms of prothrombin are produced. These abnormal forms lack a full complement of γ-carboxyglutamic acid residues and are unable to bind calcium normally; thus they are inactive in blood coagulation. The precise mechanism by which vitamin K activates the glutamyl γ-carboxylase is unclear. Vitamin K–dependent carboxylase activity is necessary for the formation of a number of proteins that contain γ-carboxyglutamic acid residues. Included are clotting factors VII, IX, and X; osteocalcin; protein S; and protein C (Fig. 6-4).

Absorption

Vitamin K is absorbed in the small intestine by an apparent saturable, energy-dependent system and is incorporated into chylomicrons. Fat malabsorption syndromes are associated with reduced vitamin K absorption.

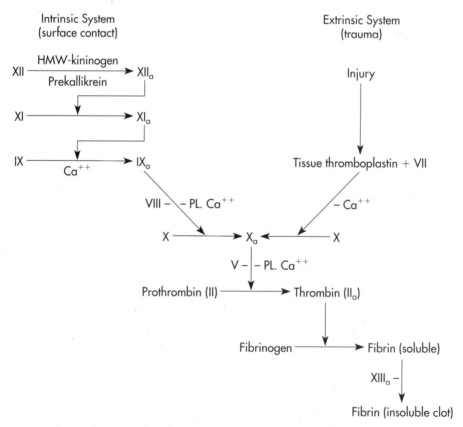

Fig. 6-4 The clotting cascade. (From Shils ME, Young VR: *Modern nutrition in health and disease,* ed 7, Philadelphia, 1988, Lea & Febiger.)

Metabolism and excretion

No specific plasma carrier has been identified for vitamin K. It is distributed to tissues via LDLs. Vitamin K is present in tissues only in small amounts, with very little long-term storage. Vitamin K localizes in various cellular membranes, particularly in the Golgi and smooth microsomal membrane fractions. Vitamin K_1 is rapidly metabolized to more polar metabolites and excreted in the urine and bile.

Recommended dietary allowance and nutrient interactions

A specific recommended allowance for vitamin K has not been established because of the variable contribution from the synthesis of the vitamin K forms by the intestinal flora. For adults a daily intake of 65 to 80 µg is suggested; for infants a daily intake of 10 µg is suggested. Mature breast milk provides approximately 15 µg of vitamin K per liter. Infant formulas usually contain a minimum of 4 µg of vitamin K per 100 kcal.

Food sources

Vitamin K is a fat-soluble compound that occurs naturally in two forms: vitamin K_1 (phylloquinone), which is present in green plants, and vitamin K_2 (menaquinones), produced by microorganisms. Green leafy vegetables are good sources of vitamin K_1, with lesser amounts provided by cereals, fruits, dairy products, and meats. The average diet is estimated to provide 300 to 500 µg of vitamin K_1 daily.

Evaluation of nutritional status

The adequacy of vitamin K intake is commonly evaluated by measuring the plasma concentration of one of the vitamin K–dependent clotting factors: prothrombin (factor II), factor VII, factor IX, or factor X. In the clinical laboratory, the one-stage prothrombin-time (PT) measurement is the standard procedure used to determine the extrinsic-pathway clotting time. Methods are available to measure the specific clotting factors but are generally not used to monitor vitamin K adequacy.

Signs, symptoms, and treatment of deficiency state

Uncomplicated cases of dietary inadequacy of vitamin K seldom occur because the vitamin can be synthesized by intestinal flora. However, excess intake of vitamin E can antagonize the action of vitamin K. Certain drug therapies such as warfarin, phenytoin, sulfa drugs, neomycin, and salicylates may interfere with vitamin K metabolism. The only known symptom of vitamin K deficiency in humans is increased PT, often associated with easy bruisability and bleeding (Fig. 6-5 and Plate 8).

Vitamin K deficiency occurs most commonly in newborns. Vitamin K does not cross the placental membrane well; thus tissue stores are low in the newborn. Newborns also lack the intestinal flora necessary to synthesize vitamin K. A single dose of 0.5 to 1 mg of vitamin K is routinely administered by injection to newborns.

In fat malabsorption syndromes, vitamin K deficiency may occur, especially if there is use of antibiotics that suppress the flora in the large bowel.

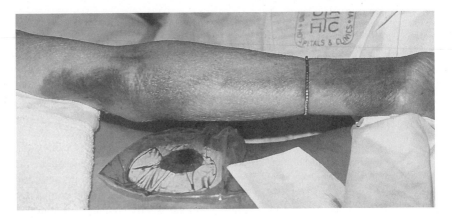

Fig. 6-5   Easy bruisability in vitamin K deficiency.   ▲

Use and effect of large doses

Patients with parenchymal liver disease may have hypothrombinemia because of an inability to use vitamin K in the biosynthesis of vitamin K–dependent clotting factors. Some patients respond favorably to a parenteral dose of 10 mg of vitamin K daily for 3 days. Vitamin K_1 (phylloquinone, phytonadione) is relatively nontoxic in humans, although rapid intravenous administration of vitamin K_1 has produced dyspnea, flushing, chest pains, cardiovascular collapse, and rarely, death. These effects may have been related to the dispersing agents rather than to the vitamin.

Excessive bleeding produced by administration of oral vitamin K antagonist anticoagulants, such as warfarin, can be corrected in a few hours by the administration of vitamin K_1 (phylloquinone). A single dose of 2.5 to 10 mg of vitamin K_1 has been used to treat a mild overdosage of anticoagulants (e.g., warfarin).

BIOTIN
Physiology and biochemical pathways

Biotin, a member of the vitamin B complex, is composed of fused tetrahydrothiophene and ureido rings with a valeric acid side chain. Covalent attachment to the apoenzyme forms the prosthetic group (biocytin). This is accomplished by the energy-dependent formation of an amide bond using the valeric acid side chain and the ϵ-amino group of a specific lysine residue in the apoenzyme. Biotin formation is catalyzed by the holoenzyme synthetase. Adenosine triphosphate (ATP)–dependent carboxylation reactions are catalyzed by holoenzymes (e.g., acetyl-coenzyme A [CoA] propionyl-CoA, B-methyl-crotonyl-CoA, geranoyl-CoA, and pyruvate carboxylases), which are involved in fatty acid, cholesterol, protein, and carbohydrate metabolism. The central intermediate in these reactions is the N'carboxybiotinyl enzyme. Some storage of the vitamin occurs in the liver.

Absorption

Absorption of the vitamin occurs in the proximal small intestine by a sodium-dependent active transport mechanism. Biotin-synthesizing bacteria live in the intestine and contribute to body pools of available biotin. Clinical experiments have demonstrated that the vitamin is also absorbed in the distal colon. Absorption of the vitamin from different foods varies considerably, although on average approximately 50% of dietary biotin is absorbed.

Metabolism and excretion

Normal activity of the holoenzyme synthetase and biotinidase (the enzyme that catalyzes the hydrolytic cleavage of biotin from the ϵ-amino group of lysine) is required for metabolism. It is therefore likely that turnover of the vitamin from one apoenzyme to another is required. Biotinidase also hydrolyzes lipoic acid from the ϵ-amino group of lysine. The principal excretory product is free intact biotin. Urinary and fecal excretion is greater than dietary intake, reflecting biosynthesis by gut flora.

Recommended dietary allowance and nutrient interactions

There is no RDA for biotin. The estimated safe and adequate daily intake is based approximately on 50 μg/1000 kcal and is shown in Table 1-2. Uncooked egg whites contain a glycoprotein, avidin, that binds the vitamin, making it unavailable for absorption.

Food sources

Good sources include liver, whole-grain rice, and eggs. Other sources include nuts, cauliflower, cowpeas, mackerel, and sardines. Biotin occurs in the free form in plant-derived food and is bound to protein in animal-derived food. The average American diet includes 100 to 300 μg/day.

Evaluation of nutritional status

Microbiologic and isotope dilution assays are most frequently used to evaluate the nutritional status of biotin. Whole blood levels and urinary levels are highly variable.

Normal whole blood levels range from 200 to 500 pg/ml. Levels below 100 pg/ml may indicate deficiency. Normal urinary excretion ranges from 6 to more than 100 μg in 24 hours.

Signs, symptoms, and treatment of deficiency state

Biotin deficiency resulting from poor dietary intake is rare. Experimental biotin deficiency is characterized by dermatitis, hair loss (Fig. 6-6 and Plate 9), atrophy of the lingual papillae, graying of mucous membranes, muscle pain, paresthesias, hypercholesterolemia, and electrocardiogram abnormalities. Some of these signs and symptoms have been observed in people eating raw eggs and in patients given long-term, high-dose antibiotics. Total parenteral nutrition solutions used for the long term (more than 8 weeks) should contain biotin. Biotin deficiency responds to 300 μg/day for several days. Holoenzyme synthetase deficiency is a rare inborn

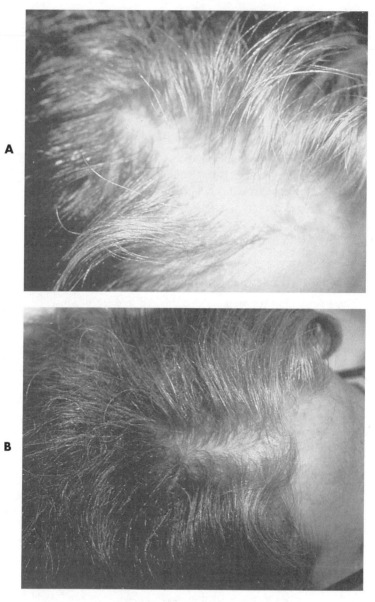

Fig. 6-6   Alopecia before **(A)** and after **(B)** biotin therapy in a patient on long-term total parenteral nutrition without biotin.   ▲

error of metabolism that is characterized by erythematous rash, persistent vomiting, and impaired immune function. The Michaelis constant (K_m) for the enzyme is reported to be 500 times higher in these patients when compared with normal. The activity of all of the carboxylases is low.

Biotinidase deficiency also is a rare inborn error that results in delayed neuromotor development, nystagmus, hypotonia, impaired immune function, ketosis, and the accumulation of lactate in the tissues. In these patients, biotinidase activity in plasma is low; however, the activity of the carboxylases is normal.

Use and effects of large doses

Holoenzyme synthetase and biocytinase deficiency respond to 10 to 100 mg of biotin per day. Up to 10 mg/day over long periods of time has no toxicity in humans.

FOLIC ACID, FOLATE
Physiology and biochemical pathways

Folate describes a group of compounds that contain a pteridine ring, para-aminobenzoic acid, and glutamic acid, and that possess the biologic activity of folic acid (pteroylglutamic acid). Most natural folates are in polyglutamate forms containing additional glutamic acid residues bound in a peptide linkage. The folate polyglutamates are the functional coenzymes in tissues, where they participate primarily in one-carbon transfers. As such, they participate in purine and pyrimidine biosynthesis, formate metabolism, and amino acid interconversions (e.g., serine and glycine interconversions; homocysteine to methionine; histidine degradation to glutamic acid). Metabolic relationships exist between folate and vitamin B_{12}. A deficiency of either folate or vitamin B_{12} results in megaloblastic anemia as a result of impaired cell maturation and division.

Absorption

The presence of the different forms of folate in foods has resulted in uncertainties as to their bioavailability. On the average, 50% of dietary folate appears to be bioavailable. Before dietary folate can be absorbed, the polyglutamate forms must by hydrolyzed to monoglutamate forms by the conjugases present in the lumen and brush border of the intestine. Folate-binding proteins, associated with the brush border, appear to be involved in the transport of folate across cell membranes. Part of the absorbed monoglutamate is converted to methyltetrahydrofolate and transferred into the portal circulation.

Malabsorption syndromes such as tropical sprue, celiac disease, and Crohn's disease adversely affect the absorption of folate. Impaired ability to absorb folate may occur in malnourished alcoholics and among users of certain drugs such as sulfasalazine.

Metabolism and excretion

5-Methyltetrahydrofolate is the predominant circulating form of folate. Pteroylglutamic acid (folic acid) is taken up by the liver and converted to 5-methyltetrahydrofolate, which is either stored in the liver (primarily in the polyglutamate form) or made available to the peripheral tissues. Patients with alcoholic cirrhosis may have reduced retention of folate in the liver. The catabolism of folate is uncertain. Only small amounts of intact folate are excreted in the urine of normal individuals.

Recommended dietary allowance and nutrient interactions

The RDA for folate takes into account the bioavailability of dietary folate and an estimate of the amount required to maintain tissue stores of the vitamin. The recommended allowance for folate is given in Table 1-1.

Food sources

Folate is present in a wide variety of foods but is particularly plentiful in fresh green vegetables, liver, and some fresh fruits. As much as 50% to 95% of the folate present in foods may be lost during food processing and cooking.

Evaluation of nutritional status

Measurement of folate levels in serum and RBCs is the most practical and commonly used procedure to evaluate folate status. Measurements are provided by microbiologic assay *(Lactobacillus casei)* or by radioassay. Plasma folate values above 6 ng/ml are considered acceptable, whereas values less than 3 ng/ml are considered deficient. RBC folate levels above 160 ng/ml are considered acceptable, whereas values less than 140 ng/ml are considered deficient. Plasma folate reflects recent dietary intake, whereas RBC folate is an indicator of tissue stores. Some antibiotics and methotrexate may interfere with the microbiologic assay. Histidine loading tests (formiminoglutamic acid excretion) and deoxyuridine suppression tests are not practical as routine indexes of folate status. Patients with a suspected folate deficiency should be evaluated further to eliminate the possibility of a coexisting biochemical vitamin B_{12} deficiency.

Signs, symptoms, and treatment of deficiency state

Folate deficiency results in megaloblastic anemia that cannot be distinguished from that caused by a deficiency of vitamin B_{12} (see Fig. 2-6). Folate deficiency rarely is associated with neurologic abnormalities that occur frequently with vitamin B_{12} deficiency. Severe folate deficiency may result in depapillation of the tongue (Fig. 6-7 and Plate 10) and alterations in intestinal function resulting from abnormalities in the rapid turnover of the cells of the intestinal villi. Before treatment of megaloblastic anemia with folate, the absence of vitamin B_{12} deficiency must be established. Therapy with folate in the presence of vitamin B_{12} deficiency will correct the hematologic abnormalities but will not prevent progression of the neurologic defects associated with vitamin B_{12} deficiency. Folic acid supplementation is recommended in the periconceptual period to prevent NTDs. Patients with megaloblastic anemia should be evaluated to determine the effects of medications and alcohol intake. For folate-deficient adult patients without sprue or intestinal malabsorption, an oral dose of 1 mg of folate per day is considered adequate. A supplement of 400 μg/day during pregnancy and 100 μg/day during lactation is suggested. (See Table 1-1.)

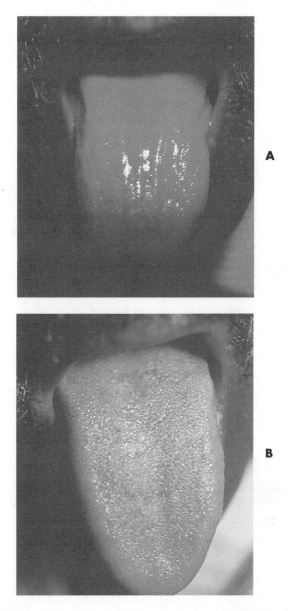

Fig. 6-7   Depapillation of the tongue. Slick tongue before (**A**) and after (**B**) folate replacement in an alcoholic patient. ▲

Use and effects of large doses

High doses of folate are rarely indicated, although oral doses as high as 15 mg/day have been used for extended periods without side effects. However, large doses may counteract the antiepileptic effects of phenobarbital, primidone, and phenytoin. Leucovorin (5-formyl tetrahydrofolic acid), a metabolite of folate, is used to reverse the effects of antifolates such as methotrexate, when used in a high dose. Daily folic acid supplements have been found to be useful to prevent toxicity during long-term, low-dose methotrexate therapy.

VITAMIN B$_3$ (NIACIN)
Physiology and biochemical pathways

Present in all cells, mainly in its amide form, nicotinamide is a structural component of the pyridine nucleotide coenzymes nicotinamide adenine dinucleotide (NAD) and nicotinamide adenine dinucleotide phosphate (NADP). Both coenzymes participate as cofactors in glycolysis and in many redox reactions or dehydrogenase systems central to tissue respiration. Tissues with high respiration rates, such as the central nervous system, are most extensively affected by niacin deficiency. Fatty acid synthesis requires NADPH, the reduced form of NADP, whereas oxidation of fatty acids requires NAD.

A new biochemical role for NAD involves the transfer of its adenosine diphosphate ribose (ADPR) moiety to a number of acceptor molecules. The reactions are catalyzed by ADP transribosylase and poly-ADPR synthase enzymes. Since most of the cell's NAD is synthesized and used in the nucleus, one of the most important functions of poly-ADPR is in the repair of DNA. When a strand break occurs in DNA, large amounts of NAD are used to create poly-ADPR to act as a signal for excision-repair enzymes.

Absorption

Niacin is absorbed from the stomach and small intestine by a carrier-mediated, sodium-dependent facilitated diffusion process at low concentrations and by passive diffusion at higher concentrations. Absorption may be impaired as a result of chronic alcoholism. Niacin is present in animal foods largely as nicotinamide nucleotides with little free nicotinic acid or nicotinamide present. The nucleotides are converted to nicotinamide at the time of absorption.

Metabolism and excretion

Nicotinic acid is converted to nicotinamide by the nicotinamide dinucleotide pathway, but direct conversion has not been demonstrated. Nicotinamide is converted to N′methylnicotinamide, much of which is converted to N′-methyl-2-pyridone-5-carboxamide (2-pyridone). Normally, adults excrete 20% to 30% of their niacin catabolites as N′methylnicotinamide and 40% to 60% as 2-pyridone. The amounts of intact niacin excreted in the urine are small and are influenced little by dietary intake of niacin or tryptophan.

Recommended dietary allowance and nutrient interactions

The RDA for niacin is expressed in terms of niacin equivalents, in which one niacin equivalent is equal to 1 mg of niacin or 60 mg of tryptophan. The RDA for niacin for adults is related to energy expenditure, in which 6.6 niacin equivalents are required per 1000 kcal. Additional allowances are made for pregnancy and lactation. (See Table 1-1.)

Food sources

Niacin is remarkably stable and can withstand considerable periods of cooking, storage, and heating. Legumes, cereals, and meats are good sources. However, niacin may be present in wheat, corn, and certain cereal products in bound forms (called *niacytin*) that are not biologically available to humans. Fish, poultry, and red meats with their high content of both niacin and tryptophan are excellent sources of niacin.

Evaluation of nutritional status

Laboratory procedures for the assessment of the nutritional status of this vitamin are limited. The only practical biochemical procedure is the measurement of the urinary levels of the niacin metabolites N′methylnicotinamide and 2-pyridone. The ratio of these values is used as an index of niacin nutritional status. Under normal conditions a ratio of 1.4 to 4.0 exists between 2-pyridone and N′methyl-nicotinamide excretion. A ratio of less than 1.0 is indicative of niacin deficiency.

Signs, symptoms, and treatment of deficiency

Niacin deficiency results in pellagra, which is characterized by diarrhea, dermatitis, dementia, and ultimately death. Early symptoms may include anorexia, weakness, irritability, insomnia, glossitis, stomatitis, numbness, burning sensation in various parts of the body, vertigo, and forgetfulness. Intermittent constipation and diarrhea may occur. The first lesions to appear are those of the mucous membranes of the mouth, tongue, and vagina. Pigmented keratotic scaling lesions are especially prominent on the areas of the body exposed to the sun, such as the face, hands, neck, feet, and forearms (Fig. 6-8 and Plate 11). Dementia is generally an advanced manifestation of the deficiency.

Treatment with either nicotinic acid or nicotinamide produces a prompt response, often within 24 hours. Nicotinamide is usually preferred to avoid the flushing reaction produced by nicotinic acid. Recommended treatment is an oral dose of 50 mg of niacin given up to 10 times daily or intravenous injections of 25 mg two or more times daily. Pellagra may occur in Hartnup disease because of impaired tryptophan utilization and in some patients with carcinoid tumors.

Use and effects of large doses

Nicotinic acid (but not nicotinamide) has been used as a vasodilator and to lower plasma cholesterol. Large doses of nicotinic acid may rapidly reduce plasma triglycerides and, more slowly, plasma cholesterol. When nicotinic acid is used alone, triglycerides may be reduced by 20% to more than 80%, and plasma LDL-C often is reduced 10% to 15%. Used in combination with a bile acid–binding resin, a 40% to 60% reduction in plasma LDL-C may be seen. High doses of nicotinic acid must be used with care because of adverse effects, such as abnormalities in hepatic function, hyperglycemia, elevated plasma uric acid, and vasodilation. Sustained-release nicotinic acid preparations are not recommended.

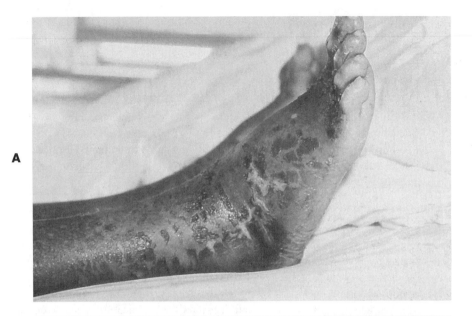

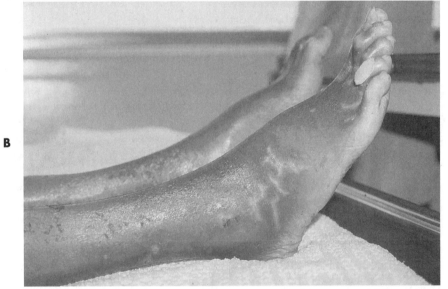

Fig. 6-8   Clinical findings of niacin deficiency before **(A)** and after **(B)** therapy in an alcoholic patient. ▲

PANTOTHENIC ACID

Physiology and biochemical pathways

Pantothenic acid is a B-complex vitamin composed of a substituted butyric acid and β-alanine joined by a peptide bond. Pantothenic acid is a vitamin precursor of CoA and 4′phosphopantetheine, the prosthetic group of acyl carrier protein (ACP). More than 70 enzymes are known to require CoA or ACP. These enzymes are involved in fatty acid synthesis; lipid, carbohydrate, and amino acid metabolism; cholesterol synthesis; and many other pathways. Both CoA and ACP are required for acyl group transfer reaction; a thiol ester is the common intermediate.

Liver and adrenal glands have the highest concentration; however, body stores are small.

Absorption

Approximately 50% of the pantothenic acid in food is absorbed. Intestinal microflora may also be a source. Cellular uptake of pantothenic acid occurs by a specific saturable mechanism in concert with the cotransport of sodium ions.

Metabolism and excretion

Pantothenic acid is phosphorylated by ATP to yield 4′phosphopantetheine acid, followed by the addition and subsequent decarboxylation of cysteine to yield 4-phosphopantetheine. The addition of the elements of adenosine monophosphate (AMP) is followed by phosphorylation of ribose convert 4′phosphopantetheine to CoA. A phosphodiester is formed linking 4′phosphopantetheine to a serine of ACP. Urinary excretion of pantothenic acid is proportionate to intake. Normal urinary excretion is 2 to 7 mg/day; 1 to 2 mg/day is lost in feces.

Recommended dietary allowance and nutrient interactions

There is no RDA for pantothenic acid. Estimated safe and adequate daily intakes are listed in Table 1-2. Higher intakes may be required for pregnancy and lactation.

Food sources

Pantothenic acid is widely distributed in foods. Good sources include meats, whole-grain cereals, and legumes.

Evaluation of nutritional status

Whole blood and urine pantothenate may be determined by microbiologic assay and by radioimmunoassay after pantotheinase treatment of the specimen. Serum levels are considered unreliable as indicators of nutriture. Average whole blood levels are 100 to 300 μg/dl. Whole blood levels less than 100 μg/dl may indicate deficiency.

Signs, symptoms, and treatment of deficiency state

There is little clinical evidence of dietary deficiency in humans. Experimentally, deficiency has been produced in subjects given ω-methylpantothenic acid (a metabolite antagonist) and in subjects consuming a semisynthetic diet deficient in the vitamin. Signs and symptoms include vomiting, malaise, abdominal distress, burning, cramps, fatigue, insomnia, and paresthesias of the hands and feet. Single, uncomplicated pantothenic acid deficiency is very rare. However, marginal deficiency may occur concurrent with other B-complex vitamin deficiencies.

Use and effects of large doses

Doses of up to 10 g/day have been given without toxicity. Diarrhea has been reported when doses of 10 to 20 g/day have been used.

VITAMIN B₂ (RIBOFLAVIN)

Physiology and biochemical pathways

Riboflavin is a water-soluble B-complex vitamin and is composed of a substituted isoalloxazine ring and a ribitol side chain. The coenzyme forms of the vitamin—flavin mononucleotide (FMN) and flavin adenine dinucleotide (FAD)—bind reversibly to the apoenzyme; FAD binds covalently to succinic dehydrogenase, sarcosine dehydrogenase, and monoamine oxidase. Riboflavin-dependent enzymes catalyze a diverse array of chemical reactions, including one-electron transfers, pyridine nucleotide-dependent and independent reactions, disulfide reductases, and oxygen reductases. These enzymes play an important role in amino acid metabolism; purine and pyrimidine metabolism; choline and fatty-acid oxidation; glycolysis; the tricarboxylic-acid cycle; and the metabolism of vitamin K, folic acid, pyridoxamine, and niacin. The vitamin is not stored effectively. The coenzyme forms FMN and FAD found in food are hydrolyzed to riboflavin by nonspecific enzymes. Free riboflavin is found in milk and eggs.

Absorption

The main site of absorption of riboflavin is the proximal intestine. The process occurs via a saturable transport mechanism involving phosphorylation and dephosphorylation. The absorption process is saturated with 25 mg of the vitamin. Substantial amounts of circulating riboflavin are bound nonspecifically by serum albumin. Lesser amounts are bound by other plasma proteins.

Metabolism and excretion

Riboflavin is converted to FMN and FAD by the action of flavokinase and FAD pyrophosphorylase. It is likely that the biosynthesis of the apoenzyme occurs before covalent attachment of FAD. Both specific and nonspecific phosphatases hydrolyze FMN to riboflavin. Riboflavin, rather than catabolites, is the major excretory product in urine and feces.

Recommended dietary allowance and nutrient interactions

The recommended allowance of riboflavin varies with age, gender, pregnancy, and lactation. The RDA is listed in Table 1-1. Riboflavin-dependent enzymes are involved in the biosynthesis of niacin from tryptophan and the transformation of coenzymes from pyridoxine, folic acid, and vitamin K.

Food sources

Good sources of riboflavin include milk, yogurt, cheese, meat, eggs, broccoli, asparagus, oranges, and whole-grain foods. The vitamin is unstable to exposure to light and heat.

Signs, symptoms, and treatment of deficiency state

The signs and symptoms of riboflavin deficiency include nasolabial seborrheic dermatitis, cheilosis, glossitis, angular stomatitis (Fig. 6-9 and Plate 12), burning and itching of the eyes, corneal vascularization, and anemia. Single uncomplicated riboflavin deficiency is rare because food sources for other B-complex vitamins are the same and nutrient interactions complicate the clinical picture. Riboflavin metabolism is altered in patients treated with chlorpromazine, tetracycline, imipramine, amitriptyline, and phenothiazine. The evidence that the use of oral contraceptives increases requirements for riboflavin is controversial. Riboflavin deficiency can usually be treated with an oral intake of 10 to 15 mg/day for 1 week. A parenteral preparation can be used when malabsorption is severe.

Evaluation of nutritional status

Erythrocyte glutathione reductase activity and stimulation by added FAD in vitro is the most common procedure. The upper limit of the normal range of stimulation is 76%. There are HPLC and spectrofluorimetric methods for detection in blood and urine. Also, egg white riboflavin-binding protein has been used to detect the vitamin in urine.

A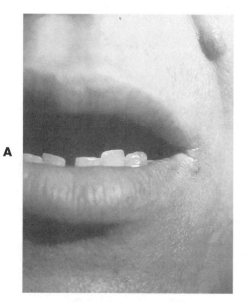 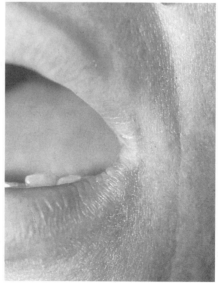B

Fig. 6-9   Angular stomatitis of riboflavin deficiency before (**A**) and after (**B**) therapy. ▲

Use and effects of large doses

There are no reports of human toxicity. Toxicity in laboratory animals is very low. Three riboflavin-responsive inborn errors of metabolism have been reported. They include carnitine deficiency with lipid myopathy, short-chain acyl-CoA dehydrogenase deficiency, and ethylmalonic-adipicaciduria.

VITAMIN B₁ (THIAMIN)

Physiology and biochemical pathways

Thiamin is a B-complex vitamin composed of a substituted pyrimidine and thiazole ring with a hydroxyethyl side chain. The coenzyme form of the vitamin, thiamin pyrophosphate (TPP), is required by enzymes involved in oxidative decarboxylation (e.g., pyruvate, ketoglutarate, and branched-chain keto acid decarboxylations) of glycolysis, tricarboxylic acid (TCA) cycle, and amino acid metabolism. TPP also is required by the transketolase enzyme in the pentose phosphate pathways.

Another important metabolic product of thiamin is thiamin triphosphate (TTP). TTP is thought to bind at or near the sodium channel in nerve membranes. Certain nerve toxins displace TTP from the nerve membrane in concert with blockage of the sodium channel. Dephosphorylation of TTP together with sodium influx may be required for nerve-impulse propagation.

Neither thiamin nor TPP is stored effectively.

Absorption

Absorption occurs in the upper small intestine by active transport at physiologic concentrations and by passive diffusion at higher concentrations. Active thiamin transport may be coupled to a sodium-dependent phosphorylation of the vitamin. There is no binding protein in circulation.

Metabolism and excretion

Intracellularly, thiamin is converted to TPP by thiamin pyrophosphokinase. The most important organ for this reaction is the liver; patients with cirrhosis have defective thiamin phosphorylation, and in these patients, erythrocyte transketolase activity does not respond to thiamin therapy. TPP is the major form in the body, accounting for approximately 80% of the body pool; 50% of this is found in muscle. The high content in muscle probably reflects its demands for carbohydrate metabolism.

More than 20 metabolites of thiamin have been detected in human urine. In general, these metabolites are substituted pyrimidine-ring and thiazole-ring compounds. Alcohol dehydrogenase oxidizes the hydroxyethyl side chain of both thiamin and its thiazole moiety.

Recommended dietary allowance and nutrient interactions

The RDA for thiamin varies with age, gender, pregnancy, lactation, and energy intake. An intake of 0.5 mg of thiamin per 1000 kcal of energy is recommended with a minimum intake of 1 mg for adults. RDAs are found in Table 1-1.

Alcohol abuse and folate deficiency result in malabsorption of the vitamin. Vitamin antagonists include caffeic acid and tannic acid found in coffee and tea. Refeeding after starvation may precipitate thiamin deficiency because vitamin stores may be insufficient to handle the metabolism of a large amount of carbohydrate.

Food sources

Good food sources include lean pork, legumes, whole-grain cereals, breads, and any enriched grain product.

Evaluation of nutritional status

The most common procedure for assessing thiamin status is the measurement of erythrocyte transketolase activity and its stimulation in vitro by added TPP. The upper limit of the normal range of stimulation is 23%; average normal stimulation is 12% to 15%. In patients with beriberi, average stimulation is 35%; in patients suffering from Wernicke's encephalopathy, the stimulation varies from 28% to 67%. Spectrofluorometric and HPLC methods are also used to determine thiamin levels in serum and urine. Average whole blood thiamin levels in control subjects are 68 ng/ml (ranges 50 to 80) and 39 ng/ml in beriberi patients. Normal urinary excretion is greater than 60 μg/g creatinine in adults and greater than 150 μg/g creatinine in children.

Signs, symptoms, and treatment of deficiency state

Classical thiamin deficiency, known as *beriberi,* is rare in this country except among alcoholics. Dry beriberi is characterized by chronic polyneuropathy with the following signs and symptoms: anorexia, ataxia, apathy, weakness, decreased attention span, calf tenderness, paresthesia, footdrop (Fig. 6-10 and Plate 13) and wristdrop, ophthalmoplegia (Fig. 6-11 and Plate 14), and nystagmus. Wet beriberi is characterized by edema and high-output cardiac failure and may be rapidly precipitated by physical exercise or infection. Signs and symptoms include palpitations, shortness of breath, chest pain, increased systolic blood pressure, and pulmonary congestion. Neuropathy resulting from thiamin deficiency may be underdiagnosed in this country because of nonspecific symptoms such as weakness, leg cramping, and burning feet. Because beriberi is a medical emergency, aggressive treatment with 100 mg of intramuscular or intravenous thiamin hydrochloride daily is indicated. Response is usually noticeable in several hours. Treatment with other B-complex vitamins also is indicated. Alcoholic polyneuropathy resulting from thiamin deficiency responds to 10 to 15 mg administered orally along with other B-complex vitamins.

Wernicke-Korsakoff syndrome may be an inborn error in metabolism resulting from a decreased affinity (high K_m of the transketolase enzyme for TPP) coupled with lower absolute levels of the transketolase. This syndrome is masked when the patient is thiamin replete and is unmasked by alcohol abuse, dietary deficiency diet, or malabsorption. Some characteristic signs and symptoms include ataxia, ophthalmoplegia, nystagmus, disorientation, severely impaired short-term

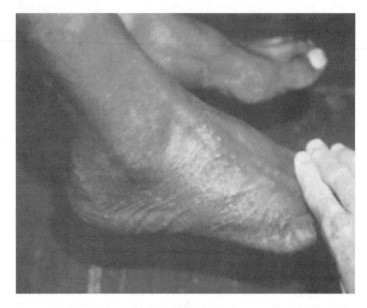

Fig. 6-10   Inability to dorsiflex the foot (footdrop) in an alcoholic patient with thiamin deficiency. ▲

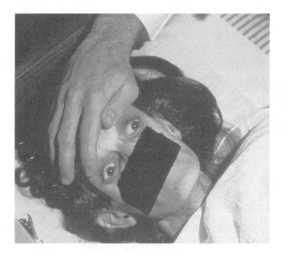

Fig. 6-11   Paralysis of external ocular muscles (ophthalmoplegia) because of thiamin deficiency and phosphorus deficiency. ▲

memory, and confabulation. These patients usually respond to 100 mg administered intramuscularly or intravenously and to 10 to 15 mg/day of orally administered thiamin.

Use and effects of large doses

Thiamin-responsive inborn errors of metabolism (in addition to Wernicke-Korsakoff syndrome) include branched-chain keto-acid decarboxylase deficiency (maple syrup urine disease), pyruvate dehydrogenase deficiency (subacute necrotizing encephalomyelopathy), and megaloblastic anemia associated with diabetes mellitus. Oral dosages of 300 mg/day are nontoxic in humans; however, parenteral dosages greater than 400 mg/day may cause anorexia, lethargy, mild ataxia, and reduced tone of the intestinal tract.

7

Minerals and Trace Elements

Calcium
Iodine
Iron
Magnesium
Phosphorus
Zinc
Other trace elements

CALCIUM

Physiology and biochemical pathways

Calcium is the fifth most abundant element in the body, with 99% present in the bones. It is also the most abundant cation in the body. Calcium is required for the formation and maintenance of skeletal tissue and teeth and is essential for the functional integrity of nerve and muscle, where it influences excitability and muscle contraction and release of neurotransmitters. Blood clotting also is dependent on calcium. Half of the plasma calcium is ionized and physiologically active and presumably under hormonal control. A significant decrease in plasma-ionized calcium will result in tetany and convulsions.

Absorption

From 25% to 50% of the calcium in the diet is absorbed from the intestine by an active transport system. Vitamin D, as 1,25-dihydroxycholecalciferol $(1,25(OH)_2D_3)$, is required for active calcium transport via the production of the vitamin D–dependent calcium-binding protein in the intestine. Passive absorption may also occur. Some dietary factors enhance the absorption of calcium, such as certain amino acids (lysine and arginine) and lactose. High oxalate and phytate, present in some foods, may decrease calcium absorption. Unabsorbed fatty acids in the intestine (those present because of fat malabsorption resulting from intestinal diseases or resection of the small intestine) bind calcium, form unabsorbable compounds, and result in negative calcium balance.

Metabolism and excretion

The metabolism of calcium is controlled by parathyroid hormone, calcitonin, and vitamin D. Vitamin D stimulates intestinal absorption of calcium and decreases renal excretion. Normally, 100 to 200 mg (2.5 to 5 mmol) of calcium are excreted daily in the urine. Calcium retention may be reduced by increased protein intake and high sodium intake.

Recommended dietary allowance and nutrient interactions

Intake of large amounts of protein and sodium may increase calcium requirements. In the United States the recommended intake of calcium is probably higher than in countries with lower usual intakes of protein-rich foods and salt. About 25% of adolescent American women and 50% of American women over 35 years of age consume less than 500 mg (12.5 mmol) of calcium per day. The RDA for calcium is shown in Table 1-1. See Chapter 2 for recommendations regarding calcium intake for the prevention and treatment of osteoporosis.

Food sources

Highly concentrated sources of calcium (300 mg or more per serving) include yogurt, milk, fortified fruit juices, Swiss cheese, and sardines with bones. Good sources of calcium (at least 200 mg per serving) include most cheeses, calcium-set tofu, and fortified cereals. Other sources of calcium (at least 100 mg per serving) include salmon with bones, collards, turnip greens, instant farina, and kale. Low-fat and fat-free dairy foods are at least as high in calcium as their higher-fat counterparts and are usually recommended. In the United States, over half of the calcium intake is from dairy products.

Evaluation of nutritional status

Suitable laboratory techniques for evaluating the adequacy of calcium intake do not exist. Serum calcium levels are closely controlled by the body over a wide range of intake. Low serum calcium values are more suggestive of a pathologic condition such as malabsorption syndrome, vitamin D deficiency, or hypoparathyroidism than of a dietary deficiency of calcium. Most cases of low serum calcium levels are a result of reduced circulating levels of albumin because about 45% of serum calcium is albumin bound. Hypoalbuminemia decreases the serum total calcium by approximately 0.8 mg/dl for each 1 g/dl decrease in albumin. In this situation the active, ionizable fraction remains normal. Normal serum calcium levels range from 8.5 to 10.5 mg/dl (4.5 to 5.5 mEq/L; 2.13 to 2.63 mmol/L). Bone x-rays, bone biopsy, and dual energy x-ray absorptiometry have been used to provide an indication of bone density and the existence of osteoporosis.

Signs, symptoms, and treatment of deficiency state

Signs and symptoms of hypocalcemia include paresthesias (pins and needles), increased neuromuscular excitability, muscle cramps, tetany, and convulsions. Bone fractures, bone pain, and loss of height may occur. These signs and symptoms are not specific to a calcium deficiency but may also be the result of a vitamin D deficiency (osteomalacia). Prolonged bed rest or immobilization can cause osteopenia (loss of bone mass) because of loss of calcium from bones and increased urinary calcium excretion.

Use and effects of large doses

Calcium preparations are used in the treatment of hypocalcemic states (reduced ionized fraction). Oral ingestion of large quantities of a calcium salt is unlikely by itself to cause hypercalcemia. High intakes of calcium (1000 to 1500 mg/day) may prevent or delay the onset of osteoporosis. For postmenopausal women, an increased intake of calcium, along with estrogen replacement and weight-bearing exercise, can be effective in preventing and treating osteoporosis. Normal blood levels of vitamin D are required for optimal calcium absorption (see Chapter 6).

IODINE

Physiology and biochemical pathways

Iodine is a trace element that is an integral part of the thyroid hormones thyroxine (T_4) and triiodothyronine (T_3). Thyroid hormones exert most if not all of their effects through the control of protein synthesis. Thyroid hormones have a calorigenic effect, a cardiovascular effect, metabolic effects, and an inhibitory effect on the secretion of thyrotropin by the pituitary.

Absorption

Iodine is readily absorbed from the diet and reaches circulation in the form of iodide. In circulation it is normally present in several forms, with 95% as organic iodine and approximately 5% as iodide. Most of the organic iodine is in thyroid hormone. Most T_4 and T_3 are transported in the plasma bound to carrier proteins. Only about 0.03% of the total thyroxine in plasma is free. Thyroxine-binding globulin is the major carrier of thyroid hormones. Some is also bound to thyroxine-binding prealbumin.

Metabolism and excretion

Iodine is metabolized in the thyroid gland by a series of steps beginning with uptake of iodide ion and ending with the release of T_4 and T_3 into the blood. T_4 is converted to T_3 in peripheral tissues. The liver is the main site of thyroid hormone degradation. In humans, approximately 20% to 40% is eliminated in the feces. Thyroxine is eliminated slowly from the body with a half-life of 6 to 7 days. The intake and excretion of iodine are maintained in close balance.

Recommended dietary allowance and nutrient interactions

The daily iodine requirement for adults is about 1 to 2 µg/kg of body weight. The RDA for iodine is given in Table 1-1. Natural goitrogens present in certain foods (e.g., cabbage, cassava, and mustard) may cause goiter in some areas.

Food sources

Seafoods and seaweeds are excellent sources of iodine. Most vegetable products are low in iodine. Dairy products and eggs have a variable content of iodine that depends on the composition of the animal feed. Depending on the process used, bread may be a source of iodine. The use of iodized salt in the United States provides a substantial source of iodine. Current levels of enrichment provide 76 µg of iodine per gram of salt. Approximately 10 to 12 g of iodized salt (or 4 to 5 g of sodium) are consumed in the United States per person per day.

Evaluation of nutritional status

The average urinary excretion of iodine in healthy adults is about 150 μg/day. Serum protein-bound iodine levels range from 4 to 8 μg/dl. Various thyroid function tests can reveal disorders of the thyroid. A serum TSH (thyrotropin) level above 6 μU/ml is strongly suggestive of hypothyroidism (<6 μU/ml = normal).

Signs, symptoms, and treatment of deficiency state

Iodine deficiency is a common worldwide cause of endemic goiter and cretinism in children. Globally, 5.7 million cretins exist. In the latter, the child is dwarfed, mentally retarded, and inactive, with a pug and expressionless face and an enlarged tongue. Successful treatment requires diagnosis long before these obvious signs appear. In the adult, reduced availability of iodine for thyroid hormone synthesis results in a compensatory enlargement of the thyroid gland (goiter). It is uncommon to see goiter resulting from iodine deficiency in the United States because of the use of iodized salt.

Various thyroid hormone preparations are available to treat hypothyroidism and simple goiter. Iodine deficiency must be corrected before pregnancy to completely prevent fetal brain damage.

Use and effects of large doses

High intake of iodine may induce goiter because organification of iodine is blocked when the plasma iodine concentration exceeds 15 to 25 μg/ml. This has been documented in the Japanese, who have a high intake of seaweed. An intake in adults between 50 and 1000 μg/day of iodine is considered safe.

IRON

Physiology and biochemical pathways

With its presence in all cells, iron participates in a number of key biochemical reactions. It is present in compounds responsible for the transport of oxygen (hemoglobin and myoglobin), enzymes responsible for electron transport (cytochromes), and enzymes responsible for the activation of oxygen (oxidases and oxygenases). A 70-kg adult man has about 2500 mg of iron in circulating hemoglobin and 500 to 1000 mg of iron in storage as ferritin or hemosiderin, largely in the liver, spleen, and bone marrow. The adult woman has about 1500 mg of iron in circulation and much lower stored iron, seldom exceeding 500 mg.

Absorption

The absorptive process is not fully understood. Iron is absorbed predominantly in the duodenum and lesser amounts in the remaining portion of the upper small intestine. Inorganic (nonheme) iron is absorbed with a low efficiency (<10%). Heme iron (from dietary hemoglobin and myoglobin) is more readily absorbed (10% to 20%). In general, healthy individuals absorb about 10% of dietary iron; iron-deficient individuals absorb between 10% and 20%. Ascorbic acid and meat in the diet will facilitate the absorption of nonheme iron. (Normal absorption is about 1 mg/day in men and 1.5 mg/day in women.) Increased uptake occurs when there is iron deficiency, when iron stores are depleted, or when erythropoiesis is increased.

Certain plant constituents such as oxalate, phytate, fiber, and tannin may reduce the absorption of nonheme iron. Reducing sugars, ascorbic acid, and heme increase the absorption of nonheme iron. Subjects with gluten-induced enteropathy or with achlorhydria absorb nonheme iron less efficiently from the diet. Antacids taken with meals also may reduce iron absorption.

Metabolism and excretion

Virtually all of the iron present in the erythrocytes is conserved and reutilized in the formation of new cells. Iron is transported in the plasma by transferrin and stored as ferritin or hemosiderin. This large protein may contain over 30% of its weight as iron. Hemosiderin represents aggregated ferritin molecules. Aside from menstrual losses in women, the daily loss of iron from skin, hair, sweat, intestinal desquamation, and urine amounts to about 0.9 mg/day in the adult. Menstrual losses average about 60 ml of blood per month, representing an additional loss of 0.5 mg/day of iron.

Recommended dietary allowance and nutrient interactions

Iron requirements are determined by obligatory physiologic losses and the needs imposed by growth. Men have a requirement of about 1 mg of absorbed iron per day, whereas the menstruating woman requires about 1.5 mg/day. Postmenopausal women have a reduced need for iron, approximating that of men. Iron requirements are higher for the infant and during the last two trimesters of pregnancy. The infant frequently has inadequate intake because of the low iron content of milk and limited body stores of iron at birth. This is corrected by the introduction of iron-enriched cereals by 4 to 6 months of age. The RDA is shown in Table 1-1.

Food sources

Diets in the United States provide iron at about 6 mg/1000 kcal. Foods high in iron include organ meats such as liver and heart, wheat germ, egg yolks, oysters, fruits, and some dried beans. Lesser amounts are present in muscle meats, fish and fowl, and most green vegetables and cereals. Milk and milk products and most nongreen vegetables are low in iron. Heme iron contributes only 1 to 2 mg of iron per day in the average U.S. diet. Hence, nonheme iron is the main source of iron in the diet.

Evaluation of nutritional status

Hematocrit and hemoglobin determinations can establish the presence of anemia, but additional measurements are required to establish iron deficiency. For this purpose, measurements of serum ferritin levels are quite useful. Approximately 1 μg of ferritin per liter of serum is equivalent to 8 mg of stored iron. Hence, low serum ferritin levels are associated with depleted iron stores. However, infection, malignancy, and inflammatory disease may cause falsely high serum ferritin levels. A common laboratory finding suggestive of iron deficiency is a low serum iron level with an elevated total iron-binding capacity (TIBC), giving a low percentage of TIBC saturation. Peripheral blood smear morphology and bone marrow iron stains are also useful. (See Chapter 2.)

Signs, symptoms, and treatment of deficiency state

Iron deficiency is one of the most common nutritional deficiencies in the world. Iron deficiency results in fatigue, pallor, tachycardia, listlessness, exertional dyspnea, burning sensation of the tongue, lingual depapillation, and a hypochromic, microcytic anemia. Fatigue and impaired cognitive function and alertness may occur in early stages of iron deficiency before anemia. Therapeutic supplementation with iron preparations is recommended when there is a clearly established iron deficiency. Orally administered ferrous sulfate is the preparation of choice in the treatment of iron deficiency. Administration for 6 months or longer is usually required to replenish bone marrow stores. Some patients may encounter gastrointestinal side effects requiring the initial dose to be reduced and then slowly increased. In some cases, ferrous gluconate has been successfully used in place of ferrous sulfate. Dietary changes should be made to include more iron-rich foods and ample intake of vitamin C to enhance iron absorption. Iron deficiency occurs most frequently in infancy and in menstruating and pregnant women. When iron deficiency occurs in men or in postmenopausal women, who have decreased iron requirements, bleeding should be investigated as a possible cause of the deficiency because chronic blood loss will produce iron loss that will eventually lead to iron deficiency and anemia.

Use and effects of large doses

Excessive intake of medicinal, dietary, or transfused iron may result in iron overload, a relatively rare condition called *hemochromatosis*. The normal person is able to control absorption of iron despite high intake. Only those with underlying disorders that augment iron absorption run the risk of hemochromatosis. However, large amounts of ferrous salts are toxic but rarely cause death in adults. Most deaths occur in the young, particularly those who are 12 to 24 months of age. For the young, as little as 1 to 2 g of iron may be fatal. Quick diagnosis and administration of deferoxamine have reduced the mortality rate from iron poisoning.

MAGNESIUM
Physiology and biochemical pathways

The magnesium content in the adult human is about 24 g, with 60% found in the skeleton, 39% in the intracellular space (20% in skeletal muscle), and 1% in the extracellular space. Magnesium is associated with more than 300 different enzyme systems. Magnesium is essential to the metabolism of adenosine triphosphate (ATP) and as such participates in glucose utilization; synthesis of proteins, fats, and nucleic acids; muscle contraction; certain membrane transport systems; and nerve impulse transmission. Magnesium is highly concentrated in the mitochondria, where it is needed for oxidative phosphorylation. Red cells contain three times more magnesium than does serum.

Absorption

On the average, 35% to 45% of dietary magnesium is absorbed in the small intestine. Vitamin D and its metabolites have little or no effect on the intestinal absorption of magnesium. Absorption may be influenced by total magnesium intake;

intestinal transit time; the amount of lactose and phosphate in the diet; and rate of water absorption. There is evidence to suggest that magnesium is absorbed by a carrier-mediated system and by simple diffusion, primarily at higher concentrations. Magnesium reenters the intestinal tract from bile and pancreatic and intestinal juices. Under normal conditions, nearly all is reabsorbed.

Metabolism and excretion

At least three different magnesium pools exist in the body, each with a different rate of turnover. The extracellular pool has a rapid turnover rate. The intracellular pool has a turnover rate about half that of the extracellular pool. The major pool, the skeleton, has a very slow turnover rate. In the plasma, 55% of the magnesium is in the free form, 13% in a complex form, and 32% in protein-bound forms. Approximately 60% to 70% of ingested magnesium is excreted in the feces, with most of the remainder excreted in the urine. An average of 1.4 mg of magnesium per kilogram of body weight is excreted daily in the urine.

Recommended dietary allowance and nutrient interactions

Magnesium and thiamin appear to interact. For example, thiamin administered to magnesium-deficient rats is not used and thiamin deficiency may develop. Calcium homeostasis is dependent on magnesium in that severe hypomagnesemia prevents the release of parathyroid hormone and can cause hypocalcemia. The RDA for magnesium is 350 mg/day for men and 280 mg/day for women. During pregnancy and lactation an extra allowance of 150 mg/day is recommended (see Table 1-1). Oriental diets and diets of vegetarians are high in magnesium.

Food sources

In the United States the average adult consumes 180 to 480 mg of magnesium daily. Dairy items, grains, and nuts are rich sources of magnesium. Meats, seafoods, and vegetables, especially green leafy types, are also good sources of magnesium. Magnesium present in the chlorophyll of plants appears readily available. Human milk contains 40 mg of magnesium per liter; cow's milk contains approximately 120 mg/L.

Evaluation of nutritional status

In magnesium deficiency, serum magnesium levels are markedly reduced and urinary excretion is low. Atomic absorption spectroscopy is the easiest method to measure magnesium levels in urine or serum specimens.

Normal adult serum levels range from 1.8 to 2.3 mg/dl (0.75 to 0.96 mmol/L; 1.5 to 1.9 mEq/L; mean 0.85 mmol/L). Urinary excretion levels for magnesium in the adult range from 36 to 207 mg/24 hours (1.5 to 9.5 mmol/24 hours; 3 to 17 mEq/24 hours).

Signs, symptoms, and treatment of deficiency state

Magnesium deficiency may cause increased neuromuscular excitability, muscle spasms, and paresthesias. Prolonged deficiency can progress to tetany, seizures, and coma. Hypocalcemia and hypokalemia often accompany hypomagnesemia.

Magnesium deficiency can be a complication of kwashiorkor. Hypomagnesemia is most often seen in alcoholics and in patients with fat malabsorption syndromes and other malabsorption syndromes.

Use and effects of large doses

Magnesium sulfate (Epsom salt) at a dose of approximately 15 g is used for its laxative effect. Milk of magnesia and magnesium hydroxide and other magnesium salts are used as gastric antacids. Because of the possibility of hypermagnesemia, their use should be avoided in individuals with impaired renal function. The normal kidney is capable of rapidly excreting large amounts of absorbed or injected magnesium.

PHOSPHORUS

Physiology and biochemical pathways

The phosphorus content of a male adult is approximately 500 g, of which about 85% is found as bone minerals, calcium phosphate, and hydroxyapatite. The remainder is in the cells and extracellular fluids as inorganic phosphate ions, phospholipids, phosphoproteins, and organic phosphoric esters. Most phosphorus is present as phosphate; no elemental phosphorus as such is present in the body. Phosphate is a constituent of nucleic acids and cell membranes and is an essential factor in all energy-producing reactions in the cells; it plays an important role in modifying concentrations of calcium in tissues, maintenance of acid-base equilibrium, and renal excretion of hydrogen ions.

Absorption

Phosphate is absorbed only from the small intestine by an active sodium-requiring transport process and to the largest extent by passive diffusion. Vitamin D stimulates phosphate absorption through a mechanism that is apparently separate from its action on calcium transport. Hence, in vitamin D deficiency, with a reduction in the availability of $1,25(OH)_2D_3$, absorption of phosphorus and calcium is reduced. When fed human milk, infants absorb 85% to 90% of the phosphorus present. When infants are fed cow's milk, which is seven times higher in phosphorus than human milk, the intestinal absorption of phosphorus is reduced to 65% to 70%. In older children and adults, with an intake of 1000 to 1500 mg of phosphorus, the efficiency of absorption is approximately 50% to 60%. Ingestion of aluminum-containing antacids reduces its absorption. The phosphorus in phytic acid, as present in cereal brans and unleavened breads, is unavailable for absorption.

Metabolism and excretion

Phosphate is present in plasma and extracellular fluids, in cell membranes, and in intracellular fluids. Serum concentrations of phosphate are higher in children than in adults. The higher serum concentration of phosphate during the growth period is important for mineralization of growing bone and cartilage. Phosphate absorbed from the intestine is readily excreted in the urine under the influence of parathyroid hormone to maintain body phosphate balance. Most of the phosphate in the plasma is in the ionic form (80%).

Recommended dietary allowance and nutrient interactions

The RDA for phosphorus, in milligrams per day, is the same as for calcium (with infants being an exception) and thereby provides a Ca:P ratio of 1.0. For the infant, evidence supports the recommendation of a dietary Ca:P ratio of about 1.5. A phosphorus intake greatly in excess of calcium, especially in the presence of a minimal intake of calcium, can reduce the availability of calcium and contribute to calcium deficiency. The recommended allowance for phosphorus is shown in Table 1-1.

Food sources

Phosphorus is abundant in the food supply. Most seafoods, nuts, grains, legumes, and cheeses are good sources (100 to 1200 mg per 100 g of food item). Most green leafy vegetables, cauliflower, brussels sprouts, okra, potatoes, yams, and milk provide low amounts of phosphorus (50 to 100 mg per 100 g of food item).

Evaluation of nutritional status

Essentially, procedures to evaluate phosphorus status have been limited to measuring serum phosphorus levels. From a nutritional standpoint, interpretation of serum phosphorus levels is difficult because of the numerous factors that may influence the serum level. In hospitalized patients, reduced serum levels occur most often because of rapid intravenous infusions of glucose. In outpatients, hypophosphatemia usually results from chronic use of aluminum-containing antacids. Other causes include alcohol abuse, rickets, hyperparathyroidism, sprue, and insulin therapy. Hypophosphatemia requires prompt diagnosis and treatment. Elevated serum phosphorus values have been observed to occur with hypoparathyroidism, renal disease, diabetes, and healing fractures. The average serum phosphate of the normal adult is 3.5 mg/dl (2.5 to 4.0 mg/dl: 0.81 to 1.29 mmol/L). Higher serum phosphate levels are observed in premature infants (7.9 mg/dl) and full-term infants (6.1 mg/dl), whereas values for children 1 to 10 years of age are lower (4.6 mg/dl). Under normal conditions, urinary phosphorus levels reflect dietary phosphorus intake.

Signs, symptoms, and treatment of deficiency state

Phosphorus is abundant in a wide variety of foods. Consequently, nutritional deficiencies are rare. However, renal hypophosphatemia may occur in people with abnormalities of renal tubular function, thereby reducing tubular reabsorption of phosphate. Fanconi's syndrome may include hypophosphatemia. The major manifestations of chronic primary hypophosphatemia are growth retardation, skeletal deformities, and bone pain resulting from defective mineralization of bones. Phosphate depletion results in diminished concentration of intracellular organic phosphoric acid esters, including ATP and 2,3-diphosphoglycerate in RBCs and ATP in muscle. Hemoglobin interacts with 2,3-diphosphoglycerate to promote oxygen release from oxyhemoglobin, which is diminished in hypophosphatemia, predisposing to tissue hypoxia. Phosphate depletion may increase the rate of hemolysis of RBCs, produce severe muscle weakness and ophthalmoplegia (see Fig. 6-11), and diminish the phagocytic function of granulocytes.

Hypophosphatemia is particularly likely to occur in starved patients and alcoholics after refeeding, in diabetic ketoacidosis patients after treatment with insulin and glucose, and in patients receiving high concentrations of glucose intravenously. In a controlled human phosphorus deficiency study, symptoms such as weakness, anorexia, debility, and bone pain occurred when the serum phosphorus levels fell to less than 1.0 mg/dl (0.3 mmol/L).

Use and effects of large doses

Phosphates are of limited therapeutic usefulness, although they may have a role in the management of the phosphate-depletion syndromes. Sodium phosphate has been used to diminish hypercalcemia. Excess phosphate salts have a cathartic effect. Phosphate preparations are also used as urine acidifiers and antacids.

ZINC

Physiology and biochemical pathways

Zinc is essential for the function of more than 200 metalloenzymes and is particularly essential for rapidly growing tissues. Deficiency will retard the synthesis of DNA, ribonucleic acid (RNA), and protein, resulting in impaired cellular division, growth, and repair. DNA polymerase and RNA polymerase require zinc. Zinc is essential for sexual maturation, fertility and reproduction, night vision, sense of taste, and immune functions.

Absorption

Zinc is absorbed by an active process in the duodenum, jejunum, and probably to a lesser extent in the ileum. Phytate and dietary fiber can reduce zinc absorption. The efficiency of zinc absorption depends on the type of meal eaten and the individual's zinc status; absorption may range from 10% to 40%. Fat malabsorption can reduce zinc absorption, and small-bowel diarrhea can result in losses of 12 to 17 mg of zinc per liter of diarrheal fluid.

Metabolism and excretion

After absorption, zinc is circulated bound to albumin (65%) and an α-macroglobulin (30%). Zinc is initially concentrated in the liver and then distributed to tissues. Zinc in the skeleton is relatively unavailable to other tissues. The adult body contains 1 to 2 g of zinc.

The turnover of zinc in the body is slow, with a biologic half-life of 250 days. However, the labile body pool of zinc is relatively small with a rapid turnover rate. Consequently, a continuous intake of zinc is necessary to prevent a zinc deficiency. The major route of excretion is in pancreatic and intestinal secretions, with only about 5% excreted daily in the urine. Depending on the ambient temperature or the presence of fever, up to 1 mg of zinc can be lost per liter of sweat.

Recommended dietary allowance and nutrient interactions

Excess zinc in the diet may decrease the absorption of copper. Recommended dietary allowances are given in Table 1-1.

Food sources

Meat, liver, eggs, and seafoods, especially oysters, are good sources of zinc. Whole-grain products (e.g., whole-wheat or rye bread, oatmeal, whole corn) contain zinc, but it is less bioavailable in these food sources.

Evaluation of nutritional status

The laboratory criteria for evaluating zinc status are not well established. Various laboratory procedures include dark adaptation, taste acuity testing, and activities of zinc metalloenzymes such as alkaline phosphatase and carbonic anhydrase. Normal ranges of values for some of the laboratory measurements for zinc are shown below:

Zinc content of	Normal ranges
Serum	80-140 μg/dl
Red cell	40-44 μg/g hemoglobin
White cell	80-130 μg/10^{10} cells
Saliva (parotid)	23-70 ng/g
Sweat	0.55-1.75 mg/L
Nail	100-400 μg/g
Hair	100-230 μg/g
Urine	230-600 μg/day

Signs, symptoms, and treatment of deficiency state

Clinical manifestations of zinc deficiency include growth retardation and hypogonadism, impaired taste or smell acuity or both, and poor wound healing. Mental lethargy, poor appetite, and dry, scaly skin may occur (Fig. 7-1 and Plate 15). A reduction in immune competence is frequently noted. Nondietary zinc deficiency may be seen in cases of acrodermatitis enteropathica, a rare inherited disorder that is responsive to zinc therapy, and with certain malabsorption syndromes.

Use and effects of large doses

Toxic effects of high doses of zinc are uncommon, although zinc may antagonize the metabolism of copper, and sickle cell anemia patients given approximately 150 mg of zinc daily may develop signs of copper deficiency. In addition, excessive oral zinc intake is a therapy for Wilson's disease, a copper overload syndrome. Plasma HDL-C levels fall after the administration of high doses of zinc, and this may not be desirable.

The use of oral contraceptives may alter the postabsorptive utilization of zinc. However, evidence indicates that the requirement for zinc is not increased in women using these agents.

OTHER TRACE ELEMENTS
Copper

Copper deficiency in humans is considered rare but is associated with Menkes' syndrome, a genetic disorder in which copper utilization is impaired. Copper deficiency has been observed in infants fed only cow's milk. The clinical manifestations of copper deficiency include neutropenia, hypochromic microcytic anemia,

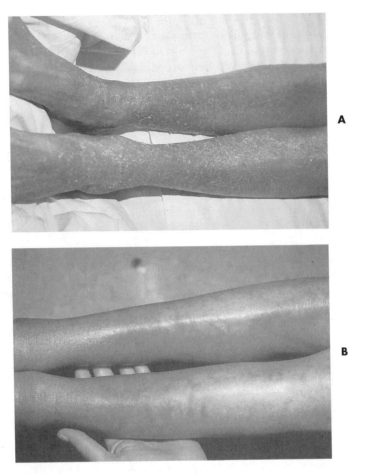

Fig. 7-1   Widespread scaling of the skin before **(A)** and after **(B)** treatment with zinc in a patient with fat malabsorption. ▲

depigmentation of skin and hair, neurologic disturbances, lethargy, and abnormalities of connective tissue accompanied by skeletal abnormalities. The anemia resulting from copper deficiency is indistinguishable from iron-deficiency anemia. In the genetic Wilson's disease, copper accumulates in the liver, kidney, and brain, producing copper toxicity. Copper is a component of a number of metalloenzymes, including ceruloplasmin, lysyl oxidase, cytochrome *c*, and superoxide dismutase. Copper plays a key role in iron absorption and mobilization. About 30% to 40% of the copper in the diet is absorbed. Liver, nuts, legumes, and oysters are good sources of copper. The copper requirement for adults is not well defined. A daily intake of 1.5 to 3 mg of copper by adults is considered safe and adequate (see Table 1-2). Normal serum levels of copper range from 90 to 125 μg/dl.

Chromium

Chromium is required for maintaining normal glucose metabolism, probably as a cofactor for insulin. Approximately 0.5% to 2% of inorganic chromium present in the diet is absorbed. Excretion is primarily in the urine. Glucose intolerance can result from chromium deficiency, such as patients on total parenteral nutrition without adequate chromium supplementation. The estimated safe and adequate daily intake for chromium for adults is 50 to 200 μg/day (see Table 1-2). There is no satisfactory test for the diagnosis of a chromium deficiency; diagnosis is based largely on documented clinical response to chromium—that is, improved glucose tolerance. For treatment, 200 μg/day of chromium as $CrCl_3$ orally or 10 g/day of brewer's yeast may be used. Meat products, eggs, cheese, whole grains, nuts, and brewer's yeast are good sources of chromium. Plasma levels of 1.6 μg/L have been reported for the normal human.

Manganese

The adult human body contains about 10 to 20 mg of manganese. Manganese-containing metalloenzymes are located primarily in mitochondria. Pyruvate carboxylase and manganese superoxide dismutase are examples of such enzymes. Manganese also functions as an enzyme cofactor and in the activation of glycosyl transferases, gluconeogenesis, lipid metabolism, and mucopolysaccharide metabolism. It may play a role in brain function through biogenic amine metabolism. About 3% to 12% of manganese is absorbed from the diet through the small intestine. Little is known of the clinical signs of deficiency, although a male subject was reported to develop weight loss, hypocholesterolemia, dermatitis, nausea and vomiting, reddening of black hair, and reduced growth rate of hair when manganese was inadvertently omitted from a purified experimental diet. Sources of dietary manganese are mainly plant foods, with tea exceptionally high in the element. The estimated safe and adequate daily intake is listed in Table 1-2. Manganese toxicity has been reported in humans resulting from inhalation of dust or fumes from mining or various industrial operations. Normal human subjects have been reported to have serum levels of 0.59 to 1.4 μg/L of manganese.

Molybdenum

Molybdenum is an essential element for animals, although the effects of molybdenum on human health are not known with certainty. Molybdenum deficiency in humans is unknown. Molybdenum is a component of the metalloenzymes aldehyde oxidase, sulfite oxidase, and xanthine oxidase. Molybdenum in foods is readily absorbed, and more than half is excreted in the urine. Diets in the United States have been reported to provide 0.05 to 0.46 mg/day. Higher intakes of molybdenum may interfere with copper metabolism. Normal human plasma has been reported to contain about 0.8 (0.28 to 1.17) μg/L of molybdenum (see Table 1-2).

Selenium

Selenium is a component of glutathione peroxidase, which protects cells and membranes against damage from peroxides when lipids are oxidized. Selenium in food is present largely in the form of amino acids, for example, selenomethionine. Selenium in food is readily absorbed. It is eliminated from the body largely by the kidney, although significant losses occur through the feces, breath, and skin. Low intakes of selenium result in lowered blood levels of selenium and may correlate with glutathione peroxidase activity in whole blood. Plasma levels of selenium below 85 μg/L (1.1 μmol/L) are considered low. Marginal intake occurs in the population of New Zealand and portions of the populations of China, Finland, and Venezuela. Individuals in areas of China where there is a low intake of selenium may develop a cardiomyopathy known as Keshan's disease, which can be prevented with selenium supplementation. Various procedures have been used to evaluate selenium status, including measuring urinary selenium levels, whole blood, erythrocyte and plasma selenium levels, and glutathione peroxidase activities of platelets or erythrocytes. No method is entirely satisfactory for assessing selenium status; thus several techniques are usually used. The RDA for selenium is 70 μg/day for men and 25 μg/day for women (see Table 1-1).

Fluorine

The importance of fluorine (known also as fluoride, the ionic form) is demonstrated in its ability to reduce dental caries and its influence on a number of biologic processes. Fluoride is a normal component of calcified tissues. The fluoride ion is incorporated into the crystalline structure of hydroxyapatite of teeth to provide increased resistance to dental caries. It is estimated that 50% to 80% of the fluoride in the human diet is absorbed. An efficient renal excretion mechanism maintains blood fluoride concentrations within a narrow range, regardless of intake. The protective effects of fluoride against caries require a total dietary fluoride intake of 1.5 mg/day or more. A range between 1.5 and 2.5 mg in adolescents and between 1.5 and 4 mg in adults has been proved safe and adequate (see Table 1-2). Higher intake may result in mottling of the teeth. The Food and Nutrition Board of the National Academy of Sciences recommends fluoridation of public water supplies at 1 ppm if natural fluoride levels are low (see Chapter 2).

8

Case Studies

Alcohol Abuse and Nutrient Deficiencies

After losing his job as a house painter, a 33-year-old man became severely depressed and spent most of his time alone. His already excessive intake of alcohol increased to the point that he was repeatedly in drunken stupors. Because of recurrent indigestion, he began taking aluminum-containing antacids throughout the day. Food intake was limited to canned soups, sodas, coffee, and four glasses or more of whole milk a day (to help relieve the indigestion). His weight remained relatively stable.

After 3 months, he was taken to the hospital by a friend who noted that he was disoriented to time and place and speaking "out of his head."

Physical examination. Weight-for-height was 90% of standard. Examination of his skin revealed no abnormalities. His tongue was slick (absence of papillae; see Fig. 6-7, *A*). He had marked generalized weakness with footdrop (inability to raise his toes; see Fig. 6-10) and ataxia (difficulty balancing while standing or walking).

Laboratory data. Hematocrit 36%, mean cell volume 106 μ^3 (normal 82 to 99), WBC count 4000/mm³ (normal 4000 to 11,000/mm³) with several hypersegmented neutrophils noted on the peripheral blood smear.

TRUE or FALSE   It is reasonable to assume that:
1. The hypersegmented neutrophils support a diagnosis of vitamin C deficiency.
2. His riboflavin intake is probably well below the RDA.
3. The alcohol intake may have contributed to the development of his neuropathy by decreasing his absorption of thiamin.
4. He most likely will be found to have abnormal vitamin B_{12} absorption as the explanation for these hematologic abnormalities.
5. He almost definitely has thiamin deficiency.
6. He almost definitely has pellagra.
7. He almost definitely has iron deficiency.
8. He almost definitely has scurvy.
9. He almost definitely has zinc deficiency.

Malabsorption Syndrome

A 50-year-old woman underwent surgical resection of most of her small intestine after a vascular occlusion. Over the ensuing months, she lost a significant amount of weight despite a good appetite and a diet consisting of a variety of foods including fruits, vegetables, starches, meats, and fats. She had six to seven bowel movements per day, which she described as large, frothy, malodorous, and difficult to flush. She took no vitamin or mineral supplements but had been on oral antibiotics for treatment of a chronic sinus infection.

She had concerns about the weight loss and recurrences of bleeding into the skin (even without evident trauma; Fig. 8-1 and Plate 16) but otherwise felt well and had no complaints. Specifically, she denied muscle spasms, paresthesia (numbness and tingling), bone pain, and symptoms suggestive of night blindness.

Under these circumstances and on the basis of this information, which of the following statements is or are true?

1. A serum carotene level of 39 mg/dl (normal 50 to 300), if found, would indicate that she could not have been eating green and yellow-orange vegetables and fruits.
2. Vitamin C deficiency can be assumed to exist.
3. Bleeding into the skin may well reflect vitamin K deficiency in this case.
4. Her illness will increase her risk of developing zinc deficiency.
5. She is at increased risk for oxalate-containing kidney stones.
6. If her terminal (distal) ileum was in fact removed, she should be given a small daily supplement of vitamin B_{12} orally to prevent deficiency.

See Appendix A for answers and discussion.

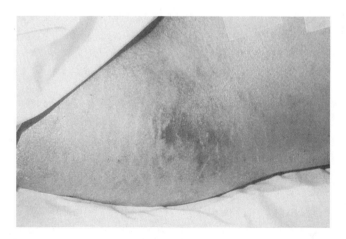

Fig. 8-1   Ecchymosis in a patient with fat malabsorption syndrome.   ▲

NUTRITION AND THE HOSPITALIZED PATIENT

9

Prevalence and Types of Malnutrition

Common types of malnutrition
Marasmus
Kwashiorkor
Marasmic kwashiorkor
Micronutrient malnutrition

Malnutrition can be either primary or secondary. *Primary malnutrition* is caused by altered or limited nutrient intakes, usually because of inadequate food supply. *Secondary malnutrition* occurs when an underlying disease process alters nutrient intake, absorption, requirements, utilization, or excretion. Although primary malnutrition is a major problem throughout the world, it is uncommon in the United States. This section will emphasize secondary malnutrition in the hospitalized patient.

In his 1974 article entitled "The Skeleton in the Hospital Closet," Butterworth focused attention on iatrogenic (physician-induced) malnutrition in the United States. Other studies since then have concluded that protein-energy malnutrition affects up to half of general medical and surgical patients. A study in 1976 revealed nutritional deterioration in 69% of general medical patients who were hospitalized for 2 weeks or longer, even if they had normal values on admission. A follow-up study in 1988 found a slightly lower likelihood of malnutrition on admission and a slight improvement in nutritional status in patients hospitalized for 2 or more weeks. These and many other studies have shown that patients with evidence of malnutrition have significantly longer hospital stays and higher mortality and morbidity rates.

In other studies, patients with reduced circulating protein levels were found to have a greater frequency of surgical complications. In addition, malnutrition reduces immune competence and increases susceptibility to infection, which are reversible with nutritional repletion. Clearly, malnutrition influences morbidity and mortality, and nutritional repletion has benefits.

COMMON TYPES OF MALNUTRITION

Malnutrition in the United States is usually caused by an underlying disease process. However, its development often results from failure to recognize and meet the increased nutritional needs of ill patients. The most common forms of malnutrition that are seen in the hospital result from protein deficiency, energy deficiency, or both. There are two main types of protein-energy malnutrition:

- Severe calorie deficiency, otherwise known as *marasmus*

- A maladaptive state with protein deficiency and metabolic stress, known as *kwashiorkor*
- There could also be a combination of the two, termed *marasmic kwashiorkor*

The features of marasmus and kwashiorkor are compared in Table 9-1, and the time course of their development is depicted in Fig. 9-1.

MARASMUS

Illnesses that produce marasmus or severe cachexia in the United States are chronic and indolent, such as cancer, chronic pulmonary disease, and anorexia nervosa. The diagnosis is based on the physical finding of severe depletion of fat and muscle in the setting of prolonged calorie deficiency. Diminished skinfold thickness reflects the loss of energy reserves (Fig. 9-2 and Plate 17). Reduced arm muscle circumference with temporal and interosseous muscle wasting reflects the resorption of protein from the skeletal muscles. This also occurs in internal organs such as the heart, liver, and kidneys.

The laboratory picture is relatively unremarkable: the serum albumin level is sometimes reduced slightly but often remains in the normal range. Despite a morbid appearance, immune competence, wound healing, and the ability to handle short-term stress are reasonably well preserved in most patients with marasmus.

Marasmus is a chronic disorder rather than an acute illness, and it should be treated cautiously to reverse the downward trend gradually. Although nutritional support is necessary, overly aggressive repletion can result in severe, even life-threatening metabolic imbalances such as hypophosphatemia. When possible, the enteral route of nutritional support is preferred. Treatment should be started slowly to allow readaptation of metabolic and intestinal functions (see Chapter 11).

KWASHIORKOR

In contrast to marasmus, kwashiorkor in the United States occurs mainly in connection with acute, life-threatening illnesses such as trauma and sepsis. The physiologic stress produced by these illnesses increases protein and energy requirements at a time when intake is often limited. In children, kwashiorkor can result

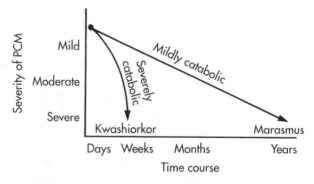

Fig. 9-1   Time course of protein-calorie malnutrition.

Table 9-1 Comparison of marasmus and kwashiorkor

Disease	Clinical setting	Time course to develop	Clinical features	Laboratory findings	Clinical course	Mortality
Marasmus	↓ Calorie intake	Months or years	Starved appearance Weight < 80% standard for height Triceps skinfold < 3 mm Midarm muscle circumference < 15 cm	Creatine-height index < 60% standard	Reasonably preserved responsiveness to short-term stress	Low, unless related to underlying disease
Kwashiorkor	↓ Protein intake during stress state	Weeks	Well-nourished appearance Easy hair pluckability Edema	Serum albumin < 2.8 g/dl Total iron-binding capacity < 200 μg/dl Lymphocytes < 1500/mm^3 Anergy	Infections Poor wound healing, decubitus ulcers, skin breakdown	High

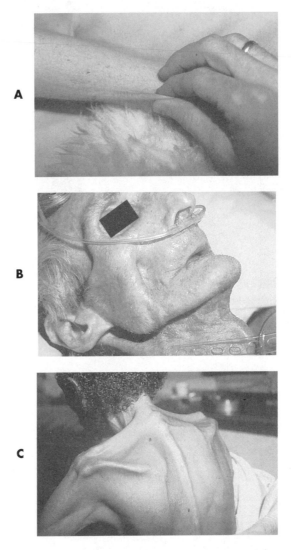

Fig. 9-2   **A** to **C**, Losses of subcutaneous fat reserves and muscle mass in patients with marasmus. ▲

when poor dietary intake is added to the stress of growth, infections, or other ill-nesses. A typical scenario in adults is the acutely ill, hospitalized patient who is re-ceiving only 5% dextrose solutions. In this setting, kwashiorkor can take as little as 2 weeks to develop. Although the etiologic mechanisms are not fully under-stood, failure of the adaptive response of protein sparing that is normally seen in fasting is an important factor. The clinical findings are often few. Fat reserves and muscle mass tend to be unaltered, which gives the deceptive appearance of ade-quate nutrition. Signs that support the diagnosis of kwashiorkor include easily

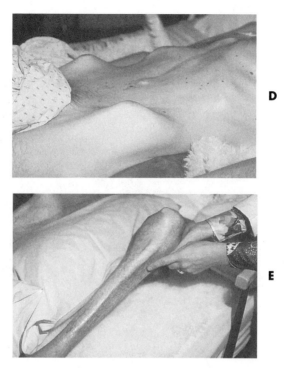

Fig. 9-2, cont'd   D to **E,** Losses of subcutaneous fat reserves and muscle mass in patients with marasmus. ▲

pluckable hair, edema, skin breakdown, and delayed wound healing (Fig. 9-3 and Plate 18). Characteristic laboratory changes include severely depressed levels of serum proteins such as albumin (<2.8 g/dl) and transferrin (<150 mg/dl) or reduced iron-binding capacity (<200 μg/dl). Associated with the fall in levels of circulating proteins is a depression of cellular immune function, reflected by lymphopenia (<1500 lymphocytes/mm^3 in adults and older children) and skin test anergy. When full-blown kwashiorkor is diagnosed in the adult, the prognosis is guarded, even with aggressive nutritional support. Dehiscence of surgical wounds may occur, host defenses are compromised, and death from overwhelming sepsis may ensue despite antibiotic therapy. Unlike treatment for marasmus, aggressive feeding should be used in an attempt to restore normal metabolic homeostasis rapidly. However, the metabolic state will not normalize until the underlying illness or other stress resolves. Although childhood kwashiorkor is often less foreboding, perhaps because of the lower degree of stress required to precipitate the deficiency state, in both adults and children it is a serious condition. Kwashiorkor can be prevented more easily than it is treated if the stress (catabolic) state is recognized early and energy and protein requirements are met.

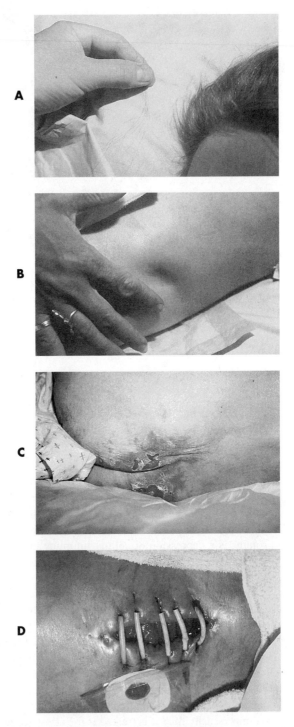

Fig. 9-3   **A** to **D,** Clinical findings in kwashiorkor, including easy, painless hair pluckability, pitting edema, skin breakdown, and delayed wound healing.   ▲

MARASMIC KWASHIORKOR

This combined form of protein-energy malnutrition can develop when acute stress, such as from surgery, trauma, or infection, is experienced by the chronically starved patient. Because it carries the high risk of infections and other complications associated with kwashiorkor, marasmic kwashiorkor can be life threatening. It is important to determine which of the 2 types of protein-energy malnutrition predominates so that an appropriate nutritional plan can be developed: the starved, hypometabolic patient is at risk of complications from overaggressive feeding, but the stressed patient with kwashiorkor is more likely to suffer from underfeeding and should receive vigorous nutritional therapy.

MICRONUTRIENT MALNUTRITION

The same illnesses and reductions in nutrient intake that cause protein-energy malnutrition can also produce deficiencies of vitamins and minerals. In addition to having reduced intake (sometimes for extended periods), patients with acute and chronic illnesses and protein-energy malnutrition often experience abnormal losses of micronutrients, such as through external secretions (zinc in diarrheal fluid or burn exudate), or metabolize or consume greater quantities, such as vitamin C in infectious illnesses. Deficiencies of nutrients having small body stores (especially the water-soluble vitamins) are most common. In the authors' experience, deficiencies of vitamin C and zinc are common in hospitalized patients. Their physical findings, and those of other deficiencies, are listed in Table 10-2. To establish the diagnosis, blood levels must be measured. For more information on specific nutrients, see Part Two.

SUGGESTED READINGS

Butterworth CE: The skeleton in the hospital closet, *Nutr Today* 9:4-8, 1974.

Coats KG, Morgan SL, Bartolucci AA, et al: Hospital-associated malnutrition: a reevaluation 12 years later, *J Am Diet Assoc* 93:27, 1993.

Torosian MH, editor: *Nutrition for the hospitalized patient,* New York, 1995, Marcel Dekker.

Torun B, Chew F: Protein-energy malnutrition. In Shils ME, Olsen JA, Shike M, editors: *Modern nutrition in health and disease,* ed 8, Philadelphia, 1994, Lea & Febiger.

Weinsier RL, Hunker EM, Krumdieck CL, et al: Hospital malnutrition: a prospective evaluation of general medical patients during the course of hospitalization, *Am J Clin Nutr* 32:418-428, 1979.

10

Nutritional Assessment

Nutritional history
Physical examination
Laboratory studies

Many physical and laboratory findings are a reflection of underlying disease, as well as nutritional status. Therefore the evaluation of a patient's nutritional status depends on an understanding of the patient's medical condition and its impact on the physical examination and the laboratory parameters. This approach helps detect nutritional problems while avoiding the conclusion that an isolated finding such as hypoalbuminemia, which can be caused by the underlying illness, indicates a nutritional problem when it may not.

Each medical and surgical subspecialty has a certain focus of its medical history and clinical and laboratory assessment that is directly relevant to that subspecialty. Similarly, clinical nutrition has a specialized history review, physical examination, and laboratory approach that are all important to a complete nutritional assessment.

NUTRITIONAL HISTORY

The nutritional history is directed toward identifying underlying mechanisms that put patients at risk for nutritional depletion or excess. These mechanisms, outlined in Table 10-1, include inadequate intake, impaired absorption, decreased utilization, increased losses, and increased requirements of nutrients.

There are many types of diet histories, but the major ones used are: dietary recalls, generally covering 24 hours; food records, in which patients write down everything eaten during a 1- to 7-day period; and food frequency questionnaires, in which patients estimate how often they eat the foods identified on a list. Each method has advantages and disadvantages. For instance, a 24-hour dietary recall may significantly underestimate usual intakes but can be easily elicited from most patients. Three-day food records provide a reasonable way to obtain a qualitative estimate of nutrient intakes, but food choices often change during recording periods and may not be representative of intake as a whole. Sometimes combinations of the various methods work best.

For routine nutritional assessment of a patient in the hospital or clinic setting, a 24-hour dietary recall provides an adequate overview of the patient's dietary pattern to determine if further detailed evaluation is necessary. In the course of the entire medical history, however, it is important to elicit information about all of the

Table 10-1 Nutritional history screen—a systematic approach to the detection of deficiency syndromes

Mechanism of deficiency	If history of	Suspect deficiency of
Inadequate intake	Alcohol abuse	Calories, protein, thiamin, niacin, folate, pyridoxine, riboflavin
	Avoidance of fruit, vegetables, grains	Vitamin C, thiamin, niacin, folate
	Avoidance of meat, dairy products, eggs	Protein, vitamin B_{12}
	Constipation, hemorrhoids, diverticulosis	Dietary fiber
	Isolation, poverty, dental disease, food idiosyncrasies	Various nutrients
	Weight loss	Calories, other nutrients
Inadequate absorption	Drugs (especially antacids, anticonvulsants, cholestyramine, laxatives, neomycin, alcohol)	See Table 12-4
	Malabsorption (diarrhea, weight loss, steatorrhea)	Vitamins A, D, K, calories, protein, calcium, magnesium, zinc
	Parasites	Iron, vitamin B_{12} (fish tapeworm)
	Pernicious anemia	Vitamin B_{12}
	Surgery	
	Gastrectomy	Vitamin B_{12}, iron
	Resection of small intestine	Vitamin B_{12} (if distal ileum), others as in malabsorption
Decreased utilization	Drugs (especially anticonvulsants, antimetabolites, oral contraceptives, isoniazid, alcohol)	See Table 12-4
	Inborn errors of metabolism (by family history)	Various nutrients
Increased losses	Alcohol abuse	Magnesium, zinc
	Blood loss	Iron
	Centesis (ascitic, pleural taps)	Protein
	Diabetes, uncontrolled	Calories
	Diarrhea	Protein, zinc, electrolytes
	Draining abscesses, wounds	Protein, zinc
	Nephrotic syndrome	Protein, zinc
	Peritoneal dialysis or hemodialysis	Protein, water-soluble vitamins, zinc

Continued

Table 10-1   Nutritional history screen—a systematic approach to the detection of deficiency syndromes—cont'd

Mechanism of deficiency	If history of	Suspect deficiency of
Increased requirements	Fever	Calories
	Hyperthyroidism	Calories
	Physiologic demands (infancy, adolescence, pregnancy, lactation)	Various nutrients
	Surgery, trauma, burns, infection	Calories, protein, vitamin C, zinc
	Tissue hypoxia	Calories (inefficient utilization)
	Cigarette smoking	Vitamin C, folate

Box 10-1   The high-risk patient

- Underweight (weight-for-height < 80% of standard) or recent loss of 10% or more of usual body weight or both
- Poor nutrient intake: anorexia, food avoidance (e.g., psychiatric condition), or NPO (nothing allowed by mouth) status for more than 5 days
- Protracted nutrient losses: malabsorption, enteric fistulae, draining abscesses or wounds, renal dialysis
- Hypermetabolic states: sepsis, protracted fever, extensive trauma or burns
- Chronic use of alcohol or medications with antinutrient or catabolic properties: steroids, antimetabolites (e.g., methotrexate), immunosuppressants, antitumor agents
- Impoverishment, isolation, or advanced age

---

areas noted in Table 10-1 (e.g., presence of alcoholism, dental disease, drug use, malabsorption) to identify potential nutrient deficiencies not elicited by the dietary recall. Individuals with the characteristics shown in Box 10-1 are at particular risk for nutritional deficiencies. The presence of any one characteristic is a warning that a patient is at increased risk for malnutrition, but the absence of these characteristics does not mean that malnutrition does not exist or cannot occur.

PHYSICAL EXAMINATION

Physical findings that suggest vitamin, mineral, and protein-energy deficiencies and excesses are outlined in Table 10-2. Most of the physical findings are not specific for an individual nutrient deficiency and must be integrated with the historical, anthropometric, and laboratory findings to make a diagnosis. For example, the finding of follicular hyperkeratosis isolated to the back of one's arms is a fairly common, normal finding. On the other hand, if it is widespread and found in a person who consumes little fruits and vegetables and smokes regularly (increasing ascorbic acid requirements), vitamin C deficiency is a very possible cause. Similarly, easily pluckable hair may be a consequence of recent chemotherapy. On the other hand, in a hospitalized patient who is not on chemotherapy and who has

Table 10-2   Clinical nutrition examination

Clinical findings	Consider deficiency of*	Consider excess of	Frequency†
Hair, nails			
Flag sign (transverse depigmentation of hair)	Protein		Rare
Easily pluckable hair	Protein		Common
Sparse hair	Protein, biotin, zinc	Vitamin A	Occasional
Corkscrew hairs and unemerged coiled hairs	Vitamin C		Common
Transverse ridging of nails	Protein		Occasional
Skin			
Scaling	Vitamin A, zinc, essential fatty acids	Vitamin A	Occasional
Cellophane appearance	Protein		Occasional
Cracking (flaking paint or crazy pavement dermatosis)	Protein		Rare
Follicular hyperkeratosis	Vitamins A, C		Occasional
Petechiae (especially perifollicular)	Vitamin C		Occasional
Purpura	Vitamins C, K		Common
Pigmentation, desquamation of sun-exposed areas	Niacin		Rare
Yellow pigmentation—sparing sclerae (benign)		Carotene	Common
Eyes			
Papilledema		Vitamin A	Rare
Night blindness	Vitamin A		Rare
Perioral			
Angular stomatitis	Riboflavin, pyridoxine, niacin		Occasional
Cheilosis (dry, cracking, ulcerated lips)	Riboflavin, pyridoxine, niacin		Rare
Oral			
Atrophic lingual papillae (slick tongue)	Riboflavin, niacin, folate, vitamin B_{12}, protein, iron		Common
Glossitis (scarlet, raw tongue)	Riboflavin, niacin, pyridoxine, folate, vitamin B_{12}		Occasional
Hypogeusesthesia, hyposmia	Zinc		Occasional
Swollen, retracted, bleeding gums (if teeth are present)	Vitamin C		Occasional
Bones, joints			
Beading of ribs, epiphyseal swelling, bowlegs	Vitamin D		Rare
Tenderness (subperiosteal hemorrhage in child)	Vitamin C		Rare

*In this table, *protein deficiency* is used to signify kwashiorkor.

†These frequencies are an attempt to reflect the authors' experience in the setting of a U.S. medical practice. Findings common in other countries but virtually unseen in usual medical practice settings in the United States (e.g., xerophthalmia and endemic goiter) are not listed.   *Continued*

Table 10-2   Clinical nutrition examination—cont'd

Clinical findings	Consider deficiency of*	Consider excess of	Frequency†
Neurologic			
Headache		Vitamin A	Rare
Drowsiness, lethargy, vomiting		Vitamins A, D	Rare
Dementia	Niacin, vitamin B$_{12}$		Rare
Confabulation, disorientation	Thiamin (Korsakoff's psychosis)		Occasional
Ophthalmoplegia	Thiamin, phosphorus		Occasional
Peripheral neuropathy (e.g., weakness, paresthesias, ataxia and decreased tendon reflexes, fine tactile sense, vibratory sense, and position sense)	Thiamin, pyridoxine, vitamin B$_{12}$	Pyridoxine	Occasional
Tetany	Calcium, magnesium		Occasional
Other			
Parotid enlargement	Protein (also consider bulimia)		Occasional
Heart failure	Thiamin (wet beriberi), phosphorus		Occasional
Sudden heart failure, death	Vitamin C		Rare
Hepatomegaly	Protein	Vitamin A	Rare
Edema	Protein, thiamin		Common
Poor wound healing, decubitus ulcers	Protein, vitamin C, zinc		Common

poorly healing surgical wounds and hypoalbuminemia, easily pluckable hair is strongly suggestive of kwashiorkor.

It is noteworthy that tissues that have the fastest turnover rates are the most likely to show signs of nutrient deficiency or excess. Thus the hair, skin, and lingual papillae (an indirect reflection of the status of the villae of the gastrointestinal tract) are particularly likely to reveal both nutrient deficiencies and excesses and should be examined closely.

Anthropometrics

Anthropometrics provide information on body muscle mass and fat reserves. The most practical and commonly used measurements are body weight, height, triceps skinfold (TSF), and midarm muscle circumference. Body weight is one of the most useful nutritional parameters to follow in patients who are acutely or chronically ill. Commonly used reference standards for normal body weight are based on weight-for-height tables. One such reference is shown in Table 2-1. Regardless of body frame type, adult patients who are 20% or more above reference standards are likely to be obese and at increased risk of comorbid conditions. Those who are 20% or more below standard weight are likely to be severely underweight and at high risk for nutritional deficiencies. Weight loss, especially if rapid and not associated with fluid loss, often reflects loss of lean body mass (muscle and organ tis-

Table 10-3, A   Triceps skinfold thickness in adults

Percent of standard	Men (mm)	Women (mm)	Calorie reserves
100	12.5	16.5	
90	11.0	15.0	
80	10.0	13.0	Adequate
70	9.0	11.5	
60	7.5	10.0	
50	6.0	8.0	
40	5.0	6.5	Borderline
30	4.0	5.0	
20	2.5	3.0	Severely depleted

Table 10-3, B   Midarm muscle circumference in adults

Percent of standard	Men (cm)	Women (cm)	Calorie reserves
100	25.5	23.0	Adequate
90	23.0	21.0	
80	20.0	18.5	Borderline
70	18.0	16.0	
60	15.0	14.0	
50	12.5	11.5	Severely depleted
40	10.0	9.0	

sue). This can be an ominous sign, since it indicates use of vital body proteins as a metabolic fuel.

Body weights may be misleading with regard to a patient's nutritional status. For instance, underfeeding of an obese patient who is hypermetabolic resulting from injury or sepsis can result in protein-energy malnutrition while the patient remains overweight and appears well fed. By contrast, weight maintenance or weight gain in a seriously ill patient may not be a favorable sign if it reflects edema and masks loss of lean body mass.

Measurement of skinfold thickness is the easiest method to estimate body fat stores, since about 50% of body fat is normally located in the subcutaneous region. The TSF is a convenient site that is generally representative of the fatness of the entire body. The TSF measurement is taken at the midpoint of the upper arm using a set of skinfold calipers (Fig. 10-1 and Plate 19). Normal values are presented in Table 10-3, A. A thickness of less than 3 mm (equivalent to about three dimes) suggests severe depletion of energy reserves.

Estimation of skeletal muscle mass is frequently accomplished using the midarm muscle circumference (MAMC). A tape measure is used to determine the upper arm circumference at the same midpoint used for the TSF (Fig. 10-2 and Plate 20). The MAMC is calculated using the following equation and is compared with reference values in Table 10-3, B.

$$\text{MAMC (cm)} = \text{upper arm circumference (cm)} - [0.314 \times \text{TSF (mm)}]$$

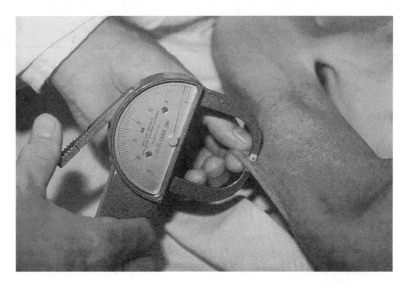

Fig. 10-1   Measurement of the triceps skinfold with skinfold calipers.   ▲

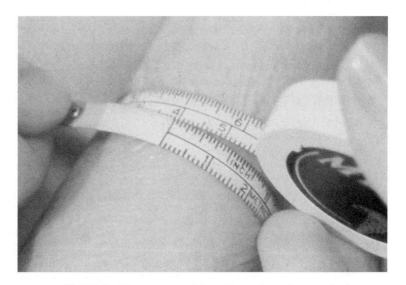

Fig. 10-2   Measurement of the midarm circumference.   ▲

LABORATORY STUDIES

A number of laboratory tests used routinely in clinical medicine can yield valuable information about a patient's nutritional status. Table 10-4 outlines relevant laboratory tests and their interpretation. Because none of these tests is specific for a nutritional problem, tips are provided in the table to help avoid assigning nutritional significance to tests that may be abnormal because of nonnutritional conditions.

Table 10-4 Laboratory tests and values*

SERUM ALBUMIN

Normal	3.5-5.5 g/dl
Nutritional use	2.8-3.5: Compromised protein status
	<2.8: Possible kwashiorkor
	Increasing value reflects positive nitrogen balance
Other causes of low value	
Common	Infection and other stress, especially with poor protein intake
	Burns, trauma
	Congestive heart failure
	Fluid overload
	Recumbency
	Severe hepatic insufficiency
	Nephrotic syndrome
Uncommon	Zinc deficiency
	Bacterial overgrowth of small bowel
Causes of normal value despite malnutrition	Dehydration
	Infusion of albumin, fresh frozen plasma, whole blood

TOTAL IRON-BINDING CAPACITY

Normal	270-400 μg/dl
Nutritional use	<270: Compromised protein status
	<200: Possible kwashiorkor
	Increasing value reflects positive nitrogen balance
	More labile than albumin
Other causes of low value	Similar to serum albumin
Cause of normal or high value despite malnutrition	Iron deficiency

BLOOD UREA NITROGEN (BUN)

Normal	8-23 mg/dl
Nutritional use	Evaluation of protein intake; if serum creatinine is normal, use BUN; if serum creatinine is elevated, use BUN/creatinine
Ratio	<8: Poor protein intake
	>12: Possibly adequate protein intake
Other causes of low value	Severe liver disease
	Anabolic state
Causes of high value despite poor protein intake	Renal failure (use BUN/creatinine ratio)
	Congestive heart failure
	Gastrointestinal hemorrhage
	Corticosteroid therapy
	Dehydration
	Shock

SERUM CREATININE

Normal	0.6-1.6 mg/dl
Nutritional use	<0.6: Muscle wasting because of calorie deficiency
Causes of high value despite muscle wasting	Renal failure
	Severe dehydration

*Actual normal value ranges will vary depending on laboratory standards.   *Continued*

Table 10-4   Laboratory tests and values—cont'd

PROTHROMBIN TIME (PT)

Normal	<1-2 sec beyond control, or 70%-100% of control activity
Nutritional use	Prolongation: vitamin K deficiency
Other causes of prolonged value	Anticoagulant therapy: warfarin (Coumadin)
	Severe liver disease

TOTAL LYMPHOCYTE COUNT (TLC)

TLC = (white blood cell count) × (% lymphocytes)	
Normal	>1500/mm^3
Nutritional use	<1500: possible immunocompromise associated with protein-calorie malnutrition, especially kwashiorkor
Significant limitation	Marked day-to-day fluctuation
Other causes of low TLC	Severe stress, e.g., infections, with left shift
	Corticosteroid therapy
	Renal failure
	Cancer, e.g., colon
Causes of high TLC despite malnutrition	Infections
	Leukemia, myeloma
	Cancer, e.g., stomach, breast
	Adrenal insufficiency

24-HOUR URINARY CREATININE

Normal	800-1800 mg/day; reflects muscle mass; standardized for height and gender
Nutritional use	Low value: muscle wasting because of calorie deficiency
Other causes of low value	Incomplete urine collection
	Increasing serum creatinine
Causes of normal or high value despite malnutrition	>24-hour collection
	Decreasing serum creatinine

24-HOUR URINARY UREA NITROGEN (UUN)

Normal	<5 g/day—depends on level of protein intake
Nutritional use	Determine level of catabolism
	Estimate nitrogen (protein) balance (EPB)
	EPB = protein intake − protein catabolic rate
	Protein catabolic rate = [24-hr UUN (g) + 4] × 6.25
Exception	Additional factors in burn patients and others with large nonurinary nitrogen losses
Causes of low UUN	Low protein intake
	Active fluid retention
	Increasing BUN
	Incomplete urine collection

Table 10-4   Laboratory tests and values—cont'd

24-HOUR URINARY UREA NITROGEN (UUN)—cont'd

Causes of high UUN	High protein intake
	Stress
	Corticosteroid therapy
	Active diuresis
	Decreasing BUN
	>24-hour urine collection

RED BLOOD CELL PARAMETERS

Normal	
Hemoglobin	Female: 12-15 g/dl
	Male: 14-17 g/dl
Hematocrit	Female: 34%-44%
	Male: 39%-49%
Mean corpuscular volume (MCV)	82-99 μ^3
Nutritional use of hemoglobin and hematocrit	Low value indicates anemia, possibly resulting from nutritional deficiency
Nutritional use of MCV	
<82 (microcytic)	Iron, copper, vitamin B_6 deficiency
82-99 (normocytic)	Kwashiorkor
≥100 (macrocytic)	Folate, vitamin B_{12} deficiency

The following are examples of tests that are of particular usefulness in assessing a patient's nutritional status.

Measurement of energy expenditure using indirect calorimetry

When it is important to have an accurate assessment of energy needs, they can be measured at the bedside using indirect calorimetry. This technique is useful in patients who are believed to be hypermetabolic from sepsis or trauma, patients whose body weights cannot be obtained accurately, or patients having difficulty weaning from a ventilator in whom energy needs should not be exceeded to avoid excessive CO_2 production.

Indirect calorimetry is based on the principles that energy expenditure is proportional to O_2 consumption and CO_2 production, and the proportion of fuels being used is reflected in their ratio, the respiratory quotient (RQ). The RQ (CO_2 produced divided by O_2 consumed) provides information on substrate utilization. Each of the three major substrates has a unique RQ (0.7 for fat, 0.8 for protein, and 1.0 for carbohydrate), and the RQ obtained from the test reflects the proportions of them being used. For example, an RQ of 0.75 suggests that the patient is relying heavily on fat as a fuel (such as when energy intake is insufficient), whereas 0.90 indicates largely carbohydrate oxidation. Inevitably, however, each of the three substrates is being used to some extent. A value of greater than 1.0 suggests that the patient is receiving excess calories and is synthesizing fat from carbohydrates. Measurement of the urinary urea nitrogen (UUN) allows one to estimate the amount of protein being catabolized; combined with the RQ, this allows relatively accurate estimates of the amount of each of the fuels the patient is utilizing.

The test entails use of a mobile metabolic cart with a clear plastic hood placed over the patient's head, or tubing connected to the patient's ventilator, to measure respiratory gas exchange for approximately 30 minutes. If the patient is not agitated and a steady state of gas exchange can be achieved even for as short a period as 5 minutes during which the patient is not hyperventilating or hypoventilating, the results are likely to be a valid reflection of energy requirements extrapolated to 24 hours.

Assessment of muscle mass using creatinine-height index

The serum creatinine level is generally used to assess renal function. However, it also reflects the patient's muscle mass, since creatine phosphate, a high-energy compound in the skeletal muscle, is normally dephosphorylated to form creatinine. A creatinine value less than 0.6 mg/dl suggests muscle wasting. The creatinine-height index, which is a better measure of skeletal muscle mass, is determined by comparing a patient's 24-hour urinary creatinine excretion with reference values from persons of the same height and gender. Since the rate of formation of creatinine from skeletal muscle is constant, the amount of creatinine excreted in the urine each 24 hours reflects skeletal muscle mass. Table 10-5 shows predicted uri-

Table 10-5   Predicted urinary creatinine values—adults

Men*		Women†	
Height	Predicted creatinine (mg/24 hr)	Height	Predicted creatinine (mg/24 hr)
5' 2" (157.5 cm)	1288	4' 10" (147.3 cm)	830
5' 3" (160.0)	1325	4' 11" (149.9)	851
5' 4" (162.6)	1359	5' 0" (152.4)	875
5' 5" (165.1)	1386	5' 1" (154.9)	900
5' 6" (167.6)	1426	5' 2" (157.5)	925
5' 7" (170.2)	1467	5' 3" (160.0)	949
5' 8" (172.7)	1513	5' 4" (162.6)	977
5' 9" (175.3)	1555	5' 5" (165.1)	1006
5' 10" (177.8)	1596	5' 6" (167.6)	1044
5' 11" (180.3)	1642	5' 7" (170.2)	1076
6' 0" (182.9)	1691	5' 8" (172.7)	1109
6' 1" (185.4)	1739	5' 9" (175.3)	1141
6' 2" (188.0)	1785	5' 10" (177.8)	1174
6' 3" 190.5)	1831	5' 11" (180.3)	1206
6' 4" (193.0)	1891	6' 0" (182.9)	1240

From Blackburn GL, Bistrian BR, Maini BS, et al: Nutritional and metabolic assessment of the hospitalized patient, *JPEN* 1:11, 1977.

80% to 100% = acceptable; 60% to 80% = moderate depletion; <60% = severe depletion.

*Creatinine coefficient (men) = 23 mg/kg of ideal body weight/24 hours.

†Creatinine coefficient (women) = 18 mg/kg of ideal body weight/24 hours.

nary creatinine values for adult men and women. Values of 80% to 100% of predicted indicate adequate muscle mass, values of 60% to 80% indicate a moderate deficit, and values less than 60% indicate a severe deficit of muscle mass.

Assessment of circulating ("visceral") proteins

The visceral compartment is composed of proteins that act as carriers, binders, and immunologically active proteins. The serum proteins that may be used to assess nutritional status include albumin, TIBC (or transferrin), thyroxine-binding prealbumin (or transthyretin), and retinol-binding protein. Since they have differing synthesis rates and half-lives (the half-life of albumin is about 21 days, whereas that of retinol-binding protein is closer to 12 hours), some of these parameters reflect changes in nutritional status more quickly than others. The general availability and stability of albumin levels from day to day make it one of the most useful tests.

Levels of circulating proteins are influenced by their rates of synthesis and catabolism, by "third spacing" (loss into interstitial spaces), and in some cases by external loss. Although adequate intake of calories and protein is necessary to achieve optimal circulating protein levels, the levels do not sensitively reflect protein intake. For instance, a drop in the serum level of albumin or transferrin often accompanies significant physiologic stress, as from infection or injury, and is not necessarily an indicator of malnutrition or poor intake. On the other hand, adequate nutritional support of calorie and protein needs is critical for their circulating levels to return to normal as the stress resolves. Thus low values by themselves do not define malnutrition but often point toward an increased risk of malnutrition resulting from the hypermetabolic stress rate. It is not unusual for protein levels to remain low despite aggressive nutritional support, as long as significant physiologic stress persists. However, if they do not rise after the underlying illness has resolved, the patient's protein and calorie needs should be reassessed to ensure that intake is sufficient.

Assessment of protein catabolic rate using UUN

Since urea is a major by-product of protein catabolism, the amount of urea nitrogen excreted each day can be used to estimate the rate of protein catabolism and to determine if protein intake is adequate to offset it. Total protein loss and protein balance can be calculated from the UUN as follows:

$$\text{Protein catabolic rate (g/day)} = [\text{24-hour UUN (g)} + 4] \times 6.25$$

The value of 4 g added to the UUN represents a liberal estimate of the unmeasured nitrogen lost in the urine (e.g., creatinine and uric acid) and in sweat, hair, skin, and feces. The factor 6.25 estimates the amount of protein represented by the nitrogen excreted because on average, nitrogen accounts for about 16% (i.e., 1/6.25) of the weight of dietary protein. When protein intake is small (e.g., less than about 20 g/day), the equation indicates both the patient's protein requirement and the severity of the catabolic state (Table 10-6). More substantial protein intakes can raise the UUN, since some of the ingested (or infused) protein is catabolized and converted to UUN. Thus at lower protein intakes the equation is useful for es-

Table 10-6   Classification of patients according to catabolic state by 24-hour urine urea nitrogen values*

Degree of catabolism	Clinical setting	Nitrogen loss
Normal		<5 g
Mild	Elective surgery	5-10 g
Moderate	Infection; major surgery	10-15 g
Severe	Severe sepsis; major burns	>15 g

*Because urea nitrogen excretion increases with increased protein intake, the values in this table apply only if intake is below the amount of the estimated protein loss by ≥10 g.

timating *requirements,* and at higher protein intakes it is useful for assessing protein *balance* (the difference between intake and catabolism).

Protein balance (g/day) = protein intake − protein catabolic rate

The UUN should not be obtained in patients with gastrointestinal hemorrhage, since it will result in a spuriously high value (the blood is a source of protein, which increases urea production). There is no accurate way to correct for this in calculating the protein catabolic rate.

Assessment of protein intake using blood urea nitrogen (BUN)

As dietary protein intake increases, the BUN level generally rises, unless the patient is unusually anabolic and using all available amino acids for protein synthesis. The converse is also true: BUN levels generally fall when protein intake is reduced. Thus, in instances where the BUN is high and there are no other causes such as renal insufficiency, dehydration, or gastrointestinal bleeding, dietary protein intake is likely to be excessive. If the BUN is low (e.g., <8 mg/dl), it suggests a low and possibly inadequate protein intake. Nondietary causes of low and high BUN levels are outlined in Table 10-4.

Assessment of immune status using total lymphocyte count (TLC)

TLC can reflect the immunocompromise associated with kwashiorkor. The value for TLC is derived mathematically from the total WBC and the differential count, where TLC = WBC $\times$ % lymphocytes. However, it is of little use in following the course of nutritional status, since many medical conditions affect TLC and since there are significant day-to-day fluctuations in both total WBC and differential counts.

Assessment of vitamin status

The detection of a vitamin deficiency by laboratory tests is desirable because a vitamin deficiency may predate more serious clinical complications. Vitamin assays also confirm clinical impressions and indicate important drug-nutrient interactions. Vitamin assays and normal values are given in Table 10-7.

Table 10-7   Reference values for vitamin levels

Carotene	79-233 µg/dl
Vitamin A	25-70 µg/dl
Thiamin	1-1.23 A/C*—acceptable
	>1.23 A/C—deficient
Riboflavin	1-1.67 A/C*—acceptable
	>1.67 A/C—deficient
Pyridoxine	1.15-1.89 A/C*—acceptable
	>1.89 A/C—deficient
Folic acid, serum	3-10 ng/ml
Folic acid, red blood cell	>160 ng/ml
Vitamin B_{12}	200-700 pg/ml
Vitamin C	0.5-1.5 mg/dl

Courtesy Clinical Vitamin Laboratory, University of Alabama at Birmingham.
*The activity coefficient (A/C) is a ratio of enzyme activity in a sample, with or without the addition of coenzyme to the system. Therefore the higher the A/C, the lower the vitamin level, and the lower the A/C, the higher the vitamin level.

SUGGESTED READINGS

Lee RD, Nieman DC, editors: *Nutritional assessment,* Madison, Wis, 1993, Brown & Benchmark.
Shils ME, Olson JA, Shike M, editors: *Modern nutrition in health and disease,* ed 8, Philadelphia, 1994, Lea & Febiger.
Torosian MH, editor: *Nutrition for the hospitalized patient,* New York, 1995, Marcel Dekker.

11

Nutritional Support

Guidelines for feeding the hospitalized patient
Therapeutic diets
Enteral feeding
Parenteral nutrition

GUIDELINES FOR FEEDING THE HOSPITALIZED PATIENT

General guidelines for feeding the hospitalized patient

Decisions about nutritional repletion, or refeeding, involve the method of eating, as well as the rapidity of refeeding and the goals for protein and calorie intake. The feeding quadrangle (Fig. 11-1) demonstrates that feeding can either be parenteral, which completely circumvents the gastrointestinal tract, or enteral. A combination of approaches, such as beginning tube feeding in a patient on parenteral nutrition, can be used.

Estimating calorie needs

The Harris-Benedict equation allows an estimation of the BEE. The formulas below or the nomograms in Fig. 11-2 can be used to calculate the BEE.

Women: BEE = 655.10 + 9.56 (W) + 1.85 (H) − 4.68 (A)
Men: BEE = 66.47 + 13.75 (W) + 5 (H) − 6.76 (A)
where W = weight in kg, H = height in cm, and A = age in years

Caloric requirements are estimated by multiplying the BEE value by a factor that allows for activity and stress of illness. For most hospitalized patients, caloric needs will be reasonably approximated in the range of BEE × 1.2 to 1.5. The lower value is used for patients without evidence of significant physiologic stress; the upper value is sued for patients with marked stress, such as from widespread infection or severe trauma. If weight gain is desired, in metabolically stable patients, then 2 × the BEE is generally prescribed. A formula for estimating 24-hour energy expenditure in burn patients, the Toronto formula, is discussed in Chapter 12. In some cases, caloric needs may be difficult to determine on an individual basis, since disease states can dramatically alter calorie requirements. A metabolic cart (indirect calorimetry) can be used to establish caloric needs.

Estimating and calculating protein needs

The optimal protein intake for nutritional support can initially be approximated based on the RDA (see Table 1-1). The amount of protein recommended for an

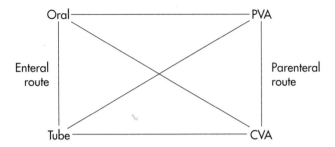

Fig. 11-1 The feeding quadrangle. PVA, peripheral venous alimentation; CVA, central venous alimentation.

average healthy adult is 0.8 g/kg/day, but requirements may be increased to 1 to 1.5 g/kg/day in situations of significant physiologic stress with normal renal and hepatic function. Higher protein needs may be seen in trauma and burns. A more precise estimate of protein needs is made on the basis of the 24-hour UUN described in Chapter 10. If a patient is receiving little or no protein, a 24-hour UUN ([UUN (g) + 4] × 6.25) gives an estimate of the amount of obligate protein breakdown per day. If the patient is consuming protein, the UUN must be viewed as a balance procedure where protein balance = protein intake − protein catabolic rate, where the latter is determined from the 24-hour UUN. Additional protein, 10 g/day, is often provided to ensure protein balance. The 24-hour urine for UUN can be affected by the completeness of the urine collection, steroid administration, renal shutdown, renal dialysis, and gastrointestinal bleeding. In patients with burns the formula to calculate the UUN is modified to account for protein losses through the burned skin: protein loss (g/day) − [UUN (g) + 4 + (0.2 g × % third-degree burn) + (0.1 g × % second-degree burn)] × 6.25.

If a UUN is not available or yields uninterpretable results, 12% to 16% of total calories as protein can be prescribed as a reasonable amount for unstressed patients. From 17% to 19% of total calories as protein is an intermediate level of protein, and 20% to 25% of calories as protein is a high-protein diet. A high-protein diet is indicated for highly stressed, hypermetabolic patients and for cachectic patients who are undergoing repletion.

Refeeding

The refeeding syndrome describes the metabolic and physiologic consequences of the depletion, repletion, and shifts in fluid, electrolytes, vitamins, and minerals as patients with malnutrition are fed. Patients with protein-calorie malnutrition (marasmus and kwashiorkor) are particularly at risk for the refeeding syndrome. Table 11-1 describes the refeeding strategies for patients with protein-calorie malnutrition.

The refeeding of a chronically starved hypometabolic patient (i.e., with marasmus) can be complicated by repletion heart failure and hypophosphatemia. Repletion heart failure occurs because atrophy of the heart parallels the loss of lean body mass. During the reintroduction of calories and fluid, the metabolic rate rises

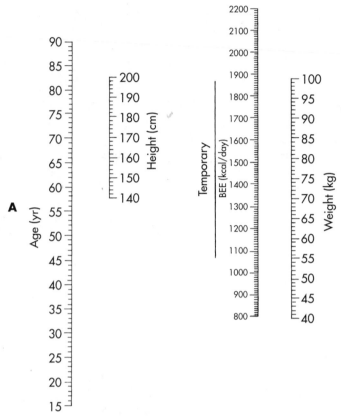

Fig. 11-2   A, Nomogram for calculating basal energy expenditure for men.

Table 11-1   Selective approaches to nutritional support

Patient type	Aim	Nutritional support	Risks of overfeeding
Hypometabolic, starved (marasmus)	Rebuild	Cautious, with a portion of fuel as fat	Hypophosphatemia, repletion heart failure
Hypermetabolic, stressed (kwashiorkor)	Replace	Aggressive but not excessive	↑ O_2 consumption, ↑ CO_2 production

together with plasma volume and afterload. If fluid and electrolyte balance is not carefully controlled, repletion heart failure may occur. Hypophosphatemia is another possible refeeding complication in patients with marasmus. Patients with marasmus use ketones and fatty acid as their major body fuels, and the rate of utilization of phosphorus is low. By contrast, the intermediary metabolism of glucose, which requires phosphorus, is markedly increased during refeeding. If sufficient phosphorus is not present in feedings, patients can become profoundly hypophosphatemic. The sequelae of hypophosphatemia include acute ventilatory failure, neuromuscular compromise, altered myocardial function, and hemolysis.

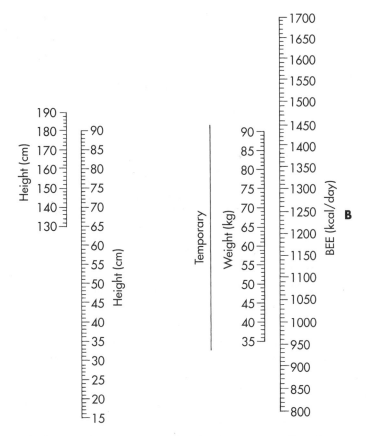

Fig. 11-2, cont'd   B, Nomogram for calculating basal energy expenditure for women. Directions: 1. Locate the height and weight on the scale, placing a straightedge (ruler) between these points, intersecting the temporary variable line. 2. Holding a pencil at the point of intersection (on temporary variable line), locate the age, and pivot ruler to this point on the age scale. The point of intersection on the BEE scale is the predicted BEE. (From Rainey-MacDonald CG, et al: The Harris-Benedict equations, *JPEN* 6;59, 1982.)

Because marasmic patients rely on fatty acid metabolism, generally a portion of the fuel prescribed is as fat.

Patients with marasmus should be refed slowly; the aim is to replete body stores. Generally, such patients are fed at 0.8 times their BEE for the first few days, carefully watching fluid balance and electrolytes. Total calories are then increased to BEE × 1.0, BEE × 1.2, and BEE × 1.5 as indicated by patient tolerance. To promote weight gain, 2 × BEE can be approached. Table 11-2 summarizes the refeeding of the hypometabolic patient.

Patients with kwashiorkor are hypermetabolic and require aggressive nutritional support to provide adequate calories and protein. If inadequate calories and protein are provided, hypermetabolic patients have large losses of lean body mass. However, overly aggressive support (excessive calories) can cause refeeding complications. Excessive caloric loads, especially with high carbohydrate mixtures,

Table 11-2   Calorie goals in refeeding the hypometabolic-starved patient

Days	Calories related to basal energy expenditure (BEE)
1, 2	BEE $\times$ 0.8
3, 4	BEE $\times$ 1.0
4-6	BEE $\times$ 1.2-1.5
6 and after	BEE $\times$ 2.0, if weight gain is desired

can increase O_2 consumption and CO_2 production and increase the resting metabolic rate. The correct approach to refeeding such patients is to provide adequate calories (generally within 1.2 to 1.5 $\times$ BEE) within 1 to 2 days of beginning nutritional support. Protein balance should be monitored. The strategy is to be aggressive but not excessive. Table 11-1 summarizes the refeeding strategy for a patient with kwashiorkor.

Vitamin and mineral allowances

The best guide to dietary adequacy of vitamins and minerals is the U.S. RDA shown in Table 1-1. However, extrapolations must be made for the malnourished or ill patient. Although no guidelines exist for prescribing supplements for patients with illness, Table 10-1 can help identify certain situations in which higher vitamin or mineral allowances should be made.

Fluid needs

There are many ways to calculate fluid needs. The RDAs indicate that 1.0 to 1.5 ml/kcal/day is a reasonable estimate of water requirements. A general guideline for patients not requiring fluid restriction is 30 to 35 ml/kg/day.

THERAPEUTIC DIETS

Diet therapy is an important approach to many disease states, complementing and perhaps even replacing drug therapy in some cases. Consultation with a registered or licensed dietitian is invaluable for assistance in the prescription and monitoring of therapeutic diets. Therapeutic diets represent permutations of the components of the general diet, which provides optimal health in patients whose condition does not require diet modification. A useful schema to understand therapeutic diets breaks the general diet into its basic components: water, carbohydrate, protein, fat, vitamins, minerals, and other substances such as alcohol. It is possible to use modifications of amounts of these components to form a therapeutic diet. For example, a diet may be altered to be low in fat, low in protein, and low in sodium. Certain disease states have commonly prescribed therapeutic diets in which the individual constituents are modified. The following are examples:

- *Water-modified:* restricted fluid intake in severe heart failure, kidney failure
- *Carbohydrate-modified:* carbohydrate-controlled diet for diabetes and hypertriglyceridemia (Box 11-1)
- *Protein-modified:* low protein for the unstressed patient with chronic kidney failure, high protein for the stressed patient (Table 11-3)

Box 11-1   Guidelines for the carbohydrate-modified (diabetic) diet

The goals for the dietary treatment of diabetes mellitus are:
1. Maintenance of near-normal glucose levels by balancing diet and insulin (exogenous or endogenous)
2. Achieving optimal serum lipid levels
3. Providing adequate calories for attainment or maintenance of reasonable body weight in adults and normal growth in children
4. Prevention and treatment of short-term (hypoglycemia, exercise-related hypoglycemia) and long-term (nephropathy, neuropathy, hypertension, cardiovascular disease) complications of insulin-treated diabetes
5. Improvement of health through optimal nutrition

Insulin therapy should be matched to the meal plan (using the Diabetic Exchange System) and should be tailored to take into account lifestyle (eating and exercise) habits. The suggested caloric pattern is:
1. Protein: 10% to 20% of calories
2. Less than 10% of calories from saturated fats
3. Up to 10% of calories from polyunsaturated fats
4. Cholesterol intake should be <300 mg/day
5. The remainder of calories from monounsaturated fats and carbohydrates; the intake of carbohydrates should be individualized based on caloric needs, eating habits, and glucose and lipid control
6. Sucrose, fructose, and sucrose-containing foods may be substituted for other carbohydrates in the meal plan; however, the substitution of simple sugars for fruits, vegetables, and whole-grain cereal products does not support the principles of the Food Guide Pyramid and may in some cases worsen diabetic control
7. Fiber intake should be in the range of 20 to 35 g/day
8. If there is hypertension, no more than 2400 mg of sodium per day
9. For insulin-requiring diabetics, <2 alcoholic beverages (= 12 oz beer, 5 oz wine, 1½ oz distilled spirits) may be ingested in addition to the usual meal plan
10. Nonnutritive sweeteners should be used in moderation

- *Fat-modified:* low total and saturated fat and low cholesterol for hypercholesterolemia, low total fat for malabsorption syndromes (Table 11-4)
- *Vitamin-modified:* restricted amounts of vitamins A and C in renal failure, increased vitamin C in the infected or injured patient
- *Mineral-modified:* low sodium, potassium, and phosphorus in kidney failure (Table 11-5)
- *Other substances:* restricted alcohol intake for hypertriglyceridemia

In addition, therapeutic diets may be modified in consistency or texture. Common examples include dental-soft diets for patients without teeth and high-fiber (high-residue) diets for patients with constipation. Box 11-2 describes diets of modified consistency. Another variation in therapeutic diets involves the sequence in which they are used.

Table 11-3   Modified diets—protein*

Daily protein intake (g)	Food limitations	Practicality
150-200	Meat, cheese, eggs: >10 oz per day (1 egg = 1 oz of meat); starches: 5 or more servings per day; vegetables: 4 or more servings per day; fruits: 3 or more servings per day. Milk, shakes, eggnogs, protein supplements may be added.	High-protein, high-fat diet. Dietitian supervision is preferable.
100-140	Meat, cheese: 10 oz per day; starches: 5-6 servings per day; vegetables: 4-5 servings per day; fruits: 3-4 servings per day. Milk included.	Average American diet; relatively high in fat and may exceed protein needs for many people.
60 (10% of total calories)	Meat, cheese: 6 oz per day; starches: 5 servings per day; vegetables: <4 servings per day; fruits: <3 servings per day; milk in limited amounts. Calories can be increased with the addition of sugar and fat.	Generally acceptable for home use; diet fairly easily manipulated according to patient preferences.
40 (6% of calories)	Meat, cheese: 4 oz per day; starches: 3 servings per day; vegetables: 4 servings per day; fruits: 3 servings per day. Calories can be increased with sugar and fat.	Difficult to follow at home unless patient is unusually cooperative.
20 (3% of calories)	Meat, cheese: essentially none; eggs: 2 per day; starches: 2 servings per day; fruits: 2 servings per day; vegetables: 2 servings per day. Calories can be increased with sugar and fat.	Should be limited to hospital use.
8-10 (trace)	Meat, cheese, eggs, milk: essentially none; starches, vegetables: severely limited (low-protein bread only). Calories are mostly from fruits, juices, sugar, and fat.	For hospital use only.

*Percentage of calories based on 2400 kcal/day. Serving sizes: most vegetables = ½ cup; most fruits = 1 piece or ½ cup; starches = 1 slice of bread or approximately ⅓ to ½ cup of cooked starch.

Table 11-4 Modified diets—fat*

Daily fat intake (g)	Food limitations	Practicality
90-110 (35% to 40% of calories)		Average American diet.
65-80 (25% to 30% of calories)	Meats limited to 8-9 oz per day (1 egg = 1 oz meat). Fats limited to 3-7 tsp butter, mayonnaise, salad dressing, oil. Whole milk in limited amounts. All products prepared with fat (biscuits, cornbread, cakes, pastries, fried foods) excluded unless fat in these products is counted as a part of the total fat allowance.	Very practical for home use; diet easily manipulated according to patient preferences.
40-50 (15% to 20% of calories)	All fried foods are excluded from the diet. Meat and eggs are limited to 6 oz of lean meat, poultry, fish, or egg daily if 3 tsp margarine or equivalent is used. 8-9 oz of meat and eggs may be used daily if no extra fat such as whole milk, margarine, butter, or mayonnaise, salad dressing, nuts, and gravies is used.	Fairly practical for home use.
20-25 (8% to 10% of calories)	Meat and eggs limited to 5-6 oz per day. All other above restrictions apply.	Generally for hospital use only.
Fat-free (approximately 2 g/day)	No meat or eggs allowed. Starches, vegetables, fruits in unlimited amounts if prepared with fat. Skim milk is allowed.	For hospital use only.

*Percentage of calories based on 2400 kcal/day. MCT oil may be added to any of these diet plans. Generally, start by adding 1 tsp per meal and gradually increase to 2 to 4 tsp per meal.

Table 11-5 Modified diets—sodium

Daily sodium (Na^+) intake	Food limitations	Practicality
5-6 g Na^+ = 12.5-15 g salt	Includes table salt, heavily or visibly salted items	Average American diet
4 g Na^+ = 10 g salt	No additional salt on tray or at table	Practical for home use
3 g Na^+ = 7.5 g salt	Food only lightly salted in preparation; restrict heavily or visibly salted items (potato chips, pretzels, crackers, pickles, olives, relishes, sauces, most commercially prepared soups), no salt on tray	Practical for home use
2 g Na^+ = 5 g salt	Above limitations plus no salt in food preparation; avoid most processed foods (canned foods with added salt, luncheon meats, bacon, ham, cheese) unless calculated into the diet; regular bread, butter, and milk in limited amounts.	Fairly practical for home use with a cooperative patient
1 g Na^+ = 2.5 g salt	Above limitations plus use of salt-free bread	Practical for home use with only an unusually cooperative patient
0.5 g Na^+ = 1.25 g salt	Above limitations plus limitations of meat (4 oz per day, eggs, some vegetables, milk (1 pint per day) and salt-free butter allowed.	Not practical for home use

Box 11-2   Diets of modified consistency

Clear liquid diet

This diet provides clear fluids that leave little residue and are absorbed with a minimum of digestive activity. It includes only broth, gelatin, strained fruit juices, clear beverages, and low-residue supplements. Since some of these have high osmolality, they may not be well tolerated by some patients. Clear liquids generally do not provide the RDA for any nutrient except perhaps vitamin C. Clear liquid diets should not be used for more than 2 to 3 days without supplementation.

Full liquid diet

This diet includes foods that liquefy at room temperature. Many foods such as whole milk, custard, pudding, strained cream soups, eggnog, and ice cream contain fat and lactose, which some patients tolerate poorly. Complete enteral supplements may be preferred in such cases or may be added to increase calories and protein (see Chapter 11). This diet can meet the RDA for all nutrients except iron for women of childbearing age. Modifications of the full liquid diet such as the high-protein, high-calorie full liquid diet can be made. A low-fat full liquid can also be ordered. If a low-lactose variation is desired, lactose-free enteral supplements and lactase-treated dairy products may be used.

Soft diet

The soft diet contains foods that are tender but are not ground or pureed. Whole meats, cooked vegetables, and fruits of moderate fiber content are allowed. This generally excludes fried foods, most raw fruits and vegetables, and very coarse breads and cereals, and is fairly low in fiber and residue. The gastrointestinal soft diet is a modification of the soft diet that omits highly seasoned and spicy foods and foods high in fiber.

Pureed or ground diet

This diet includes foods that are especially easy to masticate and to swallow. It is useful in patients who have dysphagia or dental problems.

Low-fiber, low-residue diet

This diet is intended to reduce fecal bulk and is restricted in milk, certain vegetables, fruits, and whole-grain breads and cereals.

High-fiber diet

This diet includes unrefined starches (whole-grain bread, brown rice, potatoes, corn, beans) raw fruits, and vegetables. Bran and other fibers may be added if desired.

Box 11-3   Refeeding after prolonged bowel rest*

Day 1

Clear liquids to check swallowing

Days 2-3

Lactose-free enteral feeding formula or six small feedings of 30-g-fat, low-lactose, soft diet.

Days 4-5

50-g-fat diet, progressing to regular diet as tolerated

Since tube feeding maintains the bowel in a fully functional state, tube-fed patients need not follow this regimen; rather, their adaptation to oral intake is usually determined by their ability to chew and swallow or by the underlying bowel disease, when present

---

*Prolonged bowel rest is defined as nonuse of the gastrointestinal tract for 3 weeks or more.

The *refeeding diet* is used in patients who have been without enteral feeding for an extended period and who usually have some digestive dysfunction (see Box 11-3). The refeeding regimen is a graduated approach to the reintroduction of foods into the diet. The regimen commonly used in the past, going from clear liquid diets to full liquid diets, has two inherent drawbacks: clear liquid diets are high in osmolality and nutritionally inadequate, and full liquid diets are high in fat and lactose. Both of these factors may complicate the refeeding of an impaired intestinal tract. In their place, a lactose-free formula or six small feedings of a low-fat, low-lactose soft diet may be introduced. After several days the fat content is liberalized and the size of the meals is increased. A regular diet is usually tolerated by the sixth day in patients who have no underlying intestinal disease.

ENTERAL FEEDING

For obvious reasons, oral intake is the preferred method of nutritional support. When this is not possible for more than 5 to 7 days, enteral nutrition, commonly referred to as *tube feeding,* can be initiated, as long as at least part of the gastrointestinal tract is functional. Enteral feeding should always be considered before parenteral nutrition because of its lower cost, fewer complications, and greater likelihood of maintaining gastrointestinal mucosal integrity. Its use is widespread in U.S. hospitals and fairly common in the nursing home and home setting.

Gastrointestinal access

The selection of tubes and pumps specially designed for feeding is quite broad. Because of their pliability and long-term tolerance, small-gauge feeding tubes should virtually always be used for enteral feeding (Fig. 11-3). In patients who are not at high risk for aspiration (i.e., who are alert and have a normal gag reflex), it is not necessary to confirm tube placement radiographically before beginning feed-

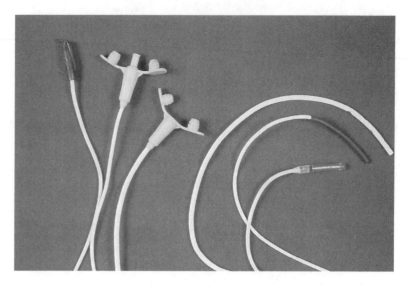

Fig. 11-3   Small-bore feeding tubes used in enteral nutrition support.

ing. Insufflation of air with auscultation over the stomach or return of bile or gastric contents after suctioning, followed by monitoring during the first hour of feeding, is usually adequate and avoids delay of feeding. Many tubes have weighted tips with the intention that they should prevent retrograde migration or facilitate nasoduodenal intubation, but such weights may actually *impede* passage of the tip through the gastric pylorus. When transpyloric feeding is desired, for example, to reduce the risk of aspiration or to bypass a gastric ileus, nasoduodenal intubation can be accomplished by several techniques. A conservative method involves giving metoclopramide 10 mg intravenously and inserting an ample length of an unweighted tube into the stomach. If this fails, various fluoroscopic and endoscopic methods can be tried.

Although soft nasogastric tubes have been used safely for months and even years in some patients, long-term tube feeding is usually best accomplished through a percutaneous endoscopic gastrostomy (PEG). This method of gastrostomy placement is preferred over surgical gastrostomies because of low morbidity and cost. A PEG tube is placed by passing an endoscope with a light source into the patient's stomach. The light is viewed through the skin, and an incision is made using local anesthesia. The PEG tube is inserted directly through the incision, or directed down the esophagus and out the incision, and secured. Because the risk of pulmonary aspiration may not be appreciably lower with gastrostomies than with nasogastric tubes, in patients at high risk for aspiration, duodenal intubation either through the nose or through a PEG is advised.

Formula selection

The choices of enteral feeding formulas have increased significantly in recent years, and formulas are sometimes promoted for features that have little physiologic significance. The most important criteria for selection of formulas are energy density, protein content, route of administration, and cost. Energy density determines the amounts of most nutrients delivered per liter, including not only the calories but also protein, water, and others. Most formulas have energy densities of approximately 1, 1.5, or 2 kcal/ml. Higher-energy formulas (1.5 to 2 kcal/ml) can result in dehydration, so the fluid status of these patients should be carefully monitored (see Complications). On the other hand, it is not necessary to use commercial starter formulas or diluted standard formulas with a density of 0.5 kcal/ml. The practice of diluting formulas is still somewhat widespread, but there is no evidence that it improves tolerance, and in fact it could increase bacterial contamination of the formula. In adults, feedings should be started at full strength unless there is no other acceptable route for giving additional fluid.

When the energy density has been selected, the formula of choice is usually determined by the protein content, the route of administration (oral or tube), and the lowest cost. Protein content should be considered not in absolute terms but relative to total energy content (such as percent of total kilocalories or calorie:nitrogen ratio). Formulas that provide more than 20% of energy as protein are considered high in protein.

Less important criteria for formula selection include osmolality, nutrient complexity, and content of fat, lactose, minerals, and residue. There is no evidence that high osmolality impairs formula tolerance. Lactose-containing formulas, which are intended for oral consumption, may not be well tolerated by acutely ill patients because they commonly have acquired lactase deficiency. Oligomeric formulas (containing small peptides or amino acids or both) have uncertain advantages over polymeric formulas (containing whole proteins) and cost considerably more.

Tube feeding methods

Continuous feeding. For hospitalized patients the continuous drip method with a closed, aseptic system is preferred. A pump should always be used to avoid accidental infusions of dangerously large volumes. Continuous feeding ensures reliable nutrient delivery and reduces the risks of diarrhea, gastric distention, and pulmonary aspiration of the feeding formula.

The initial infusion rate and the rapidity of its increase should vary depending on the patient's overall condition. Patients with impaired mental status or prolonged nonuse of the gastrointestinal tract (>2 weeks) should have feedings introduced and increased more slowly than alert patients whose intestines have been used recently.

Bolus feeding. This method involves infusing a volume of formula into the feeding tube by gravity over several minutes several times a day. It is most useful for long-term feeding in stable patients and is commonly used in homes and nursing homes. It allows mobility and reduces cost, since a pump and infusion set are not needed.

Complications

Diarrhea, a common complication of enteral feeding, has been attributed to many different causes including hypertonic feeding formulas, hypoalbuminemia, bacterial contamination of the feeding or dysentery or both, inadequate fiber in feeding formulas, infusion methods (e.g., bolus infusions or rapid advancement of the infusion rate), fecal impaction, lactose in feeding formulas, and others. The best-documented causal factors are medications, pseudomembranous colitis, and gastrointestinal dysfunction, none of which is necessarily related to tube feeding. Tube feeding itself is most often not responsible for diarrhea and should not be blamed until other causes have been ruled out. The following causes should be considered:

- Sorbitol-containing elixirs (acetaminophen, theophylline, and many others). Sorbitol is added to many liquid medications to provide texture and sweetness and is considered "inert" by the FDA. However, it causes diarrhea after 10 to 20 g—contained in as little as 2 to 3 doses of some liquid medications—have been administered. Medication package inserts do not list sorbitol content, which varies widely among manufacturers of the same medication, so at times it is necessary to contact the manufacturer or even discontinue all enteral medications to resolve a case of diarrhea.
- Magnesium-containing antacids (e.g., Maalox, Mylanta), oral antibiotics, phosphorus supplements, and other medications.
- Pseudomembranous colitis. If this is suspected, the stool *Clostridium difficile* titer should be checked.
- Gastrointestinal disorders.

Gastric retention is defined imprecisely as the presence of more than 150 to 200 ml of gastric contents 2 hours after the last feeding. Although paralytic ileus (the absence of bowel activity) is probably the most common cause, hypokalemia, effects of drugs, and intestinal obstruction must be ruled out. Parenteral feeding is required in cases of unremitting retention.

Pulmonary aspiration of gastric contents is the most feared complication of tube feeding and is the main reason to monitor gastric residual volume. Whenever possible, the patient's head should be elevated during feeding to avoid reflux.

Enteral feeding results in far fewer metabolic complications than does parenteral feeding. The most common complication is probably hyperglycemia, particularly in patients with preexisting glucose intolerance. This can be handled through tighter diabetes control and rarely requires reduction of the feeding.

As a rule of thumb, total free water intake should equal approximately 30 to 35 ml/kg/day; enteral formulas generally contain between 70% and 88% water by volume. Although fluid requirements are usually satisfied when 1 kcal/ml tube feeding formulas are used, formulas with high energy density (1.5 to 2 kcal/ml) or protein content do not contain enough water for many patients to handle their renal solute load. If a patient is fed 2000 kcal, using a 1 kcal/ml formula provides about 1700 ml water, but using a 2 kcal/ml formula provides only about 700 ml water. Patients fed with the latter formulas who are unable to regulate their fluid needs voluntarily and who do not have adequate intravenous fluid intake may become dehydrated, hyperosmolar, and hyperglycemic. The osmolality of formulas is not related to these problems because carbohydrates (the main osmotic component) are ordinarily metabolized and do not contribute to the renal solute load. The fluid status and blood glucose levels of patients at risk should be closely monitored.

PARENTERAL NUTRITION

Total parenteral nutrition (TPN), or intravenous feeding, can be administered in a central vein as central venous alimentation (CVA) or in a peripheral vein as peripheral venous alimentation (PVA). Energy is supplied by carbohydrate, usually in the form of dextrose, and by fat in the form of vegetable-oil emulsions. Protein is supplied by crystalline amino acids. Vitamins, minerals, and trace elements are added in groups or individually. Certain medications, such as insulin, cimetidine, ranitidine, heparin, and hydrocortisone, can be added to TPN solutions when necessary.

Indications for parenteral nutrition

The indications for parenteral nutrition include: (1) conditions obviating enteral access, such as bowel resection or other gastrointestinal surgery or trauma to the abdomen or head and neck, adynamic ileus not amenable to duodenal feeding, or intestinal obstruction; (2) severe malabsorption, such as short bowel syndrome; (3) intractable intolerance of enteral feeding; and (4) conditions in which bowel rest may be desirable, such as inflammatory bowel disease or intestinal fistulas. Usually, parenteral nutrition is used when oral or enteral intake is inadequate to meet a patient's needs for more than 5 to 7 days.

The contraindications to parenteral nutrition are all relative; there are no situations in which a person should *absolutely* not be fed. Relative contraindications include the presence of a functional gastrointestinal tract (surprisingly, some clinicians still tend to resort to TPN when enteral feeding could be used), intended use for less than about 5 days, and imminent death because of underlying disease. Specific exceptions to these can be cited, however, so each case should be evaluated on its own merit.

Routes of administration

To attain sufficient energy intake without giving excessive volumes of fluid, the nonprotein calories must be concentrated. This is achieved by using final concentrations of up to 35% dextrose, which results in osmolalities of roughly 1800 mOsm/kg water, which are very irritating to the venous endothelium. Therefore these solutions must be infused into central veins, where they are rapidly diluted by high blood-flow rates. Typically, the catheter tip is introduced into the superior vena cava via the subclavian or internal jugular vein (Fig. 11-4).

When central venous catheterization is undesirable, or when parenteral nutrition is desired for short periods, more dilute solutions can be infused into peripheral veins (although the shorter the intended use, the weaker the indication is). Even with final dextrose concentrations of only 10% (such as when 500 ml of 20% dextrose are admixed with 500 ml of amino acids), the osmolality of these formulas is 900 to 1100 mOsm/kg water, resulting in fairly short periods of vein patency resulting from phlebitis. To meet energy requirements, intravenous lipid emulsions should be used daily as a source of energy to compensate for the dilute dextrose. Total volumes of more than 3 L/day must often be used to meet nutritional needs through this route, exceeding the tolerance of many patients.

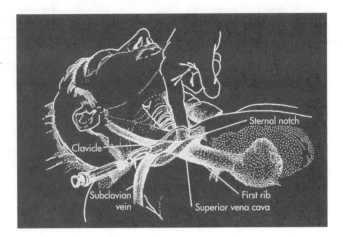

Fig. 11-4   A schematic diagram describing method and location for placement of a sub-clavian catheter for central venous alimentation.

Nonprotein calorie sources

The major source of nonprotein energy in TPN, dextrose (D-glucose), is provided in the monohydrous form, reducing its energy yield to 3.4 kcal/g rather than the 4 kcal/g from dietary carbohydrate. Supplied in concentrations up to 70%, dextrose contributes most of the osmolality of the TPN solution.

Intravenous lipid emulsions are available in 10% (1.1 kcal/ml) or 20% (2 kcal/ml) concentrations, generally derived from safflower oil, soybean oil, or a combination of the two. These emulsions can be given piggyback at the same time as the TPN solution or mixed with dextrose and amino acids in total nutrient admixtures (i.e., protein, carbohydrate, and fat in a single bag; Fig. 11-5) in a variety of concentrations, as long as certain guidelines are observed. The addition of lipids reduces the osmolality and hence the caustic nature of parenteral nutrition.

Continuous infusions of concentrated dextrose and the consequent steady elevation of insulin levels can prevent mobilization of endogenous adipose tissue stores of EFAs, thereby resulting in biochemical evidence of EFA deficiency within a week. To prevent this, lipid emulsions must be used at least weekly. However, daily and preferably continuous lipid infusion is the most physiologic and beneficial method of administration. In some patient groups this is particularly true. In diabetic patients, better glucose tolerance and lower insulin requirements can be achieved when less dextrose is infused. Patients with ventilatory failure and CO_2 retention, especially those without hypoxemia, can benefit from the lesser CO_2 production associated with lipid oxidation compared with glucose oxidation.

Intravenous lipid emulsions have very few adverse effects. Severe hypoxemia can be aggravated by rapid infusion of lipids if the clearance of circulating triglycerides is delayed. However, this complication can nearly always be prevented by infusion of the required amount over 24 hours. Significant underlying hypertriglyceridemia (greater than 500 mg/dl), especially when associated with pancreatitis, can represent a contraindication to the use of intravenous lipid. To check for

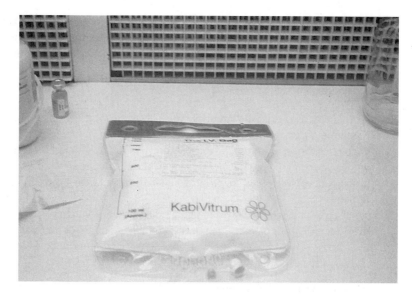

Fig. 11-5   A three-in-one admixture used for CVA.

lipid intolerance, a random serum triglyceride level should be checked at some point during the lipid infusion.

Amino acid solutions

Protein is supplied as synthetic crystalline amino acids, which are safe, effective, and available in concentrations between 3.5% and 15% (3.5 to 15 g/dl). They yield 4 kcal/g. Except in patients who are in markedly positive nitrogen balance, the protein ingested is generally assumed to replace protein that is oxidized. Thus the infused protein contributes to total energy consumption and is generally included as part of the total energy content of TPN mixtures.

Vitamins

The RDAs for micronutrients do not apply to parenteral nutrition because the absorptive process is bypassed. Guidelines for parenteral vitamin requirements have been incorporated into the commercial multivitamin preparations most commonly used in TPN. They have been shown to be adequate for maintaining vitamin status when it is already normal, but they may not be adequate to correct preexisting vitamin deficiencies or to meet the needs of ill patients with increased requirements. For example, vitamin C requirements are increased in the stress state, so it is often advisable to use added amounts, such as 500 to 1000 mg/day, as long as renal function is normal.

Minerals

The major electrolytes provided in parenteral nutrition are sodium, potassium, calcium, magnesium, and phosphorus. It is possible to make changes in the patient's mineral and acid-base status by altering the levels of these and the anions chosen for each. For example, by substituting acetate for chloride, with or without changes in sodium and potassium intake, it is possible to help correct significant acidoses. Likewise, when the patient needs more phosphorus, it can be given as the sodium or potassium salt, as desired.

Trace elements

As in the case of vitamins, multiple trace element solutions are available that satisfy the maintenance requirements of most patients. These usually include zinc, copper, chromium, and manganese. Additional zinc should be used for patients who have increased requirements, such as those who are stressed or postoperative or have increased losses resulting from small-bowel diarrhea or draining wounds or fistulas.

Iron dextran can be added to parenteral nutrition solutions when needed. However, because most patients are not on TPN long enough for poor intake to deplete their body iron stores, this is rarely necessary. Selenium can be added as well but is generally needed only by patients on long-term (home) TPN.

Management of parenteral nutrition

For CVA the catheter should be placed in the superior vena cava (see Fig. 11-4). Energy and protein requirements should be calculated as described previously in this chapter, and a decision must be made whether to use intravenous lipid daily or intermittently during the week.

The initial infusion rate should vary with different patients. Highly stressed patients who have been receiving intravenous dextrose infusions can be started at about 50 ml/hr and advanced quickly, usually about every 8 to 12 hours, to reach their full energy requirements within 24 to 48 hours. Hypometabolic-starved patients should be fed more gradually, as described previously in this chapter.

Dextrose infusion stimulates insulin secretion that persists for a short while even if the dextrose flow is interrupted. Therefore if the infusion is terminated abruptly for any reason, hypoglycemia may ensue. Although most TPN patients are protected from this by stress-induced, insulin-resistant hyperglycemia, it is wise to taper the infusion rate by 50% to 70% for 30 to 60 minutes before discontinuing parenteral nutrition. Longer tapering periods are unnecessary, and no tapering is required if the patient is being fed enterally or orally when the infusion is discontinued.

In addition to proper general medical and nursing care, careful laboratory monitoring is important during TPN. Alterations in electrolytes and other blood parameters often necessitate adjustment of the TPN formula.

Complications

Complications of parenteral nutrition fall into three main categories: technical, infectious, and metabolic. They can nearly always be avoided by careful patient management. Technical complications relate to the placement of the central venous catheter and are therefore not unique to parenteral nutrition. The most common of these, pneumothorax (air introduced into the thorax) and hemothorax (bleeding into the thorax), are best prevented by careful, unhurried insertion of the central line by an experienced physician. The catheter can become occluded (thrombosis or occlusion by components of the TPN solution such as lipid or calcium and phosphorus precipitates) if it is used for other purposes such as administering medications or is manipulated improperly.

Sepsis, when it occurs in the TPN patient, is most often caused by poor technique in catheter care and is therefore not unique to parenteral nutrition. It can be prevented by adhering to standard nursing guidelines for catheter care. The offending organisms are usually skin contaminants, but in hospitalized patients, gram-negative infections may occur. Definite catheter sepsis may require removal of the catheter, and if necessary it can be replaced in another location. Local infections at the site of catheter entry can usually be treated with meticulous site care and do not require removal of the catheter.

Metabolic complications are the most common, since metabolic requirements (e.g., electrolytes and energy) cannot be stereotyped. The most serious of these is sudden, severe hypophosphatemia induced by dextrose infusion. Although phosphorus levels drop in many patients after TPN begins, severely cachectic patients are the most susceptible to potentially lethal consequences. It is therefore important to put phosphorus in all TPN solutions unless a specific contraindication exists. The serum levels of phosphorus and other electrolytes should be monitored periodically, especially when initiating TPN. Adjustments in the TPN solution can then be made as required.

The most common, but less serious, metabolic abnormality in TPN patients is hyperglycemia. It is treated by correcting hypophosphatemia if present (a cause of glucose intolerance), adding insulin to the TPN solution, reducing the dextrose load by substituting lipid for dextrose, and ensuring that the total energy load is not excessive.

Other metabolic complications include hypokalemia and hyperkalemia, which can be prevented and treated by using appropriate amounts of potassium in the TPN. Hyponatremia and hypernatremia require assessment of both sodium and water balance and should be treated by appropriate alterations in total sodium and water intake.

Abnormalities in liver functions occur frequently in patients on parenteral nutrition. The cause is probably fatty deposits in the liver, induced by the constant dextrose infusion. It is usually benign and self-limited, requiring no intervention. If progressive increases in the tests occur, cycling the TPN (infusing the full energy load in during 12 to 18 hours and giving the liver a rest during the rest of each day) often is effective. Causes other than the TPN should always be considered before it is assumed that the TPN is responsible.

Home parenteral nutrition

Just as other modalities of therapy such as renal dialysis have been adapted for home use, home TPN enables selected patients who depend on parenteral feeding to return to a reasonably normal lifestyle. A specialized catheter is introduced through a tunnel under the skin to reduce the likelihood of infection. The catheter exits the chest at a place where the patient can care for it conveniently (Fig. 11-6 and Plate 21). Infusing the necessary solutions during the night while the patient sleeps leaves him or her free to leave the home and even work during the day. If the intestinal tract is functioning, although inadequately, TPN can be used to supplement

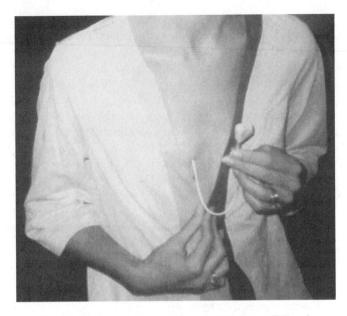

Fig. 11-6   A specialized catheter used for home CVA. ▲

oral intake, such as by infusing the TPN several nights a week rather than daily. Home TPN is expensive, but when it is used appropriately, the cost is offset by allowing the patient to be at home and in many cases to resume a productive life.

SUGGESTED READINGS

The American Dietetic Association, Signore J, editor: *Handbook of clinical dietetics,* ed 2, Hanover, Mass, 1992, Yale University Press.

A.S.P.E.N.: Guidelines for the use of parenteral and enteral nutrition in adult and pediatric patients, *J Parent Ent Nutr* 17(suppl 4):1SA-52SA,1993.

Department of Food and Nutrition Services, University of Alabama at Birmingham University Hospital: *Manual for nutritional management,* Birmingham, Ala, 1993, The University.

Edes TE, Walk BE, Austin JL: Diarrhea in tube-fed patients: feeding formula not necessarily the cause, *Am J Med* 88:91, 1990.

Franz MJ, Horton ES, Bantle JP, et al: Nutrition principles for the management of diabetes and related complications, *Diabetes Care* 17:490-518, 1994.

Johnston KR, Govel LA, Andritz MH: Gastrointestinal effects of sorbitol as an additive in liquid medications, *Am J Med* 97:185, 1994.

Position statement, nutrition recommendations and principles for people with diabetes mellitus, *Diabetes Care* 17:519-522, 1994.

Rombeau JL, Caldwell MD, editors: *Clinical nutrition: enteral and tube feeding,* ed 2, Philadelphia, 1990, WB Saunders.

Rombeau JL, Caldwell MD, editors: *Clinical nutrition: parenteral feeding,* ed 2, Philadelphia, 1992, WB Saunders.

Weinsier RL, Heimburger DC: *Handbook of clinical nutrition,* ed 3, St Louis, 1996, Mosby.

12

Nutritional Support in Special Disease States

Renal failure
Nutrition and liver disease
Nutrition and the pancreas
Nutrition and inflammatory bowel disease
Nutrition and celiac sprue
Nutrition and pulmonary disease
Critical care
Nutrition, HIV infection, and AIDS
Drug-nutrient interactions

RENAL FAILURE

The kidneys play a crucial role in maintaining an optimal metabolic environment for the body. In addition to important regulatory functions, the kidneys have synthetic, degradative, and hormonal functions. As renal function deteriorates, a wide variety of metabolic abnormalities may occur, including:
- Impaired regulation of sodium, potassium, phosphorus, magnesium, water, and hydrogen ions
- Impaired clearance of urea and other nitrogenous metabolites
- Impaired vitamin D metabolism and resultant metabolic bone disease
- Altered calcium and phosphorus metabolism
- Decreased synthesis of erythropoietin with subsequent anemia
- Increased clearance of pyridoxine (vitamin B_6)
- Accumulation of homocysteine

Symptoms and signs of uremia including nausea and vomiting, anorexia, bone pain, and loss of lean body mass are the ultimate manifestations of these metabolic derangements. The duration of the renal failure (acute or chronic) and the degree of catabolic stress associated with underlying disease states are reflected in the severity of these changes. The role of nutritional support in renal failure is to prevent or reverse malnutrition, minimize toxicity from inappropriate intake of nutrients, and minimize the progression of renal failure.

Acute renal failure

Acute renal failure (ARF) is defined as an abrupt and marked decrease in the glomerular filtration rate resulting from insults such as hypotension and shock, dehydration, infection, nephrotoxins, and trauma. Urine output can be normal (nonoliguric), reduced (oliguric), or nonexistent (anuric). Fluid and electrolyte balance becomes deranged. However, with the advent of dialysis, fluid and electrolyte abnormalities and uremic symptoms can be minimized. Patients with ARF are often catabolic because of the stress of underlying diseases. The sequelae of catabolism, including poor wound healing, infections, and increased mortality, are unaffected by dialysis alone and require appropriate aggressive nutritional support. The availability of dialysis permits full nutritional support without the buildup of toxic metabolic products.

Chronic renal failure

Chronic renal failure (CRF) is the result of injuries of a more sustained and often irreversible nature, leading to progressive nephron destruction. Reductions in renal mass cause structural and compensatory hypertrophy of the remaining nephrons, with an increase in glomerular capillary pressure and flow. Eventually this adaptation proves maladaptive. The added burden on the remaining glomeruli leads to glomerular sclerosis and ultimate destruction.

Patients with renal function of at least 50% of normal (i.e., serum creatinine <2 mg/dl) may have a stable clinical course with minimal adverse metabolic sequelae and minimal need for metabolic and nutritional interventions. The emphasis in such patients should be to maintain optimal nutritional status and prevent further renal deterioration.

For patients with 20% to 50% of normal renal function (i.e., serum creatinine 2 to 5 mg/dl), nutritional support becomes important because of retention of nitrogen, sodium, potassium, magnesium, phosphorus, and water. With progressive CRF, there is often increased malnutrition, reflected as reductions in fat and lean body mass and decreased synthesis of visceral proteins. Decreased nutrient intakes, uremic symptoms, accumulation of toxic by-products, and the stresses of underlying diseases all play important roles in CRF-associated malnutrition. With appropriate nutritional modifications, such as protein restriction, and control of blood pressure, the progression of CRF may be substantially stabilized and dialysis delayed.

Finally, patients with renal function less than 20% of normal (i.e., serum creatinine >5 mg/dl, BUN > 100) are likely to be dialyzed because nutritional support at this point is not sufficient to control uremic symptoms. With appropriate nutritional modifications and control of blood pressure, dialysis may be delayed and progression of CRF reduced. With the addition of dialysis, nutritional restrictions may be somewhat liberalized and adjusted according to individual needs (Table 12-1).

Dialysis. Up to 70% of hemodialysis and 50% of continuous ambulatory peritoneal dialysis (CAPD) patients are malnourished. Dialysis is associated with increased morbidity and mortality. Low visceral protein and cholesterol levels are indexes of malnutrition that are associated with an increased risk of mortality. Chronic dialysis patients are prone to malnutrition because of inadequate food intake, the accumulation of toxic metabolites, and several dialysis-related factors such as inadequate dialysis, increased losses of amino acids and proteins in the dialysate, and higher energy expenditures. Research indicates that intensive nutritional counseling, early initiation of dialysis, more frequent dialysis, more complete dialysis, the use of biocompatible membranes, and dialysis solutions are beneficial. Intensive nutri-

Table 12-1   General diet recommendations for renal patients*

Treatment	Pre-ESRD	Hemodialysis	Peritoneal dialysis
Protein (g/kg IBW)	0.6-0.8†	1.1-1.4	1.2-1.5
Nephrotic syndrome	0.8-1.0		
Energy (kcal/kg IBW)	35-40	30-35	25-35
Phosphorus (mg/kg IBW)	8-12‡	≤17§	≤17§
Sodium (mg/d)	1000-3000 if necessary	2000-3000	2000-4000
Potassium (mg/kg IBW)	Typically unrestricted	Approximately 40	Typically unrestricted
Fluid (ml/d)	Typically unrestricted	500-750 + daily urine output *or* 1000 ml if anuric	2000+
Calcium (mg/d)	1200-1600	Depends on serum level	Depends on serum level

ESRD, end-stage renal disease; *IBW*, ideal body weight.
*See specific guidelines for each treatment modality.
†The upper end of this range is preferred for diabetes and malnourished patients.
‡Whereas 5-10 mg/kg IBW is frequently cited in the scientific literature, 5 mg/kg IBW is practical only when used in conjunction with a very low protein diet supplemented with amino acids or ketoacid analogs.
§A diet that is higher in protein may make it impossible to meet the optimum phosphorus prescription.

tional counseling should be applied as soon as possible, ideally in the predialysis period. Other interventions under investigation include intradialytic parenteral nutrition, recombinant human growth hormone, and recombinant human insulin-growth factor-1 administration, alone or in combination.

Nutritional support in renal failure

General nutritional assessment is discussed in Chapter 10. The steps in nutrition assessment are also applicable to patients with renal disease.

Ideally, a patient's nutritional needs should be met by oral intake. However, if the patient is unable to take in an adequate amount or if nutrient demand exceeds the ability for intake, supplemental enteral or parenteral nutrition support is indicated. If the gastrointestinal tract is functioning, enteral feeding is the preferred route. If the gastrointestinal tract is nonfunctioning, parenteral nutrition may be indicated or may be used in combination with enteral feeding. Renal diets are prescribed by specifying a caloric and protein level and amounts of Na^+, K^+, $PO_4^=$, and fluid (see Table 12-1). Table 12-2 shows the renal exchange lists for diabetic and nondiabetic patients with renal failure, which are used in calculating diets.

Calorie requirements

The number of kilocalories required daily is a function of BEE (as calculated by the Harris-Benedict equation, Chapter 11), the level of activity, and the level of

Table 12-2   Average calculation figures for nondiabetic and diabetic renal diets*

Food choices	kcal	Protein (g)	Cholesterol (g)	Fat (g)	Na (mg)	K (mg)	P (mg)
NONDIABETIC							
Milk	120	4.0	12	6	80	185	110
Nondairy milk substitute	140	0.5	12	10	40	80	30
Meat	65	7.0	—	4	25	100	65
Starch	90	2.0	18	1	80	35	35
Vegetable							
Low K	25	1.0	5	Trace	15	70	20
Medium K	25	1.0	5	Trace	15	150	20
High K	25	1.0	5	Trace	15	270	20
Fruit							
Low K	70	0.5	17	—	Trace	70	15
Medium K	70	0.5	17	—	Trace	150	15
High K	70	0.5	17	—	Trace	270	15
Fat	45	—	—	5	55	10	5
High-calorie	100	Trace	25	—	15	20	5
Beverage	Varies	Varies	Varies	Varies	Varies	Varies	Varies
Salt	—	—	—	—	250	—	—
DIABETIC							
Milk	100	4.0	8	5	80	185	110
Nondairy milk substitute	140	0.5	12	10	40	80	30
Meat	65	7.0	—	4	25	100	65
Starch	80	2.0	15	1	80	35	35
Vegetable							
Low K	25	1.0 ·	5	Trace	15	70	20
Medium K	25	1.0	5	Trace	15	150	20
High K	25	1.0	5	Trace	15	270	20
Fruit							
Low K	60	0.5	15	—	Trace	70	15
Medium K	60	0.5	15	—	Trace	150	15
High K	60	0.5	15	—	Trace	270	15
Fat	45	—	—	5	55	10	5
High-calorie	60	Trace	15	—	15	20	5
Beverage	Varies	Varies	Varies	Varies	Varies	Varies	Varies
Salt	—	—	—	—	250	—	—

*To calculate a renal diet, determine the total daily calories and the amount of high-biological-value protein to be provided, as well as the amount of sodium, potassium, phosphorus, and fluid. It is recommended that at least two thirds of the protein should come from high-quality protein. First calculate the number of meat and milk exchanges necessary to meet the protein requirement. Divide the remaining protein among fruit, vegetable, starch, and nondairy milk substitute exchanges. Provide the remainder of the caloric requirement from fat and other high-calorie choices. Make sure that the sodium, phosphorus, potassium, and total fluid recommendations are followed in the dietary pattern developed.

associated catabolic stress. An unstressed patient will require daily calories at a level of 1 to 1.2 × BEE. A hypermetabolic patient may require 1.2 to 1.5 × BEE kcal/day. An adequate caloric intake is important in sparing protein breakdown. In highly stressed patients, indirect calorimetry can be a useful adjunct in the prescription of caloric needs.

Protein requirements

Adequate but not excessive protein intake is important to the nutritional management of renal failure, especially for the predialysis phase of CRF. The appropriate level of daily protein intake per kg of ideal body weight in the predialysis period may be estimated from the glomerular filtration rate (GFR): 20 to 25 ml/min—60 to 90 g/day; 15 to 20 ml/min—50 to 60 g/day; and 10 to 15 ml/min—40 to 60 g/day. For a GFR of 4 to 10 ml/min, 0.55 to 0.6 g/kg/day is indicated. When the GFR is less than 4 to 5 ml/min, dialysis is generally required. Patients on hemodialysis will require 1 to 1.2 g/kg/day of protein. Those receiving peritoneal dialysis require 1.2 to 1.5 g/kg/day of protein (see Table 12-1). The benefits of protein restriction in lessening the accumulation of nitrogenous wastes must be balanced with the possibility of net losses of somatic and visceral proteins. High-biologic-value (HBV) protein sources (i.e., animal sources containing higher proportions of essential amino acids) are recommended. HBV proteins can be combined with lower-biologic-value proteins from vegetable sources. A mixture of essential and nonessential amino acids is recommended for both enteral and parenteral formulations. Protein balance, in patients with urine output, can be calculated using the equations for 24-hour UUN or urea nitrogen appearance (UNA) (see Chapter 11).

Protein restriction and blood pressure control delay the progression of renal disease in animals. Some human studies have suggested that dietary protein restriction in predialysis patients is beneficial in delaying the progression of renal failure by decreasing hyperfiltration. However, others have shown only marginal benefits with protein restriction. Protein intake to match needs (24 UUN) will not increase urea generation.

Special renal amino acid formulations (both parenteral and enteral) that contain mainly essential amino acids or ketoacids have fairly limited indications and are for short-term use only. They may be indicated for a brief period to delay dialysis. The use of these formulas on a long-term basis is inappropriate.

In patients with nephrotic syndrome, high-protein diets are frequently prescribed; however, this regimen negatively affects residual renal function and does not improve serum albumin metabolism. Therefore modest protein restriction is recommended. Low-protein diets (i.e., 0.6 g/kg/day) have resulted in an improvement in the proteinuria level and lipid profile after 6 months of treatment.

Lipid

Lipid abnormalities, particularly hypertriglyceridemia, reduced HDL-C levels, and elevation of Lp(a) are common in end-stage renal disease, but limited data exist to support the efficacy of dietary therapy on these conditions. High cholesterol levels are associated with increased morbidity and mortality. In patients with lipid abnormalities, dietary restriction of saturated fat and cholesterol would seem prudent. When patients receive intravenous fat emulsions, it is reasonable to assess serum triglyceride levels.

Vitamins

Water-soluble vitamin deficiencies are common in patients with CRF as a result of poor oral intake, losses from dialysis, or both. Pyridoxine (vitamin B_6) requirements are increased in patients with uremia. Plasma homocysteine levels are often increased in patients with CRF, which can be associated with atherosclerosis and thrombotic cardiovascular complications. Folate, pyridoxine, and vitamin B_{12} deficiency should be ruled out as contributors to elevated homocysteine levels. Supplementation with folic acid and vitamins B_6 and B_{12} can be useful in lowering homocysteine levels. Because of impaired excretion of retinol-binding protein, vitamin A levels will be increased; therefore vitamin A is generally omitted from renal-formulation vitamins. Because of risk of oxalosis, the daily intake of vitamin C for persons with renal failure should not exceed 150 mg/day. This allows for 90 mg of dietary intake and not more than 60 mg of supplemental intake per day. Vitamin D deficiency and metabolic bone disease occur in CRF patients because the kidney is unable to hydroxylate 25-hydroxycholecalciferol to form 1,25-dihydroxycholecalciferol (calcitriol), the active form of the vitamin. Vitamin D replacement is indicated if vitamin D deficiency is present. However, to avoid the formation of calcium-phosphate precipitates in soft tissue, vitamin D should not be started if either calcium or phosphorus levels are elevated. A variety of vitamin supplements have been formulated specifically for dialysis patients. Vitamin requirements in ARF are probably qualitatively similar to those in CRF. The recommended vitamin allowances for patients with end-stage renal disease are shown in Table 12-3.

Anemia, folic acid, vitamin B_{12}, pyridoxine, and iron. The anemia associated with CRF is a serious, disabling problem. The primary cause of anemia in these patients is erythropoietin (EPO) deficiency. Other contributing factors in-

Table 12-3   Recommended daily amounts for patients with end-stage renal disease

Vitamin/mineral	RDA
Vitamin A	0
Vitamin K	0
Vitamin D	Individualized
Thiamin	1.5 mg
Riboflavin	1.7 mg
Niacin	20 mg
Pyridoxine	10 mg
Folic acid	0.8-1 mg
Vitamin B	6 μg
Biotin	300 μg
Pantothenic acid	10 mg
Vitamin C	60 mg
Elemental iron	Individualized

clude: uremic toxins, decreased survival of red cells, frequent blood sampling and blood loss from dialysis, catabolic process of dialysis or infections or both, aluminum toxicity, and deficiencies of nutrients such as vitamin B_{12}, folic acid, pyridoxine, and iron. EPO is a hormone produced in the kidney (90%) and liver (10%). EPO production increases when tissue oxygenation decreases and then stimulates the bone marrow to produce RBCs. Treatment of anemia in CRF has been dramatically changed with the development of recombinant human erythropoietin. In patients who do not respond to EPO treatment, nutritional deficiencies must be considered. Therefore it is important to monitor the levels of iron, vitamin B_{12}, and folic acid and to replace them as required. If iron replacement is necessary, 325 mg of $FeSO_4$ may be given up to three times per day.

Phosphorus, calcium, and parathyroid hormone. Disturbances in calcium, phosphorus, vitamin D, and parathyroid hormone metabolism are manifest as metabolic bone disease. These changes occur before the beginning of dialysis therapy. Abnormal vitamin D metabolism can lead to osteomalacia and also results in decreased calcium absorption, with resultant hypocalcemia. The decreased GFR elevates serum phosphorus levels. Both of these phenomena stimulate parathyroid hormone, with resultant secondary hyperparathyroidism. Therefore it is important to keep serum phosphorus levels within the normal range by reducing phosphorus intake to 600 to 1200 mg/day (see Table 12-1). Phosphate binders and calcium supplementation can also aid in controlling PO_4 levels. Most physicians no longer use aluminum hydroxide antacids as phosphorus binders because aluminum accumulation leads to neurologic disorders and osteomalacia. Calcium carbonate or calcium acetate supplementation is recommended at a dose of 1000 to 1500 mg/day. Calcium supplementation should be initiated only after serum phosphorus is normalized to prevent the formation of calcium phosphate salt deposits. Careful titration of supplemental vitamin D, often as calcitriol, is required to obtain its benefits without hyperphosphatemia or hypercalcemia. Dual energy x-ray absorptiometry and bone biopsies can be important in establishing the diagnosis of metabolic bone disease in patients with renal failure.

Fluid and electrolytes

Sodium and water. Sodium and water balance are often abnormal in CRF because of a decreased GFR or decreases in renal tubular reabsorption or both. Excessive retention of sodium and water occurs and predisposes to hypertension, edema, and congestive heart failure. In other instances, the kidney cannot retain sodium and water, disposing to dehydration, hypotension, and further reduction in renal function. Because fluid overload is more common, restriction of sodium and water is usually appropriate. An appropriate starting point for daily restriction would be 1 to 3 g of sodium per day and a fluid intake sufficient to exceed urine output by 500 ml (to cover insensible losses). Adjustments can be made according to the clinical response to the restrictions. The goal is to establish optimal body water content, normalize blood pressure and serum sodium, and eliminate edema. Frequent weighing helps monitor shifts of body water.

pH. Metabolic acidosis is often present in patients with CRF because of the retention of acids or the renal loss of bicarbonate or both. Calcium carbonate supplements may be useful for the treatment of mild acidosis. However, sodium bicarbonate given orally or intravenously may be necessary for severe acidosis. Dialysis is indicated if these measures are ineffective in controlling acidosis.

Magnesium. Magnesium is normally excreted by the kidneys and therefore is often restricted to approximately 200 mg/day in patients with CRF. Magnesium-containing medications such as antacids and laxatives should be avoided.

Potassium. The kidney is the primary route of potassium excretion. Potassium excretion is generally not impaired until creatinine clearance is less than 10 ml/min. Therefore potassium restriction of 40 to 60 mEq/day is appropriate in advanced renal failure.

NUTRITION AND LIVER DISEASE

The liver integrates a wide variety of major metabolic processes including carbohydrate, fat, and protein metabolism; vitamin storage and activation; and detoxification and excretion of both endogenous and exogenous waste products. Therefore impaired liver function can produce major imbalance of metabolic and nutritional status. Conversely, progressive impairment of nutritional status can further impair liver function.

Because the liver has an enormous functional reserve (it can perform satisfactorily with only 20% of functional liver cells and has a marvelous potential to regenerate after injury), the goal of nutritional therapy is to support liver function and to enhance the liver's ability to regenerate after injury.

Carbohydrate metabolism

The liver regulates carbohydrate metabolism by the synthesis, storage, and breakdown of glycogen. Whenever exogenous sources of glucose are insufficient for the body's requirements, the liver initially increases blood glucose level by breaking down glycogen (glycogenolysis). As the glycogen stores become depleted, the liver increases glucose availability through the process of gluconeogenesis (obtaining glucose from amino acids). With severe hepatic insufficiency, glycogen metabolism and gluconeogenesis may be impaired to the point of causing hypoglycemia.

Fat metabolism

The liver is a major site of fatty acid breakdown and triglyceride synthesis. Fatty acids from endogenous and exogenous sources are converted in the liver to acetyl CoA, which is processed by the citric acid cycle for further energy production. The breakdown of fatty acids provides ketone bodies as an alternative source of energy when glucose is unavailable, such as during starvation. This has its advantages as a gluconeogenesis-sparing process that conserves further breakdown of muscle protein sources to form glucose as an energy substrate. Thus lean body mass is conserved by using ketone bodies rather than glucose as a fuel source. Triglyceride synthesis occurs when carbohydrate intake exceeds energy requirements. Under such conditions, glucose may overwhelm the glycogen reservoir, and acetyl CoA generated by glycolysis is not needed for oxidative phosphorylation. Therefore acetyl CoA is conserved by its conversion to fatty acids and ultimately to triglycerides. The liver is also involved in cholesterol, bile acid, and lipoprotein synthesis. When there is liver insufficiency, all of these functions may be impaired. Fat malabsorption may result from diminished bile salt production and therefore is associated with fat-soluble vitamin deficiencies.

Protein metabolism

The liver plays a central role in synthesis and degradation of protein. Endogenous proteins are continuously being hydrolyzed and resynthesized. Through transamination, amination, and deamination, there is a constant interchange of amino acid substrates and the substrates of carbohydrate and fat metabolism for the eventual production of energy. Plasma proteins including albumin, coagulation factors, transferrin, and ceruloplasmin constitute about one half of the protein synthesized by the liver. Ammonia, a by-product of amino acid metabolism, is converted to urea by the liver and is eventually excreted in the urine.

Altered protein metabolism is probably the most significant consequence of liver disease. It is manifest clinically by encephalopathy and muscle wasting and is characterized by altered plasma amino acid profiles. Typically, the branched-chain amino acids (leucine, isoleucine, and valine) are decreased and the aromatic amino acids (phenylalanine, tyrosine, and tryptophan) and methionine are increased. The precise mechanisms for the development of encephalopathy are complex and multifactorial and relate to the buildup of abnormal amounts of metabolites that interfere with neurotransmitter production and function.

As hepatic insufficiency develops, the liver becomes less efficient at providing the body with glucose for energy. As a consequence, the branched-chain amino acids (BCAAs) are used locally by tissues as energy substrates. Thus the BCAA levels decrease. On the other hand, the aromatic amino acids (AAAs) are not metabolized normally by the liver, and their levels increase. At the level of the blood-brain barrier, the ratio of AAA to BCAA is increased and more AAAs cross the blood-brain barrier. The AAAs are precursors of central neurotransmitters, including the inhibitory neurotransmitter serotonin, and false neurotransmitters. Thus the inhibition of brain function (e.g., stupor, asterixis) seems to occur with increasing amounts of AAA entering the brain.

Protein synthesis by the liver is influenced by the nutritional state, as well as by hormones. Insulin, glucagon, and glucocorticoids are particularly important. Insulin and steroids stimulate the synthesis of hepatic proteins, whereas glucagon inhibits synthesis and promotes their degradation.

Vitamin and trace element metabolism

Because the liver is involved in the storage and activation of many vitamins and synthesizes the carrier proteins involved for many of the vitamins, disturbances in vitamin metabolism are present in hepatic insufficiency. The reasons for these deficiencies include poor oral intake, increased needs associated with the increased catabolic stress of hepatic insufficiency, malabsorption of fat-soluble vitamins, and decreased liver storage (i.e., folic acid). By similar mechanisms, there is impaired metabolism of zinc, copper, potassium, magnesium, molybdenum, cadmium, and selenium.

Chronic liver disease

Many studies have shown a high incidence of malnutrition in patients with alcoholic liver disease and other chronic liver diseases (CLD). Severe protein-calorie malnutrition (marasmus) is almost universal in advanced liver disease, seriously undermining the capacity for the liver to regenerate and restore its function. The more severe the malnutrition, the worse the prognosis.

Nutritional assessment in patients with CLD is important so that the type and degree of malnutrition are identified and appropriate therapy is devised. In CLD the appetite may be affected and eating habits may be poor. The underlying disease may damage the function of other digestive organs, such as the pancreas and intestine, thereby amplifying the possibility of malnutrition. In the history and physical examination, attention should be paid to signs and symptoms of malabsorption, gastrointestinal bleeding, encephalopathy, and fluid retention. Signs of vitamin deficiency such as glossitis, cheilitis, and anemia are often evident but overlooked. Fluid status should be estimated on the basis of blood pressure, jugular venous pressure, urine output, skin turgor, serum sodium and creatinine, and the presence of peripheral edema or ascites or both. Body weight is not a sensitive parameter because of sodium and water retention. Patients with decompensated CLD often have inadequate intravascular volume despite gross excesses in total body sodium and water. Studies using the tracer isotope dilution techniques demonstrate that extracellular fluids might be increased even in patients with cirrhosis without ascites. Triceps skinfold thickness provides an estimate of body fat reserves, and midarm muscle circumference is an estimate of muscle mass. These measurements are reasonably accurate, even in the presence of excess body water. These parameters also show a progressive reduction as liver function deteriorates.

Serum albumin is not a sensitive indicator of malnutrition in patients with CLD. Hypoalbuminemia is due to an increased volume of distribution and an increased catabolic rate without a compensatory increase in albumin synthesis. Other measures of visceral proteins such as serum prealbumin, retinol binding protein, and transferrin can be difficult to interpret in CLD because they are also synthesized by hepatocytes.

Malnutrition is closely correlated with abnormalities in immune system function. Altered skin test reactivity has been seen in 60% of patients with cirrhosis and in 93% of patients with fulminant hepatic failure.

In patients with cirrhosis, certain amino acids become *conditionally essential* (i.e., choline, cysteine, taurine, and tyrosine). These amino acids are not essential in normal subjects because they can be synthesized from precursors. In cirrhotic patients, acquired defects in metabolic pathways may create insufficiencies in production. Thus their essentialness is conditional on the cirrhotic state.

Treatment

Hepatic insufficiency creates a treatment dilemma for the clinician. On the one hand, protein intolerance manifest clinically as encephalopathy may occur with even normal amounts of protein intake. On the other hand, protein insufficiency will produce inadequate protein synthesis and result in significant reductions in the function of organ systems, especially the immune system. Therefore the therapeutic strategy for hepatic insufficiency is to provide both the estimated energy requirements and sufficient protein to establish nitrogen balance without precipitating or exacerbating encephalopathy.

Keeping these principles in mind, the following guidelines may be used to formulate nutritional support:

- BEE is generally considered to be no different in patients with liver disease unless there is evidence of acute stress. If there is evidence of fluid retention, indirect calorimetry may be useful in estimating caloric needs. For most patients, caloric needs are initially approximated by feeding 1.2 × BEE.
- A 24-hour UUN collection is useful to provide an estimate of the degree of catabolism and estimate the appropriate level of protein intake (gastrointestinal bleeding, diuretics, and dehydration can alter the 24-hour UUN). Standard sources of dietary protein and general amino acid mixtures for enteral or parenteral support are generally first prescribed. The use of general amino acid mixtures is suggested initially if hepatic encephalopathy is not present. Protein intake can be started at a dose of 0.5 to 0.7 g/kg of *dry* weight per day and may be increased to 1 g/kg/day as tolerated. If the patient is encephalopathic, reversible causes (i.e., gastrointestinal bleeding, excessive use of diuretics, infections, etc.) should first be excluded. A trial of BCAAs is then appropriate.
- Fluid and sodium restriction should be instituted in the presence of ascites, edema, or both.
- Dietary fat restriction is unnecessary unless fat malabsorption is present. Approximately 30% to 35% of total energy should be given as fat. Serum triglyceride levels may be monitored as an index of fat tolerance in parenterally fed patients.
- The preferred route of administration of nutrients is oral/enteral, unless contraindicated.
- Vitamin and mineral replacement therapy should be initiated and monitored periodically. Special attention should be given to fat-soluble vitamins in patients with evidence of hepatic cholestasis. Zinc deficiency can decrease oral intake because of impaired smell or taste. Since copper is hepatically excreted, copper levels should be monitored.
- Electrolyte disturbances should be treated as they occur.

Hepatobiliary complications of total parenteral nutrition

The advent of TPN has permitted long-term independent survival of patients with intestinal failure. With refinements in infusion solutions, vitamins, and trace elements, and advances in catheter design and placement techniques, the metabolic and septic complications of TPN have become less frequent. TPN-related hepatic dysfunction is difficult to diagnose because patients receiving TPN often have co-morbid conditions that are also associated with liver function disorders.

TPN-related liver dysfunction is manifest clinically by hepatomegaly, jaundice, or both, and biochemically by elevated enzymes and bilirubin levels. Peak enzyme levels usually occur between 1 and 4 weeks after starting TPN. The incidence of abnormal liver enzyme levels is not consistent; levels vary from 25% to 100% above normal. Enzyme elevations are usually mild and often transient. Most studies report either a fall or a normalization of elevated enzyme levels despite continuance of TPN.

The predominant hepatic histologic abnormality is steatosis in adults and cholestasis in children. It has been suggested that steatosis is an early, transient effect of TPN administration. Cholestasis supervenes later and usually persists as long as the TPN is continued. Steatosis is a consequence of carbohydrate-lipid imbalance, and cholestasis is related to amino acid excess in experimental studies. In long-term home TPN patients, CLD has been observed in 15% to 20% of patients. Patients with massive bowel resection appear to have the highest risk of developing this complication.

The mechanism leading to TPN-related liver dysfunction is unclear. It has been suggested that alterations in bile-acid metabolism, such as biliary stasis, and the increased production of hepatotoxic bile acids from small bowel overgrowth are involved. Other gastrointestinal-related complications from TPN are acalculous cholecystitis, biliary sludge, gallbladder distention, and gallstones. The incidence of these complications is closely related to the duration of TPN. In many instances, TPN may contribute to or exacerbate rather than initiate such complications.

The following measures should be followed to prevent TPN-related hepatic dysfunction:

- Avoid excessive total calories. If necessary, indirect calorimetry can be used to assess patient needs.
- Provide a portion of nonprotein calories as fat. Do not avoid fat. TPN solutions providing high content of carbohydrates have been associated with the development of steatosis of the liver.
- Avoid continuous infusions. Cycle the TPN to allow for an unfed state during part of the day.
- Resume the oral/enteral route as soon as possible.
- Avoid hepatotoxic drugs and omit copper from TPN solutions in patients with hepatic cholestasis.
- Avoid excessive protein loads by evaluating nitrogen requirements periodically.
- Consider a short course of metronidazole for bacterial overgrowth of the small bowel.

NUTRITION AND THE PANCREAS

The pancreas has endocrine and exocrine functions. Endocrine pancreatic function includes the secretion of insulin, glucagon, and somatostatin. Exocrine pancreatic function involves the secretion of digestive enzymes and bicarbonate into the duodenum. The pancreatic enzymes amylase, lipase, and trypsin are essential for the digestion of carbohydrates, lipid, and protein, respectively. Amylase cleaves polysaccharides to yield oligosaccharides and disaccharides. Lipase hydrolyzes triglycerides to fatty acids and monoglycerides. Trypsin and other enzymes (chymotrypsin) cleave proteins into smaller oligopeptides and amino acids. The acinar cells of the pancreas secrete active phospholipase A, cholesterol esterase, carboxypeptidase, and aminopeptidases. Autodigestion of the pancreas is prevented by storage of the proteases in precursor forms and the synthesis of protease inhibitors. Bicarbonate in the pancreatic juice neutralizes gastric acid delivered to the duodenum and maintains an optimal pH for digestive enzyme function.

A number of hormones are known to modulate pancreatic secretion. Excitatory hormones include vasoactive intestinal peptide (VIP), secretin, cholecystokinin (CCK), and gastrin. Inhibitory hormones include somatostatin, pancreatic polypeptide, and glucagon. Secretin stimulates water and bicarbonate secretion, whereas cholecystokinin increases pancreatic enzyme secretion.

Acute pancreatitis

Acute pancreatitis develops when premature activation of pancreatic enzymes occurs and the balance between activated proteases and protease inhibitors is disrupted. Alcohol, gallstones, and idiopathic pancreatitis account for approximately 90% of cases. Other causes include complications of endoscopic retrograde cholangiopancreatography (ERCP), perforated peptic ulcer, trauma, drugs (furosemide, 6-mercaptopurine), pancreatic outflow obstruction, hypertriglyceridemia, hypercalcemia, and infections.

Acute pancreatitis is classified as mild or severe on the basis of clinical features, laboratory evaluation, and pathologic changes. Serum amylase and lipase values are elevated. Many imaging techniques are used to evaluate acute pancreatitis and to identify complications. Dynamic contrast-enhanced computerized tomography is considered the method of choice for evaluating acute pancreatitis and its complications. However, ultrasonography, plain computed tomography, and ERCP are also useful.

The medical treatment of acute pancreatitis is supportive. There are no specific therapies that have been proved effective. Patients with mild pancreatitis require only hydration, analgesics, and NPO status for a few days. Patients with moderate and severe pancreatitis require intensive monitoring of electrolytes, volume replacement, and management of complications.

Malnutrition of the kwashiorkor type is reported in 80% to 100% of patients with protracted, severe pancreatitis. Hypermetabolism is a consistent finding in patients with acute pancreatitis, with measured energy expenditures ranging up to 14% above predicted. Patients with severe acute pancreatitis also have increased protein breakdown and resultant negative nitrogen balance. Gluconeogenesis, in the setting of pancreatitis, is not suppressed by intravenous glucose infusions as in metabolically normal individuals (see Chapter 11).

The nutritional goals in the treatment of pancreatitis are to reduce the amount of pancreatic stimulation, correct fluid and electrolyte imbalances, provide adequate amounts of calories and protein, and avoid overfeeding. Patients with mild pancreatitis should be able to tolerate low-fat oral feeding within 5 days of the onset of symptoms. Aggressive early enteral or parenteral support reduces mortality in patients with moderate-to-severe pancreatitis.

Recent reviews make a compelling argument for the use of jejunal feedings in acute pancreatitis. The degree of pancreatic stimulation depends on where the enteral formula is infused in the gastrointestinal tract. An elemental diet that is infused more distally in the small bowel will cause less pancreatic secretions because of bypass of phases of pancreatic stimulation. Human studies have shown that continuous jejunal feeding does not increase exocrine pancreatic secretion to a significant degree. Enteral feeding also has the advantages of safety, lower cost, and maintenance of gut flora and mucosal integrity by preventing subsequent bacterial translocation. Therefore enteral access beyond the ligament of Treitz should be achieved early in the course of the illness.

When enteral feeding is not possible or is contraindicated, the use of TPN should be considered. Parenteral infusions of dextrose, amino acids, and lipid emulsions do not stimulate pancreatic secretion to a significant degree. When hyperlipidemia is thought to be the cause of pancreatitis, intravenous lipids should be used with caution and serum triglyceride levels should be monitored frequently.

Chronic pancreatitis

Chronic pancreatitis refers to permanent damage to the glandular anatomy of the pancreas with or without significant changes in function. The most common cause of chronic pancreatitis is excessive alcohol intake. Chronic pancreatitis is characterized by a relentless and progressive loss of parenchymal tissue. In most cases, both exocrine and endocrine functions are lost, although the loss of endocrine function appears later in the course of the disease. Greater than 90% of the pancreas must be damaged before maldigestion of fat and protein occurs.

Serum amylase and lipase concentrations may be normal or slightly elevated, particularly if the gland is compromised by extensive fibrosis. Fecal fat excretion is elevated and can be detected by Sudan black B fat staining of the feces or quantified by the 3-day measurement of fecal fat excretion while consuming 100 g of fat per day (normal fecal fat excretion is <6 g/day). The composition of the fecal fat is mainly neutral fat, not fatty acids, as is seen in the malabsorption of bowel wall disease. Duodenal intubation to measure bicarbonate secretion during intravenous secretin stimulation is considered the gold standard to document pancreatic function. Pancreatic calcifications, which are pathognomonic (diagnostic) of chronic pancreatitis, may be seen in up to 30% of patients on plain abdominal radiographs. ERCP is considered to be the most effective imaging procedure for diagnosing chronic pancreatitis. Ultrasound and CT scanning are additional tools used to diagnose chronic pancreatitis and its complications.

Patients with chronic pancreatitis may have presenting symptoms of abdominal pain, malabsorption, and diabetes mellitus. Patients may have bouts of recurrent acute or continuous abdominal pain. The pain is not necessarily accompanied by symptoms of malabsorption. Pain that is related to eating can lead to significant malnutrition and weight loss. The weight loss is a reflection of depleted fat stores and muscle mass. These patients often have presenting symptoms of marasmic physiology.

Fat malabsorption (steatorrhea) can be another cause of significant weight loss. The level of exocrine pancreatic reserve and the type of diet tolerated define the severity of this disease. Patients may be able to digest a low-fat diet but become markedly symptomatic on a high-fat diet. Fat malabsorption can be treated with oral pancreatic enzyme supplementation and, if steatorrhea persists, a low-fat diet (<40 g/day). MCTs can also be prescribed. MCTs represent a source of fat but generally do not produce symptoms because their absorption does not require the presence of bile acids and depends on minimal amounts of pancreatic enzymes. Therapy is initiated with large doses of enzymes before meals and snacks. Enteric-coated and nonenteric-coated supplements are available. The additions of

H_2 blockers and antacids can prevent the degradation of the supplemental enzymes. Sodium bicarbonate or aluminum-containing antacids are the most commonly used. Deficiency of fat-soluble vitamins (A, D, E, and K) is prevalent, especially in patients with steatorrhea.

Another challenge in treating chronic pancreatitis is controlling abdominal pain. Abstinence from alcohol and the use of analgesic medication and nerve blocks are useful for pain control. Oral pancreatic enzyme supplements aid in the analgesic effect by blocking the stimulation of endogenous CCK secretion, leading to reduced pancreatic secretion, thus putting the pancreas at rest.

NUTRITION AND INFLAMMATORY BOWEL DISEASE

Inflammatory bowel disease (IBD) refers to idiopathic chronic inflammatory conditions of the intestine and colon, principally Crohn's disease and ulcerative colitis. Crohn's disease is a transmural granulomatous enteritis that may involve any part of the intestine but primarily the distal small intestine and the colon. Ulcerative colitis is an inflammatory condition of the mucosa of the colon.

Malnutrition is a significant problem in patients with IBD. The incidence of malnutrition ranges from 33% to 48% in Crohn's disease and 58% to 72% in ulcerative colitis. A large percentage of hospitalized patients with IBD have lost greater than 10% of their body weight, have hypoalbuminemia or anemia, and are in negative nitrogen balance.

Malnutrition in chronic IBD is multifactorial. Mechanisms leading to malnutrition include: decreased nutrient intake, malabsorption of nutrients, excessive nutrient losses, increased nutrient requirements, and drug-nutrient interactions that deplete macronutrients and micronutrients.

1. *Decreased nutrient intake* can arise because of abdominal pain, nausea, or diarrhea. These symptoms are frequently exacerbated by food intake.
2. *Malabsorption.* Patients with extensive mucosal involvement of the small bowel (Crohn's disease) or prior small bowel resections are predisposed to malabsorption. Large ileal resections may result in bile salt depletion and therefore malabsorption of triglycerides, fat-soluble vitamins (A, D, E, and K), and minerals. Ileal resection can also lead to impaired vitamin B_{12} absorption. Small bowel resection, stenotic bowel segments, and enteroenteric fistulae can all contribute to abnormal function of the small intestine. Stasis of the intestinal contents can lead to bacterial overgrowth with bacterial utilization of nutrients (vitamin B_{12}) and toxic effects of bile salts that have been deconjugated by bacteria.
3. *Excessive nutrient losses.* IBD is an exudative enteropathy; therefore protein losses across the inflamed intestinal mucosa can occur, leading to hypoalbuminemia. IBD can also lead to losses of electrolytes (sodium, potassium, and magnesium) and minerals (zinc, calcium, and copper). Iron depletion and subsequent anemia may occur as a result of acute and chronic blood loss.
4. *Increased nutrient requirements.* Patients with IBD may have increased caloric and nutrient requirements, especially during acute exacerbations of their disease. Increased requirements may be secondary to inflamma-

tion and infection. However, two studies using indirect calorimetry have shown that some patients with active Crohn's disease had BEEs that were not significantly higher than the predicted energy expenditure estimated from the Harris-Benedict equation.

5. *Drug-nutrient interactions.* Several of the medications used to treat IBD can affect nutritional status. Corticosteroids have beneficial systemic and local effects on the intestinal mucosa; however, they also decrease intestinal calcium absorption and eventually lead to osteopenia. In addition, corticosteroids can contribute to negative protein balance. Sulfasalazine (sulfapyridine and 5-aminosalicylic acid) and methotrexate can produce folate deficiency and also cause gastric irritation and abdominal pain, contributing to diminished food intake. The newer products of 5-aminosalicylic acid (5-ASA) have an enteric coating, thereby reducing its systemic and local side effects.

Malnutrition can increase the morbidity and mortality from IBD. Therefore it is important to recognize deficiencies at an early stage and to promptly initiate appropriate therapy. Nutritional management in IBD involves three aspects: replacement of malabsorbed and deficient nutrients, reduction of symptoms and nutrient losses with dietary manipulations, and assistance with disease activity control.

1. *Replacement of nutrients* is usually not difficult, except in the cases of growth failure in children and adolescents. TPN and enteral formulas and vitamin and mineral supplements are effective in replacing nutrient deficiencies in hospitalized and nonhospitalized patients.

2. *Dietary manipulations* include lactose restriction for patients with lactose intolerance; fat restriction for steatorrhea; and restriction of hard, indigestible, fibrous food for patients with small bowel strictures. Fat restriction in patients with steatorrhea can reduce diarrhea and improve calcium balance, and in patients with hyperoxaluria can reduce urinary oxalate. In patients with partial bowel obstruction, nuts, seeds, large amounts of insoluble fiber, and foods producing gas such as dried beans and peas and cruciferous vegetables are often avoided.

3. *Assistance with disease activity control.* The role of enteral or parenteral nutrition support in IBD therapy remains controversial. Active Crohn's disease can improve when nutritional status is restored with TPN or elemental diets. Possible mechanisms include adaptive responses to bowel rest, immunologic effects (decreased dietary and bacterial antigen uptake, improved cell-mediated immunity), and nutritional effects (correction of macronutrient and micronutrient deficiencies). Enteral nutrition and TPN seem to be equally effective in correcting the nutritional deficiencies seen in IBD. Short-term courses of either TPN or enteral formulas have been associated with remission rates of 60% to 80%. Elemental formulas (containing amino acids, glucose, etc.) have been as effective as corticosteroids in inducing short-term remission in patients with acute exacerbation of Crohn's disease in some studies, whereas treatment with oligomeric formulas (containing small peptides) appears to be less effective than methylprednisolone and sulfasalazine therapy in others. Long-term remission of

disease activity by enteral or parenteral nutritional support alone is even less clear; therefore nutritional support as the sole long-term treatment for patients with IBD is generally not recommended.

Enteral feeding is the preferred method of nutritional support for patients with acute exacerbations of Crohn's disease, except in the presence of high-output enteral fistulae, bowel obstruction, or unacceptable gastrointestinal symptoms. Enteral feeding generally results in a cost savings over parenteral nutrition and maintains the integrity of the gut mucosa, which decreases bacterial and toxin translocation.

Nutritional management in ulcerative colitis has a more limited role than in Crohn's disease. Macronutrient deficiencies are related to decreased intake and to protein-losing enteropathy. TPN may benefit patients with acute exacerbations of ulcerative colitis when surgery is being considered and when preservation of lean body mass and functional capacity with enteral feeding is impossible. TPN, however, does not influence disease activity in patients with severe acute exacerbations of ulcerative colitis, and it does not reduce the need for a colectomy in patients with refractory disease.

Although some controversial issues remain, there are several conclusions about the nutritional support of patients with IBD: (1) nutritional status should be assessed and macronutrient and micronutrient deficiencies replaced; (2) bowel rest is not necessary when restoring nutritional status; (3) polymeric formulas (containing whole proteins) are as effective as elemental and oligomeric formulas in managing disease exacerbations; (4) standard pharmacotherapy (steroids alone or steroids and sulfasalazine) is better than enteral nutrition with defined formula diets alone in inducing clinical remissions; (5) TPN remains a valuable tool in supporting patients with Crohn's disease who cannot meet their nutritional needs, and it is essential for patients with gut failure, extensive disease, and in some patients with short bowel syndrome.

NUTRITION AND CELIAC SPRUE

Celiac disease (celiac sprue, nontropical sprue, gluten-sensitive enteropathy) is a chronic sensitivity to gluten, a protein found in wheat, rye, oats, and barley. Ingestion of gluten leads to atrophy of the small intestinal villi, decreased activity of enzymes in the surface epithelium, and poor absorption of nutrients, resulting in malabsorption and diarrhea.

Most patients are white, with ancestors from northwestern Europe, and Asians from India and Pakistan. Celiac disease is nonexistent in Africans, Japanese, and Chinese. The family clusters of celiac disease imply a genetic predisposition; a gene in the HLA-DP region seems to predispose to celiac disease.

The disease is caused by the proximal bowel's response to gluten ingestion, specifically the gliadin component. The mechanism of injury is probably an immune-mediated process, suggested by the diffuse infiltration of the lamina propria with plasma cells and lymphocytes, and the presence of antigliadin, antijejunum, antireticulin, and antiendomysial antibodies. The pathogenesis of celiac disease involves various environmental factors superimposed on the appropriate genetic susceptibility. Environmental factors include an immunologic sensitivity to dietary gluten and possibly prior infection with adenovirus serotype 12.

The onset of celiac disease has two peaks. The first peak is in early infancy, when cereals become a significant part of the diet. The second peak is during the fourth or fifth decade of life. In infancy the most common presentations are failure to thrive, chronic diarrhea, and weight loss. In adulthood, loss of weight, diarrhea (acute or chronic), and malabsorption (steatorrhea) are prominent symptoms. Symptoms may be mild, in spite of severe mucosal damage, or full-blown malabsorption may occur. Celiac disease can also present as iron deficiency and hypocalcemia or evidence of deficiencies of fat-soluble vitamins (A, D, E, and K). Because lactase is present in the brush border epithelium, most patients have symptomatic lactose intolerance. Lactase activity returns to normal when the mucosal integrity is restored. The pathologic findings of celiac disease are atrophy of the intestinal villi, hyperplasia of the crypts, and distortion of the surface epithelium.

The diagnosis of celiac disease should be suspected in patients with manifestations of malabsorption. Useful tests to make the diagnosis of malabsorption include the D-xylose tolerance test, a serum carotene level, and a 24-hour stool test for fecal fat. Other causes of malabsorption, such as pancreatic and biliary defects, infectious diseases, and effects of drugs on absorption, should be ruled out. The diagnosis of celiac disease is most rapidly established by a small bowel biopsy, with the findings of the characteristic flat mucosal pattern. Antiendomysial antibodies are almost 100% specific and 85% sensitive; they disappear when an individual is placed on a gluten-free diet. Antibodies against gliadin, gluten, and reticulin are helpful, particularly in children. Radiologic studies, such as the small bowel follow-through, are helpful but nonspecific. Electrolytes, trace elements, and vitamin levels should be assayed and replaced as indicated. The diagnosis is also confirmed by the therapeutic response to gluten restriction in the diet. The small bowel histologic findings should normalize 3 to 6 months after gluten restriction.

Strict adherence to a gluten-free diet must be continually emphasized, since even the smallest indiscretion can result in rapid and serious decompensation. Wheat, oats, rye, and barley and derivatives of these grains are omitted from the diet. A variety of specialty products are available for patients with gluten-sensitive enteropathy. Vitamin supplementation should be tailored to match the patient. Products that may be substituted include corn, potato, tapioca, arrowroot, rice, and soy flours. Reading labels to determine the presence of gluten-containing ingredients is important. The services of a registered dietitian or joining a support group can be invaluable.

A few patients (<10%) are resistant to a gluten-free diet alone and may benefit from a course of corticosteroid therapy. Most patients with celiac disease do extremely well on a lifelong gluten-free diet. Unfortunately, various complications can supervene, including dermatitis herpetiformis, intestinal lymphoma, carcinoma of the esophagus, and ulcerations of the jejunum and ileum, which can perforate. Therefore lifelong adherence to the diet, as well as careful follow-up, is recommended.

NUTRITION AND PULMONARY DISEASE

The evaluation of nutritional status is important in the assessment and management of patients with acute respiratory failure and chronic obstructive pulmonary disease (COPD). The main adverse effects of malnutrition are altered respiratory muscle structure and function, diminished ventilatory drive, and impaired host immune defenses. Other sequelae such as altered lung structure and repair after injury and decreased surfactant production probably also occur, but these events are less clearly defined. Depletion of muscle and fat mass is reported in up to 20% of stable outpatients and 50% of hospitalized patients with pulmonary disease. Therefore patients with previously normal pulmonary function who develop respiratory failure and patients with acute respiratory failure superimposed on underlying COPD have a high risk for the development or exacerbation of malnutrition.

Patients with COPD often have anthropometric measurements consistent with marasmus, including reductions in body weight, fat reserves, and muscle mass. These changes in muscle mass are reflected in all muscle groups, including the diaphragm and other muscles of respiration (Fig. 12-1 and Plate 22). COPD increases work of breathing, which can increase caloric needs. Thus COPD can produce a cycle in which poor respiratory function promotes weight loss and weight loss further hinders respiratory function. Weight loss is an independent adverse prognostic factor in patients with COPD.

Patients with acute ventilatory failure often have kwashiorkor physiology. These patients respond differently to the provision of excess calories than normal or marasmic patients (see Chapter 11). Overfeeding can increase O_2 consumption and CO_2 production. Attention to the nutritional care of these patients is essential.

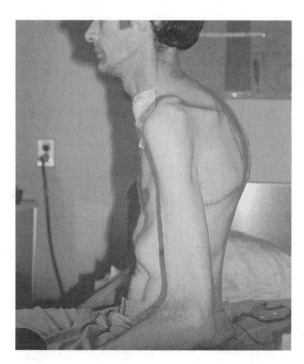

Fig. 12-1   Cachexia in a patient with chronic obstructive pulmonary disease. ▲

The goal is to prevent or minimize the loss of respiratory muscle mass and function, and therapy is directed at improving the underlying pulmonary pathology. Patients who have adequate nutritional support (e.g., calories, protein, and micronutrients) are more readily weaned from mechanical ventilation than patients receiving protein-free, energy-deficient diets.

Effects of nutrition and respiratory system

There are many levels at which nutrition affects patients with pulmonary disease (Table 12-4).

Ventilatory drive. The normal response to hypoxia is to increase the ventilatory drive (V_E). However, patients who are underfed (marasmic physiology) have a depressed ventilatory response to hypoxia. These changes tend to normalize with refeeding and are prevented if semistarvation is avoided in the first place. Therefore underfeeding has a detrimental effect on the respiratory system.

Respiratory muscles and lung tissue. Malnutrition causes impaired function of the diaphragm and muscles of respiration. Muscle wasting is an important determinant of respiratory impairment in patients with COPD, independent of the degree of airflow obstruction. Inadequate nutritional support may prolong mechanical ventilation in critically ill patients.

Undernutrition affects the pulmonary parenchyma by causing diminished collagen synthesis and increased proteolysis. This may be manifest as decreased surfactant production and alveolar collapse. Strategies such as enteral or parenteral nutritional support can be used to promote weight gain, which predominantly causes expansion of fat mass but no improvement in physiologic function.

The use of anabolic steroids to promote tissue growth remains controversial, although promising results have been reported using a short-term course of nandrolone decanoate with nutritional supplementation. This regimen increased fat free mass and improved respiratory muscle function without side effects.

Effect of total calories. In patients with COPD, decreased dietary intakes and elevated resting metabolic rates contribute to weight loss. The caloric level selected and the substrate burned affect the metabolic rate, O_2 consumption, and CO_2 production. Optimization of total calories is the first important principle of nutritional therapy. Feeding acutely stressed patients who have respiratory insufficiency with excessive calories, particularly carbohydrates, should be avoided because it increases the resting metabolic rate and work of breathing (see Chapter 11).

Table 12-4   Respiratory quotients from the oxidation of various substrates

Substrate	RQ
Carbohydrate	1.0
Fat	0.7
Protein	0.8
Lipogenesis (an RQ > 1.0 indicates lipogenesis)	8.0

Effects of substrates on ventilation. The substrates burned (i.e., carbohydrate, fat, and protein) have effects independent of the total number of calories provided. The oxidation of these substrates requires O_2 and produces CO_2, H_2O, and energy. When each of these substrates is oxidized, there is a characteristic ratio of liters of CO_2 produced to liters of O_2 consumed. This ratio is called the *respiratory quotient* (RQ). The RQ for carbohydrate is 1.0, for fat is 0.7, and for protein is 0.8. The synthesis of fat from carbohydrate yields an RQ greater than 1.0. Thus more CO_2 is produced from the oxidation of carbohydrate than from an equal amount of fat or protein. Knowledge of the RQ can be used to aid in the nutritional support of patients with hypercapnic respiratory insufficiency. The maintenance of steady-state arterial blood CO_2 levels depends on the rate of CO_2 production and its efficiency of elimination. CO_2 production is increased in hypercatabolic conditions (e.g., trauma, burns, sepsis) and in patients who are being fed excessive carbohydrate calories. Excessive carbohydrate calories may precipitate ventilatory failure or prolong mechanical ventilation by increasing CO_2 production and the work of breathing to maintain a steady level of CO_2 in the arterial blood. Substituting fat for carbohydrate calories can help patients wean from or avoid mechanical ventilation by reducing CO_2 production. The synthesis of fat from excessive carbohydrate calories is also associated with the production of large amounts of CO_2. In patients with limited pulmonary reserves, this may also precipitate respiratory failure and CO_2 retention.

Data indicating that rapid infusion of intravenous lipid can impair pulmonary O_2 diffusion has created some concern over the use of lipid emulsions in patients with hypoxemic lung disease. However, this generally has not proved to be of clinical significance when the lipid is infused over 12 to 24 hours. The use of lipids as a fuel source also affects lung function because prostaglandins and leukotrienes formed from EFAs have the ability to affect bronchial and vascular smooth muscle function and alter immune response.

Indirect calorimetry. Indirect calorimetry is a method of determining caloric expenditure. The CO_2 and O_2 levels in inspired and expired air are measured and used to calculate the REE. Indirect calorimetry also provides a measure of substrate utilization as reflected in the RQ. Therefore the caloric prescription and substrate mix can be optimized (see Chapter 11).

Hypophosphatemia. Hypophosphatemia can have a profound effect on respiratory muscle function. Decreased 2,3-diphosphoglycerate levels in RBCs and diminished levels of ATP may complicate acute respiratory failure. Reduction in levels of these compounds impairs tissue oxygen delivery and respiratory muscle function. Hypophosphatemia also impairs diaphragmatic contractility. Therefore hypophosphatemia should be anticipated and vigorously treated (see Chapter 11).

Immune system. Immune system impairment is another adverse effect of malnutrition. Malnutrition is associated with decreased cell-mediated immunity, decreased immunoglobulin production, and defects in alveolar macrophage function. All these factors increase the risk of infections associated with pulmonary disease.

Management of nutritional support

Before nutritional support is initiated, the patient's metabolic and nutritional status should be assessed (see Chapters 9 and 10). The presence of sepsis or injury affects the metabolic and nutrient requirements. Nutritional support must be individualized to the metabolic state.

Total calories provided is one of the most important factors in adequate nutritional support. Generally, calories in the range of 1.0 to 1.5 × the BEE will be adequate. A marasmic patient should be refed slowly (see Chapter 11). When there is a question about actual caloric needs or the effect of nutritional support on gas exchange, indirect calorimetry is a useful test. In nonhypercapnic patients, calories may be distributed with 50% to 60% as carbohydrate, 20% to 30% as fat, and 15% to 20% as protein. In patients with CO_2 retention, a greater percentage of calories from fat can be prescribed. Reduction of the caloric intake to the level of the BEE for short periods of time may facilitate weaning from the ventilator, but this should be avoided in catabolic patients.

If weight gain is desired (e.g., in the marasmic patient) and the patient is stable and ambulatory, intake may be increased to 2 × the BEE as long as respiratory function is not impaired.

Fluid, electrolytes, protein, and micronutrient balance are other factors that should be monitored in patients with respiratory failure. Nutritional support can significantly reverse many of the metabolic, biochemical, and physiologic alterations found in respiratory insufficiency.

Summary

To provide the optimal support for the patients with respiratory failure, the following should be done:
- Perform a complete nutritional assessment.
- Evaluate and administer the proper number of calories (do not overfeed or underfeed).
- Check protein catabolic rate (i.e., measure 24-hour UUN), and ensure protein balance.
- Monitor fluid and electrolyte levels, especially phosphorus status.
- Evaluate vitamin and mineral status as indicated.
- In patients with hypercapnia, use high-fat feedings.

CRITICAL CARE

Various critical illnesses, such as those resulting from trauma or severe sepsis, share many metabolic and nutritional features. Whether septic or not, many critically ill patients exhibit a constellation of systemic inflammatory responses that impair immune function and tissue healing and can lead to dysfunction of the lungs, kidneys, and liver (multiple organ failure syndrome) and to prolonged hospitalizations and high mortality rates.

Metabolic response to injury and infection

The three major components of the metabolic response are: (1) hypermetabolism, (2) proteolysis and nitrogen loss, and (3) accelerated gluconeogenesis and glucose utilization. The degree of substrate mobilization is closely related to the extent and severity of the insult and is mediated through the release of cytokines and counterregulatory hormones. Tissue responsiveness to insulin is severely blunted. Regardless of the nutritional support, only when the critical illness has subsided do the hormone levels return to normal. Fig. 12-2 shows the increases in resting metabolism and nitrogen excretion that occur with various degrees of stress.

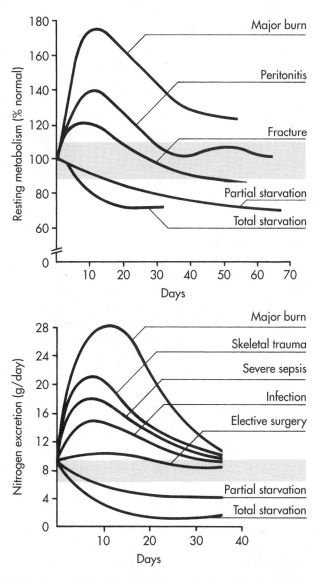

Fig. 12-2   Changes in metabolic rate and nitrogen excretion with physiologic stress. Normal ranges are indicated by shaded areas. (From Long CL, Schaffel N, Geiger JW, et al: Metabolic response to injury and illness: estimation of energy and protein needs from indirect calorimetry and nitrogen balance, *JPEN* 3:452, 1979.)

The stress response is systemic so that even when an injury is localized to one area of the body, increased oxygen consumption occurs throughout the body. Glucose is the major fuel used by injured tissues and by the cells involved in repair and immune processes. Proteolysis, which provides substrates for gluconeogenesis, is reflected in an increased UUN, which is derived largely from muscle. Hence, healing depends on the organism's ability to cannibalize its muscle protein to provide glucose by way of gluconeogenesis. Exogenous glucose administered to the critically ill patient produces little if any reduction in the rate of protein breakdown.

Without adequate nutritional support, profound weight loss and erosion of essential body compartments characterize critical illness. Lean body mass is the main component wasted, and this is accompanied by losses of potassium, phosphorus, magnesium, and zinc. Reduced circulating levels of proteins such as albumin and transferrin (or TIBC) occur. This is not necessarily an indication of malnutrition, but it reflects the severity of the stress and the magnitude of the nutritional support that may be needed. Only with adequate nutritional support and resolution of the stress can protein levels return to normal.

Nutritional support of the critically ill patient

The general principles of nutritional support require little alteration in critically ill patients. However, the advantages of enteral over parenteral nutrition are particularly important in these patients. Although it is not conclusively proven in humans, enteral feeding may maintain a healthier intestinal mucosa and thus help prevent the translocation of intestinal bacteria and toxins and reduce the risk of multiple organ failure syndrome. Given its other proven benefits, every effort should be made to feed critically ill patients enterally.

Nutrient requirements. The metabolic response to stress is essentially unaltered by nutritional support, but if sufficient nutrients are provided, the losses can be offset. The energy requirements of most injured or septic patients are in the range of 1.2 to 1.5 × their calculated BEE. Only in cases of extensive injury such as burns covering more than 40% of the body surface area (BSA) do energy requirements rise above this range. Energy needs for burned patients can be estimated as shown in Box 12-1.

Protein requirements should be calculated using the 24-hour UUN excretion. For patients with burn injury the UUN calculation can be modified as shown in Box 12-2 to account for protein lost directly through the skin.

The serum levels of many micronutrients decrease in critically ill patients because they are either consumed, excreted, or sequestered in the liver and reticuloendothelial system. Zinc and vitamins C and A should be amply supplied, whereas iron supplementation may increase the risk of infection by placing free iron in circulation and should usually be postponed until the stress has resolved and TIBC has risen to near-normal levels.

Specialized nutritional support. Much research has been done on developing nutritional formulas specially designed for critically ill patients. The amino acid glutamine, which is mobilized in large quantities from skeletal muscle and lung in critical illness, performs many functions including providing energy for

---

Box 12-1   Toronto formula for estimating 24-hour energy expenditure in burn patients (kcal/day)

$$-4343 + (10.5 \times \% \text{ TBSA}) + (0.23 \times \text{CI}) + (0.84 \times \text{BEE}) + (114 \times \text{temp}) - (4.5 \times \text{PBD})$$

where

TBSA = percent total body surface area burned (*whole number,* not decimal), estimated on admission and corrected, where needed, for amputation

CI   = number of calories received in the previous 24 hours, including all dextrose, TPN, and tube feeding

BEE = basal energy expenditure estimated by the Harris-Benedict equation

Temp = average of hourly rectal temperature in the previous 24 hours, ° C

PBD = number of days postburn on the *previous* day

From Allard JP, Pichard C, Hoshino E, et al: Validation of a new formula for calculating the energy requirements of burn patients, *JPEN* 14:115, 1990.

Box 12-2   Protein catabolic rate in burn patients (g/day)

$$[\text{UUN} + 4 + (0.2 \text{ g} \times \%3°) + (0.1 \text{ g} \times \%2°)] \times 6.25$$

where

UUN = measured urinary area nitrogen, in g

%3° = percent body surface area with third-degree (full-thickness) burns

%2° = percent body surface area with second-degree (partial-thickness) burns

---

enterocytes. Glutamine-enriched enteral formulas are commercially available, but their therapeutic role is not yet clear.

The knowledge that amino acids are more rapidly absorbed by the gastrointestinal tract when provided as small peptides rather than whole proteins has led some manufacturers to market enteral formulas containing such peptides. Several nutrients and dietary substances such as arginine, nucleotides, and fish oil have improved immune function and reduced infection rates in injured animals. A clinical trial of an enteral formula that contains these nutrients demonstrated a reduction in length of hospital stay and frequency of acquired infections in critically ill patients. Because of their high cost and lack of proven superiority in other patients, however, their use should be restricted to critically ill patients. Before committing to use any costly specialized formula, clinicians should require evidence of safety and efficacy from randomized, controlled clinical trials.

Monitoring the patient. The same parameters should be followed during the course of nutritional support of critically ill patients as in other patients, including body weight, adequacy of nutrient delivery, nitrogen balance, and serum albumin. Additional information is obtained from serial measurements of electrolytes, BUN, creatinine, phosphorus, magnesium, and anthropometric measurements.

NUTRITION, HIV INFECTION, AND AIDS
Two phases of the same disease

HIV chronically infects cells of the immune system. Classic HIV infection has two principal phases. Paradoxically, the initial phase of this ultimately fatal infection is largely asymptomatic. Infected individuals appear to be healthy, they maintain their normal body weight, and virus replication can be reduced substantially with antiviral drugs (such as zidovudine [AZT] and, more recently, viral protease inhibitors), thus slowing the progression of the disease. Later, after the infection has caused significant damage to the immune system, patients develop what has been termed the *acquired immunodeficiency syndrome,* or AIDS. AIDS is the second phase of HIV infection. It is characterized by repeated bouts of acute infection by a variety of opportunistic pathogens that, in the absence of HIV infection, would be easily controlled by a healthy immune system. This stage of the disease is dominated by infections, as well as increasingly severe direct manifestations of HIV infection, such as dementia. It is also characterized by the consequent development of malnutrition, with loss of body fat, loss of lean body mass, and decreased serum concentrations of a variety of micronutrients. As discussed below, the goals of nutritional support during HIV infection are determined by the stage of the disease.

Overview: goals of nutritional support during HIV infection

There are two principal goals of nutritional support during HIV infection:
1. Prevent the development of nutrient deficiencies that can impair immune function.
2. Prevent loss of lean body mass because this loss increases the risk of death in patients with AIDS.

These goals should be pursued through a systematic approach involving periodic nutritional assessment, dietary evaluation, and counseling by a dietitian. The concrete benefits of specific interventions have not yet been widely investigated for HIV infection, but results thus far in HIV patients, as well as in patients with other acute and chronic diseases, suggest that proper nutritional support will lengthen survival and enhance the quality of life.

Nutritional deficiencies and immune function

Protein-calorie malnutrition. Protein-calorie malnutrition (PCM) impairs the cell-mediated response to infection. HIV infection also impairs the cell-mediated immune response by specifically infecting and depleting T-helper cells (also known as CD4 cells), thus impairing the immune response to pathogens that are normally controlled by a T cell–mediated immune response. As HIV infection progresses to frank AIDS, peripheral blood CD4 cell concentrations decrease, indicating depletion of this pool of cells throughout the body. PCM also affects T cells and can independently diminish peripheral blood CD4 counts. During PCM in children, the T cell regions of the thymus and other lymphoid organs are specifically depleted. Thus fewer mature T cells are produced in the thymus and exported to peripheral blood and lymphoid tissue. Classic work done in the 1960s and 1970s in children with kwashiorkor and marasmus showed that the types of infections that are found in these children were often the same as the opportunistic infections that were later found to plague patients with AIDS in this country. These infections are caused by pathogens that are normally controlled by a T cell–mediated immune response. The list of such infections is long but includes *Pneumocystis carinii* pneumonia, oral candidiasis, herpes infections, and tuberculosis. The similar effects of PCM and AIDS on cell-mediated immunity suggest that the development of wasting malnutrition in patients with AIDS could exacerbate the already diminished T cell–mediated immune response. Correction of PCM can rapidly restore the cell-mediated immune response. In the case of acute PCM in children (kwashiorkor), provision of high-protein, high-energy foods and treatment of intercurrent infections can restore cell-mediated immunity within 1 week, as measured by delayed-type hypersensitivity skin test response to recall antigens. Thus prevention and treatment of wasting in AIDS patients can be expected to be of direct benefit in maintaining immune function.

Micronutrient deficiencies. As with PCM, micronutrient deficiencies can also impair the T cell–mediated immune response. In particular, deficiencies in vitamin A, zinc, and iron can impair cell-mediated immunity. Providing supplements to patients with documented deficiencies of these nutrients can restore immune function. The mechanisms by which these nutrients affect immune function differ. Iron is a transition metal that is a key component of cytochromes, which are important in cellular energy metabolism, and enzymes involved in cell proliferation and the immune response. Thus the metabolism and proliferation of lymphocytes is impaired by iron deficiency. Zinc is also a transition metal and is important in the activity of many enzymes, DNA-binding proteins, and the thymic hormone thymulin. Thus zinc deficiency impairs lymphocyte function by a number of mechanisms. Vitamin A specifically regulates the production of cytokines (molecules that regulate the immune response) by cells of the immune system. Vitamin A is required for the maintenance of normal, healthy mucosal epithelial surfaces, which are a first line of defense against pathogenic organisms in the respiratory, gastrointestinal, and urogenital tracts. Thus vitamin A deficiency can compromise two important aspects of host defenses. Deficiencies in antioxidant nutrients (e.g., vitamins E and C and selenium) can impair the immune response, presumably by allowing greater oxidative damage than would normally occur to cells of the immune system, thereby impairing immune function. Deficiencies in B complex vitamins such as folic acid can also compromise immune function because they function as cofactors in DNA synthesis. Without efficient DNA synthesis, the rapid production of the new lymphocytes that are needed during an immune response will be slowed, impairing the immune response.

HIV and the development of nutritional deficiencies

Body weight, particularly lean body mass, and biochemical indicators of nutritional status should be closely monitored during HIV infection. Weight loss, particularly sudden, rapid weight loss, is a poor prognostic indicator and is a common feature in AIDS. Rapid weight loss is usually associated with an opportunistic infection. However, even during periods when body weight is stable, care must be taken to maintain lean body mass and ensure that muscle is not being replaced by fat. This section first discusses the problems associated with measuring micronutrient status during HIV infection and then the mechanisms by which infection can adversely affect nutritional status.

Biochemical indicators of nutritional status. During the early stages of HIV infection before the development of AIDS, active virus replication occurs in lymph nodes. Such replication presumably triggers some aspects of the acute phase response, which can make serum markers of nutritional status difficult to interpret. This is particularly true for the micronutrients iron, zinc, copper, and vitamin A. Decreased serum levels of these micronutrients in otherwise healthy individuals indicate decreased body stores. Serum levels of iron, zinc, retinol, and retinol-binding protein (RBP; the transport protein for retinol) decrease during the acute phase response while serum copper levels increase. In addition, serum albumin and prealbumin (also known as *transthyretin*) may be decreased during the acute phase response. During the early stages of HIV infection when opportunistic infections have not yet begun and weight is stable, albumin levels should not be affected by HIV infection, although prealbumin, iron, zinc, copper, and retinol serum concentrations may be altered. During the acute phase response, the serum concentration of proteins involved in the body's response to infections (e.g., C-reactive protein) is elevated as a part of the systemic response to an infectious agent. Thus when the nutritional status of a patient with HIV infection or AIDS is being evaluated, low serum micronutrient concentrations (particularly retinol, iron, and zinc) may not indicate low body stores, particularly if serum markers of the acute phase response are elevated at the same time. It is possible, however, that decreased serum concentrations of some micronutrients during the acute phase response reflect decreased transport of these nutrients to peripheral tissues.

Decreased food intake. Maintaining food intake early in HIV infection is usually not a problem because the patient often feels well and can maintain a normal, active life. Basal metabolic rate is increased in such individuals, however, and at least one study indicates that food intake is not increased to compensate. However, voluntary physical activity appears to be slightly decreased, a compensation that maintains energy balance, thus preserving body weight. Decreased physical activity during this phase of HIV infection may eventually lead to loss of muscle mass. Such losses should be avoided because they are closely and independently associated with higher risk of death in patients with AIDS. In contrast to early HIV infection, food intake decreases dramatically during the acute febrile illnesses that occur during AIDS. This decreased intake is not accompanied by a decrease in BEE, which normally occurs during fasting in otherwise healthy children or adults. Thus decreased intake without any compensating decrease in basal metabolic rate is the primary reason for the precipitous loss in weight that accompanies the opportunistic infections of AIDS. The best way to prevent this weight loss is to prevent the opportunistic infections by using appropriate prophylactic drug regimens, and the best way to minimize the weight loss once an infection has developed is to treat the infection. Such treatment will also allow compensatory weight gain to begin as soon as the infection is controlled. Of all the interventions tested to prevent rapid weight loss during AIDS, the most effective has been to treat the infection. Nutritional interventions can prevent some loss of lean body mass during acute metabolic stress, but no intervention can totally prevent such loss. Decreased intake will also be a problem during oral infections, such as thrush or herpes, when lesions in the mouth and throat make eating painful. Nutritional counseling to maintain intake during such episodes (e.g., through making foods more palatable) is essential.

Decreased absorption. Early in HIV infection, malabsorption of fat and carbohydrates may occur, even in the absence of an obvious underlying cause such as diarrhea. This malabsorption may be due to HIV infection of the gastrointestinal tract. Decreased micronutrient, fat, and carbohydrate absorption are documented problems during and after diarrhea (and to a lesser extent during nonenteric infections) and will contribute to weight loss. Such malabsorption, along with decreased intake, appears to be a principal reason for the development of "slim disease" common in central African patients with AIDS.

Increased excretion. Nitrogen excretion as a result of net catabolism of muscle is part of the stereotypic response to metabolic stress, including infection and trauma. Loss of other nutrients resulting from increased excretion may occur. For example, retinol (bound to RBP) and zinc are excreted in the urine during severe metabolic stress, such as major surgery or serious infection. Urinary loss of these nutrients will thus be significant during some episodes of opportunistic infections but appear not to be a problem during early stages of HIV infection.

Increased requirements. Basal metabolic rate is increased during asymptomatic HIV infection. Thus energy requirements are increased slightly. To maintain stable body weight, energy intake must increase or voluntary activity must decrease. As discussed previously, it is important over the long term to maintain lean body mass. Thus patients with HIV infection should be educated as to how to maintain a proper, balanced diet, possibly with increased intake of high-protein, high-energy foods so that they can maintain normal levels of activity. It is possible that the requirements for some micronutrients may increase during HIV and other infections, but data for this are sparse. If basal metabolism is increased, requirements for certain nutrients like B vitamins and antioxidant nutrients such as vitamin C might be increased. This does not mean that nutritional supplements are required, but depending on the composition of the patient's diet, standard, RDA-level multivitamin and mineral supplements (replacement vitamins) may be recommended (see Chapter 1 and Appendix C). Such supplements provide approximately 100% of the RDA of most nutrients. Slightly higher levels of some nutrients (e.g., antioxidant nutrients such as vitamins E and C) may also be of benefit. Megadose supplements have not been demonstrated to be of value and are not recommended. Continued ingestion of doses substantially above the RDA for vitamin A and zinc should be discouraged and have been associated with shorter survival in one study of adult AIDS patients in the United States.

Altered metabolism. Altered metabolism accounts for the difficulties of relying on serum levels of iron, zinc, copper, and retinol during HIV and other infections, as discussed previously. Chronic inflammatory diseases that cause long-term perturbations in the metabolism of these nutrients can affect nutritional status. The best documentation of this is the anemia that can develop during chronic inflammatory diseases such as rheumatoid arthritis. This is apparently due to de-creased iron transport to erythrogenic tissue in favor of sequestering it in phago-cytic cells. This response is apparently beneficial during acute bacterial infections but detrimental during chronic inflammation. Other examples of altered micronu-trient metabolism are not so clearly beneficial or detrimental. Changes in energy utilization occur, including increased glucose utilization and decreased fatty acid oxidation, and are important factors during opportunistic infections. Protein me-tabolism is also dramatically altered during acute illness in that muscle tissue is ca-tabolized and acute phase proteins are synthesized in the liver. This results in a net negative nitrogen balance, which depletes lean body mass.

Prevention of micronutrient deficiencies and maintenance of lean body mass through nutrition education and intervention

Nutrition education and intervention should be an integral component of the pre-ventive health care planning and treatment of patients with HIV infection. This component of the medical care should be carried out by a physician or a regis-tered dietitian. Such care should begin immediately with the diagnosis of HIV in-fection and include a complete nutritional status assessment and identification of risk factors for malnutrition. This evaluation should include assessment of lean body mass as a benchmark against which to monitor subsequent changes in body weight and composition. Based on the initial and follow-up assessments, an indi-vidualized nutrition care plan can be developed to correct nutritional deficiencies and to address other risk factors for developing malnutrition. This plan should ad-dress healthful eating principles, food safety issues regarding foodborne pathogens (particularly important for those with HIV infection), and alternative feeding methods (e.g., use of nutritional supplements, tube feeding, and parenteral nutri-tion). Counseling should also address food fads and unproven nutritional ap-proaches that are often directed at patients with HIV infection. Finally, vigorous nutritional support strategies may become necessary when frank AIDS develops with bouts of opportunistic infections and may involve temporary use of oral nu-tritional supplements, enteral tube feeding, or parenteral nutrition. These inter-ventions are designed to minimize loss of lean body mass and recoup lean body mass lost to opportunistic infections. For example, use of gastrostomy tube sup-plementation in children with AIDS who were undergoing continued weight loss caused increases in body weight, and in the children who had the greatest increase in body weight, the risk of death during the next 40 months was reduced 2.8-fold. Thus maintenance of body weight, and particularly lean body mass, is crucial and should be the principal focus of nutritional support during AIDS. The guidelines briefly discussed here are outlined in the position paper from the American and Canadian Dietetics Associations listed in Suggested Readings at the end of this chapter.

Other strategies for prevention of loss of lean body mass during AIDS

Prevention and treatment of opportunistic infections. As discussed previ-ously, prevention and treatment of opportunistic infections is the most important factor in preventing rapid weight loss during AIDS. Prophylactic use of drugs to prevent infections and the development of effective drug regimens to treat infections has been the most important factor in prolonging the life of AIDS patients. A factor contributing to increased survival is maintenance of lean body mass above the critical level of 55% to 60% of ideal, below which death becomes a near certainty.

Increasing appetite. Megestrol acetate is a synthetic progestational agent that has been used in treatment of metastatic breast cancer and has been found to stimulate appetite and allow weight gain in anorectic patients. It has been evaluated in AIDS patients with weight loss and anorexia. Weight gain, increased appetite, and an enhanced sense of well-being have been reported. Studies differ on the composition of the resulting weight gain, variously reporting increased fat mass only and increased lean body mass. Thus the efficacy of megestrol acetate in improving lean body mass, and survival, is still under investigation. In addition, dronabinol, a synthetic form of an active ingredient in marijuana, is a proven antiemetic and has been shown to increase appetite and decrease nausea in AIDS patients with anorexia. Anorexia associated with weight loss in AIDS patients is an FDA-approved indication for dronabinol use.

Anabolic hormones. Human growth hormone is being tested to promote maintenance and recovery of lean body mass. Preliminary data indicate that protein catabolism can be reversed and gain of lean body mass promoted. Such effects have been seen in healthy subjects and HIV-infected individuals. The results of these short-term studies are promising, but data are not yet available on the long-term use of human growth hormone in AIDS patients.

DRUG-NUTRIENT INTERACTIONS

Numerous interactions can occur between drugs and nutrients or foods. Some are more significant than others and can result in adverse reactions to drugs, drug toxicity, or therapeutic failure of a drug regimen. Food can have a marked effect on drug effectiveness by increasing, decreasing, or simply delaying absorption. Food can also influence the rate of drug metabolism by either increasing or decreasing the production of drug-metabolizing enzymes or by influencing splanchnic-hepatic blood flow. For example, varying the protein/carbohydrate ratio in a diet, consuming a diet high in charcoal-broiled beef or cruciferous vegetables (cabbage, brussels spouts, etc.), or consuming grapefruit juice with certain medications all influence the metabolism of some drugs. Loss of therapeutic efficacy for a drug occurs when a food delays or prevents a drug from being absorbed or accelerates the rate of drug metabolism or elimination. A toxic reaction from a drug is possible when a food increases the absorption of a drug or prevents its metabolism or elimination. In general, drugs should not be taken with meals unless the drug causes significant gastrointestinal upset. Box 12-3 reviews the influence of food on drugs when they are taken together and provides recommendations concerning the administration times of these drugs.

Drugs that are inhibitors of monoamine oxidase, such as isocarboxazid, pargyline, phenelzine, and tranylcypromine, can produce a hypertensive crisis when taken in conjunction with high-tyramine-containing foods. The severity of the response is related to the drug dosage and the level of tyramine in the particular

Box 12-3   Drug-nutrient interactions

Nutrient effects on drugs

Decreased absorption
Avoid taking these drugs with food.
Take at least 1 hour before or 2 hours
after a meal:
  Alendronate
  Ampicillin
  Atenolol
  Azithromycin
  Captopril
  Cephalexin
  Cloxacillin
  Erythromycin stearate
  Furosemide
  Hydralazine
  Iron
  Isoniazid
  Levodopa/carbidopa
  Methotrexate
  Midazolam
  Penicillin G
  Penicillin V
  Propantheline
  Quinidine
  Tetracycline
  Zidovudine
  Zinc sulfate

Increased absorption
Food will alter the amount of the drug
absorbed; therefore the drug should be
taken at the same time(s) or way each
day:
  Atovaquoné
  Carbamazepine

  Diazepam
  Dicumarol
  Griseofulvin
  Labetalol
  Lithium
  Melphalan
  Methoxsalen
  Metoprolol
  Metronidazole
  Nitrofurantoin
  Phenytoin
  Propafenone
  Propranolol
  Spironolactone
  Sulfadiazine

Delayed absorption
Food will delay the absorption of these
drugs but not the overall amount
absorbed. These drugs should be taken
at least 1 hour before or 2 hours after a
meal:
  Acetaminophen
  Aspirin
  Cimetidine
  Doxycycline
  Hydrochlorothiazide
  Hydrocortisone
  Indomethacin
  Ketoprofen
  Pentobarbital
  Pentoxifylline
  Sulfisoxazole
  Suprofen
  Tocainide

food. Foods high in tyramine include pickled herring, beef or chicken liver, broad
beans, Chianti wines, beer, and cheese.

Drugs can induce nutritional deficiencies also. Nutrient deficiencies associated
with chronic drug intake can be due to decreased nutrient intake, malabsorption,
hyperexcretion of nutrients, increased nutrient catabolism, or impaired nutrient utilization. Whether or not a drug produces a clinically significant nutrient deficiency
depends on the level of depletion and whether or not the patient is predisposed to a
nutritional deficiency at the time of the drug exposure. The dose and duration of
use of the drug is very important in the drug's ability to induce a deficiency. Table
12-5 lists drugs that have been found to induce nutritional deficiencies.

Table 12-5   Drug effects on nutrients

Drug	Nutrient effect
ANTIINFECTIVE DRUGS	
Aminosalicylic acid	Decreased vitamin B_{12} absorption
	Decreased fat absorption
Amphotericin B	Hypokalemia, hypomagnesemia, and hyperkaluria
Capreomycin	Hypokalemia, hypomagnesemia, and hypocalcemia
Cycloserine	Decreased serum folate
Gentamicin, tobramycin, amikacin, and sisomicin	Hypokalemia, hypomagnesemia, hypocalcemia; increased urinary potassium and magnesium loss
Isoniazid	Pyridoxine deficiency
Neomycin	Decreased absorption of vitamin A, amino acids, fat, xylose, sucrose, lactose, calcium, potassium, and sodium
Pyrimethamine	Folate deficiency
Sulfasalazine	Decreased serum folic acid
ANTICOAGULANTS	
Warfarin, indanedione derivatives	Decreased vitamin K–dependent coagulation factors
CARDIOVASCULAR DRUGS	
Hydralazine	Pyridoxine deficiency
Sodium nitroprusside	Decreased levels of serum B_{12}
CENTRAL NERVOUS SYSTEM DRUGS	
Aspirin	Decreased total serum and protein-bound serum folate
	Decreased plasma, leukocyte, and platelet ascorbic acid levels
Phenytoin, phenobarbital, primidone, and carbamazepine	Decreased serum calcium, decreased serum 25-hydroxycholecalciferol
	Decreased serum folate
Phenytoin, barbiturates, and primidone	Decreased vitamin K–dependent coagulation factors (II, VII, IX, and X) in neonates
ELECTROLYTE DRUGS	
Potassium chloride slow release	Decreased vitamin B_{12} absorption
GASTROINTESTINAL DRUGS	
Aluminum hydroxide	Decreased serum phosphate
Cholestyramine	Decreased absorption of vitamins B_{12}, A, E, D, K, and folic acid; decreased fat absorption
Cimetidine	Decreased absorption of food-bound or protein-bound vitamin B_{12}
Mineral oil	Decreased absorption of vitamins A, D, E, and K
Sucralfate	Decreased serum phosphate

Continued

Table 12-5   Drug effects on nutrients—cont'd

Drug	Nutrient effect
HORMONES	
Oral contraceptives	Decreased serum folate
	Riboflavin deficiency
	Pyridoxine deficiency
Glucocorticoid steroids	Decreased serum 25-hydroxycholecalciferol, decreased serum calcium
OTHER AGENTS	
Colchicine	Increased fecal loss of sodium, potassium, fat, and nitrogen; decreased absorption of D-xylose and vitamin B_{12}
D-penicillamine	Pyridoxine deficiency
Methotrexate	Folate deficiency, decreased serum vitamin B_{12}, decreased D-xylose absorption

The active ingredient in the drug dosage formulation is usually the agent involved in drug-nutrient interactions. By contrast, sorbitol is used as a base in many liquid preparations and is generally not considered to be a pharmacologically active agent. It enhances the palatability of many medicinal preparations, improves the solution's stability, and does not crystallize like other syrup vehicles. It is also a "sugar-free" product that can be used as a substitute for sugar in diabetic patients, since it does not raise blood glucose levels. This presumably inert agent can induce osmotic diarrhea in patients receiving 20 to 30 g of sorbitol syrup (83%) or about 50 g of crystalline sorbitol. In many patients who are receiving enteral feedings, liquid drug preparations containing sorbitol are also given. Diarrhea developing while a patient is on tube feedings can be wrongly associated with the tube feeding instead of the sorbitol content of the liquid medicinal preparations. In the presence of a stool osmotic gap (stool osmotic gap = [stool osmolality] $-$ 2 $\times$ [stool Na^+ + stool K^+]) greater than 140 mmol/L, contributory osmotic medications or medication additives should be suspected as potential causes of diarrhea. Table 12-6 lists some common medications and their sorbitol content. Caution should be used in reviewing the sorbitol content of the medications listed. Sorbitol is an excipient, it is not an active agent, and its content is not listed on the label. When used as an excipient in drug products, drug manufacturers can change the sorbitol content in a product without disclosing it.

Table 12-6 Sorbitol content of selected drug preparations

Active ingredient	Dosage form	Brand name	Manufacturer	Sorbitol content (g/ml)	Sorbitol content per common dose of active ingredient
Acetaminophen		Generic	Roxane Laboratories, Inc.	0.35	7.1 g/650 mg
	Elixir	Tylenol	McNeil Pharmaceutical	<0.2	<4 g/650 mg
	Solution	Tylenol	McNeil Pharmaceutical	0	0 g/650 mg
Acetaminophen with codeine			Carnick Laboratories, Inc.	0.06	0.9 g/15 ml
			Roxane Laboratories, Inc.	0	0 g/15 ml
Aluminum hydroxide and magnesium carbonate	Suspension	Gaviscon	Marion Merrell Dow	0.073	1.1 g/15 ml
Aluminum hydroxide and magnesium hydroxide	Suspension	Maalox	Rhone-Poulene Rorer Pharmaceuticals	0.045	0.675 g/15 ml
		Maalox TC	Rhone-Poulene Rorer Pharmaceuticals	0.15	2.25 g/15 ml
		Maalox Plus Extra Strength	Rhone-Poulene Rorer Pharmaceuticals	0.1	1.5 g/15 ml
Amantadine	Solution	Symmetrel	Du Pont	0.72	7.2 g/100 mg
Aminocaproic acid	Syrup	Amicar	Lederle Laboratories	0.26	5.2 g/5 g
Aminophylline			Roxane Laboratories, Inc.	0.136	1.3 g/200 mg
Calcium carbonate	Suspension		Roxane Laboratories, Inc.	0.28	1.4 g/500 mg
Carbamazepine	Suspension	Tegretol	Ciba-Geigy	0.17	1.7 g/200 mg
Charcoal, activated	Syrup		Paddock Laboratories	0.4	48 g/25 g
Chloral hydrate	Syrup		UDL Laboratories	0.4	2 g/500 mg
			Roxane Laboratories, Inc.	0.14	0.7 g/500 mg
Chlorpromazine			Roxane Laboratories, Inc.	0.035	0.03 g/25 mg
Cimetidine	Solution	Tagamet	Smith Kline Beecham	0.5	2.5 g/300 mg
Codeine phosphate			Roxane Laboratories, Inc.	0.28	1.4 g/15 ml

Continued

Table 12-6   Sorbitol content of selected drug preparations—cont'd

Active ingredient	Dosage form	Brand name	Manufacturer	Sorbitol content (g/ml)	Sorbitol content per common dose of active ingredient
Dexamethasone		Hexadrol	Organon Inc.	0.51	3.86 g/0.75 mg
Diazepam	Solution		Roxane Laboratories, Inc.	0.24	1.84 g/0.75 mg
Diphenoxylate and atropine	Solution	Lomotil	Roxane Laboratories, Inc.	0.21	1.05 g/5 mg
			G.D. Searle	0.21	1.05 g/5 ml
Doxepin			Roxane Laboratories, Inc.	0.455	2.275 g/5 ml
Doxycycline		Vibramycin	Warner Chilcott Laboratories	0.257	1.93 g/75 mg
Furosemide		Lasix	Pfizer Laboratories	0.7	7 g/100 mg
			Hoechst-roussel Pharmaceuticals, Inc.	0.35	1.4 g/40 mg
Guaifenesin	Syrup		Roxane Laboratories, Inc.	0.49	0.49 g/40 mg
Hydroxyzine			Roxane Laboratories, Inc.	0.11	0.53 g/5 ml
Hydromorphone			Pfizer Laboratories	1.16	5.8 g/25 mg
Indomethacin		Dilaudid	Knoll Pharmaceuticals	0.13	2.6 g/4 mg
Lithium		Indocin	Merck Sharp & Dohme	0.35	1.75 g/25 mg
		Cibalith-S	Ciba Pharmaceutical Co.	0.77	3.86 g/300 mg
Methadone	Syrup		Roxane Laboratories, Inc.	0.54	2.7 g/300 mg
	Solution		Roxane Laboratories, Inc.	0.14	0.7 g/10 mg
Metoclopramide	Syrup		Roxane Laboratories, Inc.	0.28	2.8 g/10 mg
		Reglan	Wyeth-Ayerst Laboratory	0.35	3.5 g/10 mg
			Warner Chilcott Laboratory	0.42	4.2 g/10 mg
Milk of magnesia			Roxane Laboratories, Inc.	0.2	6.09 g/30 ml
Milk of magnesia with cascara			Roxane Laboratories, Inc.	0.11	0.53 g/5 ml
Minocycline		Minocin	Lederle Laboratories	0.1	1.03 g/100 mg
Molindone	Concentrate	Moban	Du Pont Multisource Products	0.26	0.65 g/50 mg
Nalidixic acid		NegGram	Winthrop Pharmaceuticals	0.7	7 g/500 mg

Table 12-6   Sorbitol content of selected drug preparations—cont'd

Active ingredient	Dosage form	Brand name	Manufacturer	Sorbitol content (g/ml)	Sorbitol content per common dose of active ingredient
Nortriptyline		Aventyl	Eli Lilly and Co.	0.64	8 g/25 mg
Oxybutynin	Syrup	Ditropan	Marion Merrell Dow	0.26	1.3 g/5 mg
Perphenazine	Solution	Trilafon	Schering Laboratories	0.2	0.5 g/4 mg
Potassium chloride	Solution		UDL Laboratories	0.18	0.45 g/10 mEq
Propranolol			Roxane Laboratories, Inc	0.63	3.15 g/20 mg
Pseudoephedrine	Syrup	Sudafed	Burroughs Wellcome	0.35	1.75 g/30 mg
Pseudoephedrine and triproli-dine	Syrup	Actifed	Burroughs Wellcome	0.49	2.45 g/5 ml
Pyridostigmine	Syrup	Mestinon	ICN Pharmaceuticals	0.14	0.7 g/60 mg
Ranitidine	Syrup	Zantac	Glaxo Pharmaceuticals	0.1	1 g/150 mg
Sodium polystyrene sulfonate	Suspension		Roxane Laboratories, Inc.	0.235	14.7 g/15 g
Sulfamethoxazole		Gantanol	Roche Laboratories	0.143	0.72 g/500 mg
Tetracycline	Suspension	Sumycin	Bristol-Myers Squibb	0.23	2.3 g/250 mg
Theophylline		Slo-Phyllin 80	Rorer Pharmaceuticals	0.4	3.7 g/300 mg
			Roxane Laboratories, Inc.	0.455	25.6 g/300 mg
		Aerolate	Fleming and Co.	0.304	9.12 g/300 mg
Thiabendazole		Mintezol	Merck Sharp & Dohme	0.28	1.4 g/500 mg
Thiothixene		Navane	Roerig	0.6	0.6 g/5 mg
			Lemmon Company	0.5	0.5 g/5 mg
Trihexyphenidyl	Syrup	Artane	Lederle Laboratories	0.83	4.15 g/2 mg
Valproate sodium	Solution	Depakene	Abbott Laboratories	0.15	1.5 g/250 mg
Vitamin E		Aquasol E	Astra Pharmaceutical Products	0.2	0.04 g/10 IU

SUGGESTED READINGS

Renal failure

Avram MM, Goldwasser P, Erroa M, et al: Predictors of survival in continuous ambulatory peritoneal dialysis patients: the importance of prealbumin and other nutritional and metabolic markers, *Am J Kidney Dis* 23:91-98, 1994.

Bergström J: Why are dialysis patients malnourished? *Am J Kidney Dis* 26:229-241, 1995.

Bergström J, Lindholm B: Nutrition and adequacy of dialysis: how do hemodialysis and CAPD compare? *Kidney Int Suppl* 43(Suppl 40):S39-50, 1993.

Consensus Development Conference Panel: Morbidity and mortality of renal dialysis: an NIH Consensus Conference statement, *Ann Intern Med* 121:62-70, 1994.

D'Amico G, Gentile MG: Effects of dietary manipulation on the lipid abnormalities and urinary protein loss in nephrotic patients, *Mineral & Electrolyte Metabolism* 18(2-5):203-6, 1992.

Goldwasser P, Mittman M, Antignani A, et al: Predictors of mortality on hemodialysis, *J Am Soc Nephrol* 3:1613-1622, 1993.

Hruska K, Teitelbaum S: Renal osteodystrophy, *N Engl J Med* 333:166-174, 1995 (review article).

Ikizler TA, Wingard RI, Hakim RM: Interventions to treat malnutrition in dialysis patients: the role of the dose of dialysis, intradialytic parenteral nutrition, and growth hormone, *Am J Kidney Dis* 26:256-265, 1995.

Klahr S, Levey AS, Beck GJ, et al: The effects of dietary protein restriction and blood pressure control on the progression of chronic renal disease, *N Engl J Med* 330:877, 1994.

Kopple JD: Nutrition, diet, and the kidney. In Shils ME, Olson JA, Shike M, editors: *Modern nutrition in health and disease,* ed 8, Philadelphia, 1994, Lea & Febiger.

Nygard O, Vollset SE, Refsum H, et al: Total plasma homocysteine and cardiovascular risk profile. The Hordaland Homocysteine Study, *JAMA* 274:1526-1533, 1995.

Oldrizzi L, Rugiu C, Maschio G: Nutrition and the kidney: how to manage patients with renal failure, *Nutrition in Clinical Practice* 9:3-10, 1994.

Owen WF, Lew NL, Liu Y, et al: The urea reduction ratio and serum albumin concentration as predictors of mortality in patients undergoing hemodialysis, *N Engl J Med* 329, 1993.

Pedrini MT, Levey AS, Lau J, et al: The effect of dietary protein restriction on the progression of diabetic and nondiabetic renal diseases: a meta-analysis, *Ann Intern Med* 124:627-632, 1996.

Sanders HN, Rabb H, Bittle P, et al: Nutritional implications of recombinant human erythropoietin therapy in renal disease, *J Am Diet Assoc* 94:1023-1029, 1994.

Nutrition and liver disease

Buchmiller CE, Kleiman-Wexler R, Ephagrave KS, et al: Liver dysfunction and energy source: results of a randomized clinical trial, *JPEN* 17:301-306, 1993.

Doweiko JP, Nompleggi DJ: The role of albumin in human physiology and pathophysiology, *JPEN* 15:207-211, 1989.

Ito Y, Shils ME: Liver dysfunction associated with long-term total parenteral nutrition in patients with massive bowel resection, *JPEN* 15:271-276, 1991.

Keaarns PJ, Young, H, Garua G, et al: Accelerated improvement of alcoholic liver disease with enteral nutrition, *Gastroenterology* 102:200-205, 1992.

Koehn V, Beranrd B, et al: Prevalence of malnutrition in alcoholic and nonalcoholic medical inpatients: a comparative anthropometrics study, *JPEN* 17:35-40, 1993.

Korsten MA, Lieber CS: Nutrition in pancreatic and liver disorders. In Shils ME, Olson JA, Shike M, editors: *Modern nutrition in health and disease,* ed 8, Philadelphia, 1994, Lea & Febiger.

Loguercio C, Sva E, Marmo E, et al: Malnutrition in cirrhotic patients: anthropometric measurements as a method of assessing nutritional status, *Br J Clin Pract* 44:98-101, 1990.

Marchesini G, Dioguardi FS, Bianchi GP, et al: Long-term branched-chain amino acid treatment in chronic hepatic encephalopathy, *J Hepatol* 11:92-101, 1991.

McCullough AJ, Mullen KD, Kalhan SL: Measurements of total body and extracellular water in cirrhotic patients with and without ascites, *Hepatology* 14:1102-1111, 1991.

Mendenhall CL, Moritz TE, Roselle GA, et al: A study of oral nutritional support with oxandrolone in malnourished patients with alcoholic hepatitis: results of a Department of Veterans Affairs Cooperative Study, *Hepatology* 17:564-568, 1993.

Muller MJ, Lantz HU, Logmann B, et al: Energy expenditure and substrate oxidation in patients with cirrhosis: the impact of cause, clinical staging and nutritional state, *Hepatology* 15:782-794, 1992.

Nompleggi DJ, Bonkovsky HL: Nutrition supplementation in chronic liver disease. An analytical review, *Hepatology* 19:518-533, 1994.

Nutritional status in cirrhosis. Italian multicentre cooperative project on nutrition in liver cirrhosis, *J Hepatol* 21:317-325, 1994.

Quigley EMM, Marsh MN, Shaffer JL, et al: Hepatobiliary complications of total parenteral nutrition, *Gastroenterology* 104:286-301, 1993.

Quigley EMM, Zetterman RK: Hepatobiliary complications of malnutrition and malabsorption, *Semin Liver Dis* 8:218-228, 1988.

Robertson JFR, Garden OJ, Shenkin A: Intravenous nutrition and hepatic dysfunction, *JPEN* 10:172-176, 1986.

Nutrition and the pancreas

Balthazar EJ, Feeny PC, vanSonnenber E: Imaging and intervention in acute pancreatitis, *Radiology* 193:297-306, 1994.

Bodoky G, Harsanyi L, Pap AM, et al: Effect of enteral nutrition on exocrine pancreatic function, *Am J Surg* 161:144-148, 1991.

Brandley EL III: A clinically based classification system for acute pancreatitis: summary of the international symposium on acute pancreatitis, *Arch Surg* 128:586-590, 1993.

Layer, P, Yamamoto H, Kalthoff L, et al: The different courses of early and late onset idiopathic and alcoholic pancreatitis, *Gastroenterology* 107:1481-1487, 1994.

Marulendra S, Kirby D: Nutrition support in pancreatitis, *Nutrition in Clinical Practice* 10:45-53, 1995.

Soergel KH: Acute pancreatitis. Sleisenger MH, Fortrand JS, editors: *Gastrointestinal diseases: pathophysiology/diagnostic management, vol 2,* ed 5, Philadelphia, 1993, WB Saunders.

Nutrition and inflammatory bowel disease

Afdhal NH, Kelly J, McCormick PA, et al: Remission induction in refractory Crohn's disease using a high calorie whole diet, *JPEN* 13:362-365, 1989.

American Society for Parenteral and Enteral Nutrition Board of Directors: Guidelines for the use of parenteral and enteral nutrition in adult and pediatric patients, *JPEN* 17(suppl):1SA-52SA, 1993.

Chan ATH, Fleming CR, O'Fallon WM, et al: Estimated versus measured basal energy requirements in patients with Crohn's disease, *Gastroenterology* 91:75-78, 1989.

Fernandez-Banares F, Cabre E, Esteve-Comas M, et al: How effective is enteral nutrition in inducing clinical remission in active Crohn's disease? A metanalysis of the randomized trials, *JPEN* 19:356-364, 1995.

Fleming CR: Nutrition in patients with Crohn's disease: another piece of the puzzle, *JPEN* 19:93-94, 1995.

Greenberg GR, Fleming CR, Jeejeebhoy KN, et al: Controlled trial of bowel rest and nutritional support in the management of Crohn's disease, *Gut* 29:1309-1315, 1988.

Guidelines for the use of parenteral and enteral nutrition in adult and pediatric patients with IBD, *JPEN* 17:1SA-52SA, 1993.

Lindor KD, Fleming CR, Burnes JU, et al: A randomized, prospective trial comparing a defined formula diet, corticosteroids, and a defined formula diet plus corticosteroids in active Crohn's disease, *Mayo Clin Proc* 101:881-888, 1992.

Malchow H, Steinhardt HJ, Lovenz-Meyer H, et al: Feasibility and effectiveness of a defined-formula diet regimen in treating active Crohn's disease, *Scand J Gastroenterol* 25:235-244, 1990.

Meguid MM, Muscaritoli M: Current uses of total parenteral nutrition, *Am Fam Physician* 47:383-394, 1993.

Royall D, Greenberg GR, Allard JP, et al: Total enteral nutrition support improves body composition of patients with active Crohn's disease, *JPEN* 19:95-99, 1995.

Rosenberg IH, Mason JB: Inflammatory bowel disease. In Shils ME, Olson JA, Shike M, editors: *Modern nutrition in health and disease,* ed 8, Philadelphia, 1994, Lea & Febiger.

Sax HC, Souba WW: Enteral and parenteral feeding: guidelines and recommendations, *Med Clin North Am* 5:863-880, 1993.

Sitrin MD: Nutrition support in inflammatory bowel disease, *Nutrition in Clinical Practice* 7:53-60, 1992.

Stokes MA, Hill GL: Total energy expenditure in patients with Crohn's disease: measurement by the combined body scan technique, *JPEN* 17:3-7, 1993.

Nutrition and celiac sprue

Connon JJ: Celiac disease. In Shils ME, Olson JA, Shike M, editors: *Modern nutrition in health and disease,* ed 8, Philadelphia, 1994, Lea & Febiger.

Egan LJ, Walsh SV, Stevens FM, et al: Celiac-associated lymphoma. A single institution experience of 30 cases in the combination chemotherapy ear, *J Clin Gastroenterol* 21:123-129, 1995.

Saltzman JR, Clifford BD: Identification of the triggers of celiac sprue (review), *Nutrition Reviews* 52:317-319, 1994.

Schultz SM, Stroebel J, Shutz EM, et al: Celiac sprue. Diagnosis and diet; keys to recovery, *North Carolina Medical Journal* 55:32-36, 1994.

Stegna-Guidetti C, Grosso S, Bruno M, et al: Comparison of serum anti-gliadin, anti-endomysium, and anti-jejunum antibodies in adult celiac sprue, *J Clin Gastroenterol* 20:17-21, 1995.

Trier JS: Celiac sprue, *N Engl J Med* 325:1709-1719, 1991.

Vazquez H, Sugai E, Pedreira S, et al: Screening for asymptomatic celiac sprue in families, *J Clin Gastroenterol* 21:130-133, 1995.

Nutrition and pulmonary disease

Annemie M, Schols WJ, Soeters PB, et al: Physiologic effects of nutritional support and anabolic steroids in patients with chronic obstructive pulmonary disease. A placebo-controlled randomized trial, *Am J Respir Crit Care Med* 152:1268-1274, 1995.

Chin R, Haponik E: Nutrition, respiratory function, and disease. In Shils ME, Olson JA, Shike M, editors: *Modern nutrition in health and disease,* ed 8, Philadelphia, 1994, Lea & Febiger.

DeMeo MT, Van De Graaf W, Gottlieb K, et al: Nutrition in acute pulmonary disease, *Nutr Rev* 50:320-328, 1992.

Donahoe M, Mancino J, Constantino J, et al: The effect of an aggressive nutritional support regimen on body composition in patients with severe COPD and weight loss, *Am J Respir Crit Care Med* 149:A3-13, 1994.

Engelen MA, Schols AM, Baken WC, et al: Nutritional depletion in relation to respiratory and peripheral skeletal muscle function in an outpatient population with chronic obstructive pulmonary disease, *Eur Respir J* 7:1793-1797, 1994.

Laaban JP, Kouchakji B, Dore MF, et al: Nutritional status in patients with chronic obstructive pulmonary disease and acute respiratory failure, *Chest* 103:1362-1357, 1993.

McClave S, Snider HL: Use of indirect calorimetry in clinical nutrition, *Nutrition in Clinical Practice* 7:5, 1992.

McMahon MM, Farnell MB, Murray MJ: Nutritional support of critically ill patients, *Mayo Clin Proc* 68:911-920, 1993.

Rochester DF, Braun NMT: Determinants of maximal inspiratory pressure in chronic obstructive pulmonary disease, *Am Rev Respir Dis* 132:42-47, 1995.

Talpers SS, Romberg DJ, Bunce SB, et al: Nutrition associated increase carbon dioxide production. Excess total calories vs high proportion of carbohydrate calories, *Chest* 102:551-555, 1992.

Wilson DO, Rogers RM, Wright E, et al: Body weight in chronic obstructive pulmonary disease, *Am Rev Respir Dis* 139:1435-1438, 1989.

Critical care

Bower RH, Cerra FB, Bershadsky B, et al: Early enteral administration of a formula (Impact®) supplemented with arginine, nucleotides, and fish oil in intensive care unit patients: results of a multicenter, prospective, randomized, clinical trial, *Crit Care Med* 23:436, 1995.

Souba WW, Wilmore DW: Diet and nutrition in the care of the patient with surgery, trauma, and sepsis. In Shils ME, Olson JA, Shike M, editors: *Modern nutrition in health and disease,* ed 8, Philadelphia, 1994, Lea & Febiger.

Torosian MH, editor: *Nutrition for the hospitalized patient,* New York, 1995, Marcel Dekker.

Nutrition, HIV infection, and AIDS

Anonymous: Position of the American Dietetic Association and the Canadian Dietetic Association: nutrition intervention in the care of persons with human immunodeficiency virus infection (published erratum appears in *J Am Diet Assoc* 94:1254, 1994 (review), *J Am Diet Assoc* 94:1042-1045, 1994.

Grunfeld C: What causes wasting in AIDS? *N Engl J Med* 333:123-124, 1995 (editorial; comment).

Macallan DC, Noble C, Baldwin C, et al: Energy expenditure and wasting in human immunodeficiency virus infection (see comments), *N Engl J Med* 333:83-88, 1995.

Miller TL, Awnetwant EL, Evans S, et al: Gastrostomy tube supplementation for HIV-infected children, *Pediatrics* 96:696-702, 1995.

Semba RD, Caiaffa WT, Graham NM, et al: Vitamin A deficiency and wasting as predictors of mortality in human immunodeficiency virus-infected injection drug users (see comments), *J Infect Dis* 171:1196-1202, 1995.

Tang AM, Graham NM, Saah AJ: Effects of micronutrient intake on survival in human immunodeficiency virus type 1 infection, *Am J Epidemiol* 143:1244-1256, 1996.

Von Roenn JH, Armstrong D, Kotler DP, et al: Megestrol acetate in patients with AIDS-related cachexia (see comments). *Ann Intern Med* 121:393-399, 1994.

Drug/nutrient interactions

Grapefruit juice interactions with drugs, *Med Lett Drugs Ther* 37:73-74, 1995.

Johnston KR, Govel LA, Andritz MH: Gastrointestinal effects of sorbitol as an additive in liquid medications, *Am J Med* 97:185-191, 1994.

Kirk JK: Significant drug-nutrient interactions, *Am Fam Physician* 51:1175-1182, 1995.

Lutomski DM, Gora ML, Wright SM, et al: Sorbitol content of selected oral liquids, *Ann Pharmacother* 27:269-273, 1993.

Williams L, David JA, Lowenthal DT: The influence of food on the absorption and metabolism of drugs, *Med Clin North Am* 77:815-829, 1993.

13

Case Studies

Protein-Calorie Malnutrition

Patient A is a 52-year-old woman with a 4-year history of weight loss and fatty stools. She formerly weighed 56 kg but now weighs 41 kg and is 165 cm tall (less than 75% of standard weight-for-height). After a "normal" meal, she frequently experiences cramping and greasy, foul-smelling stools. She denies having fever, bloody stools, or other complicating illnesses. She has been admitted to the hospital and has had minimal food intake over the past several days (Fig. 13-1, *A* and Plate 23, *A*).

Patient B is a 68-year-old male smoker with previously stable chronic lung disease and bronchitis. He has no history of weight loss or significant illness. Before admission, he had sudden onset of fever, chills, and respiratory failure, which necessitated hospitalization and mechanical ventilatory support. His problems include septic shock (circulatory collapse resulting from severe infection) and respiratory failure. His weight is 63 kg; his height is 175 cm. He has been in the hospital for 2 weeks without appreciable nutrient intake (Fig. 13-1, *B* and Plate 23, *B*).

Decide whether the numbered statements below refer to Patient A, Patient B, both, or neither.

1. Likely to have a reduced metabolic rate (resting energy expenditure)
2. Likely to excrete 15 g/day UUN (normal is < 5 g with recent low intake of protein)
3. Likely to have marked elevation of circulating epinephrine
4. Likely to excrete less than 600 mg creatinine per day in the urine (normal 800 to 1800 mg)
5. Likely to have a serum albumin level of 1.8 g/dl (normal > 3.5)
6. Likely to have a triceps skinfold measurement at 20% of standard
7. Probably relatively well adapted to the energy-deprived state
8. Particularly susceptible to heart failure on refeeding with carbohydrate

Nutritional Assessment and Support

A 63-year-old woman was hospitalized for therapy of cervical cancer. She consumed a diet consisting primarily of cornbread, grits, mustard greens (cooked by boiling for several hours), and cereals. She denied eating fresh fruit or vegeta-

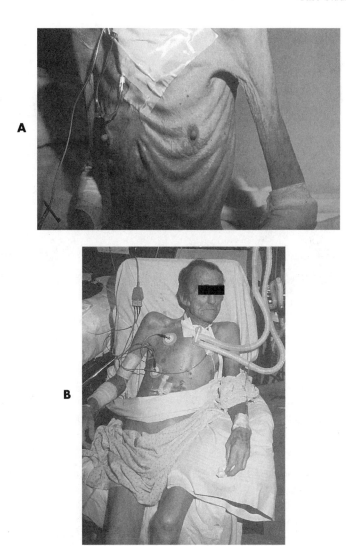

Fig. 13-1   A, Patient A: history of weight loss. **B,** Patient B: history of respiratory failure. ▲

bles, and she had no teeth. Her appetite was poor, and her weight fell from 54 kg to 47 kg over the past 2 months.

In the hospital, she ate relatively little and was maintained only on intravenous saline solutions. Five days after undergoing total pelvic exenteration (removal of lower abdominal organs as treatment for the cancer), she was noted to have bloody fluid leaking from an evidently poorly healing surgical wound (Fig. 13-2 and Plate 24).

Physical examination. There was easy and painless hair pluckability. There were perifollicular petechiae (pinpoint hemorrhages around hair follicles) over the lower extremities, large areas of bleeding into the skin at needle puncture sites,

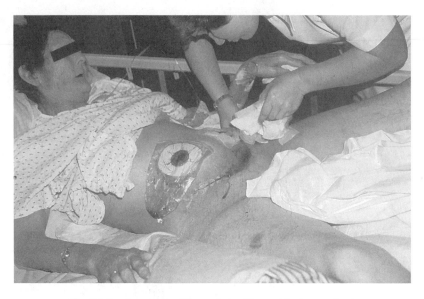

Fig. 13-2   A woman with poorly healing surgical wound. ▲

and widespread pitting edema. Her temperature was elevated at 39.5° C. Weight was 63 kg, height 150 cm (reference ideal weight is 47 kg).

Laboratory data. She had a severely reduced lymphocyte count (120 cells/mm^3), BUN of 6 mg/dl, and serum albumin of 2 g/dl. 24-hour UUN excretion was 16 g.

TRUE or FALSE:

1. On oral examination, the physician would be likely to find swollen, bleeding gums.
2. She has a clear case of kwashiorkor.
3. She is most likely obese.
4. The low BUN in this case suggests that her recent intake of protein was relatively low and possibly inadequate.
5. A reasonable estimate of her protein needs (i.e., amount needed to be in protein balance) is 185 g/day.
6. Glucose is the only endogenously produced fuel that can be used by this patient's damaged, unoxygenated tissues.

Because of poor oral intake of food and gastric retention on nasogastric tube feeding, central venous alimentation was instituted. The regimen included 500 g dextrose, 100 g protein, 2.5 mg zinc, and routine amounts of electrolytes and vitamins infused continuously over each 24-hour period.

TRUE or FALSE:

7. The glucose content of the parenteral alimentation fluids will effectively decrease protein breakdown to a basal (nonstress) level.

8. An intravenous source of essential fatty acids will not be required in this case, even if none are taken by mouth, because her fat reserves should adequately supply her needs for a number of months.
9. She will be receiving 1700 kcal/day from dextrose.
10. She should be given a larger amount of zinc.

See Appendix A for answers and discussion.

Appendix

A

Case Study Answers

Obesity

1. *False.* There is no question that some individuals (perhaps including this patient) are *predisposed* to greater weight gain because of their hereditary background. However, to date there is no evidence that genetic factors are the sole or even primary cause of obesity generally seen in humans. Regardless of genetic predisposition, whether or not someone becomes obese appears to be the direct result of dietary and physical activity patterns.

2. *False.* As is true with essentially all overweight individuals, REE tends to be higher, not lower, than in their lean counterparts. The reason is that higher body weights are associated with greater amounts of lean body mass, since more muscle and organ tissue is required to support (structurally and metabolically) the increased adipose mass, and REE is determined primarily by the absolute amount of lean body mass. Corrected for the amount of lean body mass, her REE will be similar to that of lean women her height and age.

3. *False.* It is possible that she could have a neuroendocrine cause for her obesity, but playing the odds, it is unlikely—for two reasons. One, less than 1% of overweight persons are found to have a neuroendocrine disorder; two, among such causes, marked degrees of obesity (as in this case) are even less likely to occur.

4. *True.* Her pattern of fat distribution would be classified as android or "apple" shaped. Compared with other women of the same body weight who have a gynecoid fat pattern, the presence of increased visceral or intraabdominal adipose tissue places her at greater risk for hypertension, insulin resistance, diabetes, dyslipidemia, and coronary heart disease.

5. *True.* Total cholesterol, LDL-C, and triglycerides tend to be higher, and HDL-C lower, in obese persons. Obesity can contribute to dyslipidemia by increasing secretion of VLDL, which is followed by an increased conversion of VLDL to LDL. Weight reduction, *when sustained,* is expected to have beneficial effects on the lipoprotein profile and, in turn, cardiovascular disease risk.

Hyperlipidemia

1. *False.* Using the equation LDL-C = TC − TG/5 − HDL-C, his calculated LDL-C level is 163 mg/dl, which is in the "high risk" category.

2. *True.* All patients with total cholesterol levels greater than 240 mg/dl or HDL-C levels less than 35 mg/dl or both, and those with total cholesterol between 200 and 239 mg/dl and with two risk factors for CHD should have lipoprotein levels measured. He fits the latter criteria (i.e., his total cholesterol is greater than 200 and he has two risk factors for CHD).

3. *True.* Secondary causes of high LDL-C levels should certainly be considered and ruled out if strongly suspected. Such secondary causes include diabetes mellitus, hypothyroidism, nephrotic syndrome, and cholestatic liver disease. Although medications such as anabolic steroids, thiazide diuretics, and β-blockers should also be considered, this patient admits to taking no medications.

4. *True.* Homocysteine is an amino acid produced by the demethylation of methionine, an essential amino acid derived primarily from animal protein. Folic acid is involved in recycling homocysteine back to methionine, and even a marginal deficiency of folic acid can result in elevated homocysteine levels. High levels of homocysteine appear to increase risk of CHD. This patient's dietary habits contribute to hyperhomocysteinemia in that he has a high intake of meat (a rich source of methionine) and a poor intake of folic acid (found in fruits and vegetables).

5. *False.* His diet would certainly be improved with a decrease in saturated fat. However, the goal should not be to *replace* all of his saturated fat with polyunsaturated fat. Recall that no population has ever consumed high amounts of polyunsaturated fat for long periods with proven safety. Rather, his aim should be to *reduce* his total fat intake (which is excessive) and to partially replace it with carbohydrates (such as whole grains, unrefined starches, fruits, and vegetables) and monounsaturated fat (such as olive oil).

6. *True.* Regular physical activity can increase HDL-C levels by 5% to 15%. It can also lower triglycerides, enhance insulin sensitivity, and reduce risk for hypertension and obesity. He is particularly likely to benefit from increased activity, since the greatest health benefits seem to accrue to physically inactive people who introduce some physical activity into their daily lives.

7. *False.* On the basis of current evidence, nondrinkers (as is this patient) and even established light or moderate drinkers should *not* be advised to increase their alcohol consumption to reduce their CHD risk. Alcohol intake carries with it other health risks.

CASE
STUDY **3**   *Alcohol and Nutrient Deficiencies*

1. *False.* Hypersegmented neutrophils are not associated with vitamin C deficiency but are a classic manifestation of folate or vitamin B_{12} deficiency.

2. *False.* The RDA for riboflavin for this person is 1.6 mg/day. His riboflavin intake from milk alone will be at least this amount.

3. *True.* Alcohol is known to decrease the absorption of thiamin. Ethanol intake of 1.5 to 2 g/kg body weight has been shown to decrease absorption by 40%.

4. *False.* Although there is some evidence to suggest a decrease in the production of intrinsic factor and hence a decrease in vitamin B_{12} absorption with alcohol intake, the clinical relevance is unclear. The more likely explanation for these hematologic abnormalities is folate deficiency, which is not uncommonly seen in alcoholism (up to 90%) because of poor intake and impaired absorption and utilization.

5. *True.* The history of alcohol abuse; the poor dietary intake; the use of antacids (which decrease thiamin absorption); and the clinical manifestations of Korsakoff's psychosis, ataxia, weakness, and peripheral neuropathy are all compatible with thiamin deficiency.

6. *False.* Although there is increased risk of pellagra in alcoholics, this is still uncommonly seen in the United States, and this patient has no clinical manifestations of pellagra (recall the four Ds: dementia, diarrhea, dermatitis, and death).

7. *False.* Although alcoholics may have increased iron loss from bleeding, iron deficiency is not often seen in this group because of increased absorption of iron, bone-marrow suppression (reducing requirements), and the presence of iron in certain alcoholic beverages such as red wine. In this patient, there is no hematologic evidence of iron deficiency such as microcytic (small-celled) anemia. The slick tongue that occurs as a result of iron deficiency may be seen rarely, but it is more likely due to folate deficiency in this case.

8. *False.* His diet is certainly low in vitamin C. However, without laboratory documentation or clinical evidence of scurvy such as unemerged coiled hairs, perifollicular petechiae, gum changes, and so on, it would be impossible to make the diagnosis.

9. *False.* Renal excretion of zinc is increased by alcohol intake, and zinc deficiency is more common in the alcoholic. However, without laboratory confirmation or clinical manifestations such as altered sense of taste or smell, dry scaly skin, or reduced wound healing, the diagnosis cannot be confirmed.

CASE
STUDY **4**   *Malabsorption Syndrome*
___

1. *False.* Normally, a low serum carotene level is indicative of a poor intake of green and yellow-orange fruits and vegetables (sources of carotene, the provitamin form of vitamin A). On the other hand, since carotene is fat soluble, fat malabsorption often results in a low serum carotene level, regardless of the amount eaten.

2. *False.* Even in cases of significant fat malabsorption, vitamin C intake and absorption are often adequate. Intake in this case appears to be good, and there is no clear evidence of vitamin C deficiency. Bleeding into the skin is not a finding specific for vitamin C deficiency, in contrast to perifollicular petechiae (pinpoint hemorrhages around hair follicles).

3. *True.* In light of this history, which is compatible with fat malabsorption, this patient has an increased risk of fat-soluble vitamin deficiency, includ-

ing vitamin K deficiency. In most instances, however, vitamin K deficiency does not actually develop because vitamin K is still produced by the flora of the large intestine. In this case, use of oral antibiotics may have suppressed the intestinal flora, thereby decreasing vitamin K production; and with poor absorption this may have resulted in vitamin K deficiency and its associated bleeding into the skin.

4. *True.* In a person with fat malabsorption, free fatty acids can be expected to be released from dietary fat (triglycerides) through the action of pancreatic lipase. However, without adequate small-bowel function for absorption of the free fatty acids, there will be binding of the fatty acids with divalent cations (including calcium, magnesium, and zinc) and loss of these minerals as soaps in the stool.

5. *True.* In fat malabsorption and short-bowel syndromes, oxalate absorption is increased. This may be explained in part by increased efficiency of absorption in patients with shortened small bowel and in part by the unavailability of calcium for precipitation of oxalate in the bowel (since calcium is now bound to the unabsorbed fatty acids). The increased oxalate absorption results in increased excretion and risk of kidney stones.

6. *False.* The terminal ileum is required for the absorption of the intrinsic factor–bound vitamin B_{12}. In the absence of the terminal ileum, vitamin B_{12} should be given by injection to prevent a deficiency that may otherwise develop over the course of 2 or 3 years.

CASE STUDY 5   *Protein-Calorie Malnutrition*

1. *Patient A.* This patient evidently has malabsorption, severe weight loss, and marasmus (chronic starvation). In this situation and in the absence of acute stress, the metabolic rate is reduced as the body attempts to conserve energy. By contrast, Patient B will be hypermetabolic resulting from the septic state.

2. *Patient B.* The rate of urea nitrogen excretion is proportional to the degree of gluconeogenesis as the body breaks down protein in an attempt to produce glucose in response to the stressed state. This certainly applies to Patient B, whereas Patient A is semistarved and will be expected to have a relatively low rate of gluconeogenesis.

3. *Patient B.* Circulating catecholamines and urinary catecholamines tend to be elevated in the presence of acute stress such as that from sepsis or trauma. This is part of the fight-or-flight response.

4. *Patient A.* Urinary creatinine excretion is generally proportional to one's muscle mass because creatinine is formed from creatine, which is derived from the muscle. Patient A has lost a significant amount of weight (currently she is about 75% of her ideal weight) and most likely has reduced muscle mass.

5. *Patient B.* An albumin level of 1.8 g/dl is significantly reduced and in the case of Patient B is a reflection of the severely stressed state. There is of-

ten a small reduction in serum albumin with chronic starvation, although a level this low would not be expected.

6. *Patient A.* A triceps skinfold measurement at 20% of standard (about 3 mm) indicates extreme loss of fat reserves, compatible with the status of Patient A.

7. *Patient A.* In the absence of intervening stress, chronic energy deprivation results in a relatively well-adapted physiologic state. Circulating levels of visceral proteins tend to be maintained near normal, metabolic rate and oxygen consumption are reduced, and protein losses are minimized (as reflected by a low rate of gluconeogenesis). In this situation the patient is more susceptible to nutritional complications of overzealous refeeding than to continued chronic inanition.

8. *Patient A.* As recognized by the noted physiologist Ancel Keys, the heart is more likely to go into failure during early recovery than during starvation. The heart muscle shrinks with starvation. With the introduction of carbohydrate, stimulation of insulin production increases renal sodium reabsorption and fluid retention. At the same time, the carbohydrate load stimulates catecholamine production and oxygen consumption and increases cardiac rate and cardiac output. The combination of volume expansion and cardiac demand predisposes semistarved individuals (such as Patient A) to heart failure if they are refed too aggressively.

CASE
STUDY **6**   *Nutritional Assessment and Support*

1. *False.* Although the dietary intake pattern and the finding of perifollicular petechiae in this patient substantiate a diagnosis of scurvy, scorbutic gum changes are only seen when teeth are present.

2. *True.* She has numerous findings that support the diagnosis of kwashiorkor: a predisposing history of poor protein intake accompanied by stress (in this case, major surgical); clinical findings of widespread edema; easy, painless hair pluckability and a poorly healing surgical wound; and laboratory findings of reduced levels of serum albumin and lymphocytes.

3. *False.* Her present weight of 63 kg is spuriously high because of the edema. Based on her history of weight loss to 47 kg (her "ideal" weight), she is not now obese.

4. *True.* A low BUN does point toward a low recent intake of protein. When large and excessive amounts of protein are ingested, BUN rises, reflecting the increased rate of deamination and urea formation.

5. *False.* Based on the 24-hour urinary excretion of urea nitrogen of 16 g/day, her estimated protein needs are 125 g/day (16 g + 4 g allowance for stool and nonurea urine nitrogen losses, multiplied by 6.25 to estimate protein from nitrogen).

6. *True.* Glucose is considered the fuel of reparation, since it is the only fuel that can be utilized by hypoxic tissues, young fibroblasts, and phagocy-

tizing WBCs. The need for glucose in the stressed state is a logical explanation for the increased rate of gluconeogenesis.

7. *False.* Despite the increased need for glucose in the stressed patient, an exogenous source will help meet energy requirements but will not effectively suppress endogenous glucose production (gluconeogenesis). This is in contrast to the fasting, nonstressed patient, in whom an exogenous source of glucose will suppress the rate of endogenous production.

8. *False.* Although a small proportion (about 10%) of our fat reserves are composed of essential fatty acids, this reserve may not be available if lipolysis is suppressed by the continuous infusion of glucose, as in this case. Intermittent, or cycled, parenteral alimentation will allow mobilization of stored essential fatty acids and prevent the development of essential fatty acid deficiency, even if none are provided for many months.

9. *True.* Intravenous dextrose solutions are made up of the monohydrous form of dextrose that contains 3.4 kcal/g. This is in contrast to dietary carbohydrate, which contains 4.0 kcal/g. Thus 500 g dextrose $\times$ 3.4 kcal/g = 1700 kcal.

10. *True.* Zinc infused at a level of 2.5 mg/day would be expected to cover the needs of the stable adult. With the increased requirements resulting from infection and wound healing, intake should be increased in this case to at least 6 mg/day.

Appendix

B

Normal Laboratory Values

	Normal values
HEMATOLOGY	
Hematocrit	
Men	39%-49%
Women	34%-44%
Hemoglobin	
Men	14-17 g/dl
Women	12-15 g/dl
Children	12-14 g/dl
Newborns	14.5-24.5 g/dl
Mean corpuscular volume	82-99 μ^3
Mean corpuscular hemoglobin	27-32 pg
Mean corpuscular hemoglobin concentration	32%-36%
Platelets	150,000-400,000/mm^3
Reticulocytes	0.5%-1.5%
White blood cells	4000-11000/mm^3
Differential	
Lymphocytes	15%-52% (higher in children)
Neutrophils	35%-73% (lower in children)
Monocytes	2%-14%
Eosinophils	0%-5%
Basophils	1%-2%
Serum iron (Fe)	60-180 μg/dl
Transferrin	212-405 mg/dl
Iron-binding capacity	
Total, serum	250-450 μg/dl
% saturation	15%-55%
Serum ferritin	
Males 18-30 years	30-233 ng/ml
Males 31-60 years	32-284 ng/ml
Premenopausal females	6-81 ng/ml
Postmenopausal females	14-186 ng/ml
Prothrombin time	70%-100% of control

BLOOD CHEMISTRY

Alkaline phosphatase	
1-3 mo	150-475 U/L
To 10 yr	120-320 U/L
Puberty	120-540 U/L
Adults	25-115 U/L
Ammonia (NH_3)	11-35 μmoles/L
Bilirubin	
Total	0-1.2 mg/dl
Direct	0.1-0.3 mg/dl
Calcium (Ca^{++})	8.4-10.2 mg/dl
Carbon dioxide content ($HCO_3{}^-$)	20-30 mEq/L
Carotene	79-233 μg/dl
Chloride	95-108 mEq/L
Creatinine	0.6-1.6 mg/dl
SGOT (AST, serum aspartate amino- transferase)	7-40 U/L
SGPT (serum glutamic pyruvic trans- aminase)	0-45 U/L
GGT (gamma glutamyl transpeptidase)	0-65 U/L
Glucose, fasting	65-110 mg/dl
LDH (lactic dehydrogenase)	120-240 U/L
Magnesium (Mg^{++})	1.8-2.4 mg/dl
Osmolality	280-305 mOsm/kg plasma
Phosphorus	
Children	4.0-7.0 mg/dl
Adults	2.5-4.8 mg/dl
Potassium (K^+)	3.5-5.2 mEq/L
Proteins	
Total	6.4-8.4 g/dl
Albumin	3.9-4.8 g/dl
α_1 globulin	0.15-0.4 g/dl
α_2 globulin	0.5-0.9 g/dl
β globulin	0.7-1.1 g/dl
γ globulin	0.5-1.5 g/dl
Sodium (Na^+)	135-145 mEq/L
Urea nitrogen (BUN)	8-23 mg/dl

URINE TESTS (24-HOUR EXCRETION; VARIES WITH INTAKE)

Calcium	30-250 mg (2-13 mEq)
Creatinine	800-1800 mg
Magnesium	150-300 mg (12-25 mEq)
Phosphorus	0.7-1.5 g
Potassium	0.8-3.9 (20-100 mEq)
Sodium	3-8 g (130-360 mEq)
Urea nitrogen (UUN)	See Table 10-6

STOOL TESTS

Fat

Total	<6 g/24 hr (with dietary fat intake >50 g/day); <30% of dry weight
Neutral	1%-5% of dry matter
Free fatty acids	1%-10% of dry matter
Combined fatty acids (as soap)	1%-12% of dry matter
Nitrogen	<2 g/24 hr or 10% of urinary nitrogen

FUNCTION TESTS

D-xylose absorption test: after overnight fast, 25 g xylose taken by mouth; urine collected for following 5 hr	Urine xylose 4-9 g/5 hr (or >20% of ingested dose); serum xylose 25-40 mg/dl 2 hr after oral dose
Schilling test: orally administered radio-labeled vitamin B_{12} after "flushing" parenteral injection of B_{12}; normalization of B_{12} excretion with exogenous intrinsic factor is diagnostic of intrinsic factor deficiency in patient with pernicious anemia and gastric atrophy	Excretion in urine of >10% of oral dose/24 hr

Appendix C

Multiple Vitamin Preparations

Name	Mfr	Vita-min A (5000 IU)*	Vita-min D (400 IU)	Vita-min E (30 IU)	Vita-min C (60 mg)	Thia-min (Vita-min B₁) (1.5 mg)	Ribo-flavin (Vita-min B₂) (1.7 mg)
REPLACEMENT VITAMINS							
Adavite	Hudson	5000	400	30	90	3	3.4
One-A-Day Men's	Bayer	5000	400	45	200	2.25	2.55
Therapeutic tablets	Goldline	5000	400	30	90	3	3.4
Theragran	Mead Johnson	5000	400	30	90	3	3.4
Theravim	Nature's Bounty	5000	400	30	90	3	3.4
One-A-Day Essential	Bayer	5000	400	30	60	1.5	1.7
Dayalets	Abbott	5000	400	30	60	1.5	1.7
Unicap	Upjohn	5000	400	30	60	1.5	1.7
LIQUID REPLACEMENT VITAMINS (PER 5 ML)							
Syrite	Barre-National	2500	400	15	60	1.05	1.2
Daily Vitamins	Rugby	2500	400	15	60	1.05	1.2
Vi-Daylin Multivitamin	Ross	2500	400	15	60	1.05	1.2
REPLACEMENT VITAMINS WITH MINERALS							
Decagen	Goldline	5000	400	30	60	1.7	2
Theravee-M	Vangard	5000	400	30	120	3	3.4
Adavite-M	Hudson	5000	400	30	90	3	3.4
Theravim-M	Nature's Bounty	5000	400	30	90	3	3.4
Optilets-M-500	Abbott	5000	400	30	500	15	10
Unicap T	Upjohn	5000	400	30	500	10	10
Avail	Menley & James	5000	400	30	90	2.25	2.55
Myadec	Parke Davis	5000	400	30	60	1.7	2
One-A-Day Maximum Formula	Bayer	5000	400	30	60	1.5	1.7
Centrum	Lederle	5000	400	30	60	1.5	1.7
Centrum Jr. + Iron	Lederle	5000	400	30	60	1.5	1.7
Unicap M	Upjohn	5000	400	30	60	1.5	1.7
THERAPEUTIC VITAMINS WITH OR WITHOUT MINERALS							
Quintabs-M	Freeda	10000	400	50	300	30	30
Generix T	Goldline	10000	400	5.5	150	15	10
Total Formula	Vitaline	10000	400	30	100	15	15
Nova-Dec	Rugby	5000	400	30	60	1.7	2
Centrum Silver	Lederle	5000	400	45	60	1.5	1.7
Theragran-M	Apothecon	6250	400	30	90	3	3.4
LIQUID THERAPEUTIC VITAMINS (PER 5 ML)							
Theragran	Mead Johnson	5000	400		200	10	10
Theravite	Barre-National	10000	400		200	10	10

*Amounts in parentheses indicate 100% of the RDI for each nutrient; however, RDIs are not established for all nutrients listed.

Niacin (Vitamin B$_3$) (20 mg)	Pyridoxine (Vitamin B$_6$) (2 mg)	Folate (400 μg)	Vitamin B$_{12}$ (6 μg)	Beta carotene (IU)	Iron (18 mg)	Magnesium (400 mg)	Iodine (150 mcg)	Zinc (15 mg)	Calcium (1000 mg)	Phosphorus (1000 mg)
30	3	400	9	1250						
20	3	400	9							
20	3	400	9							
20	3	400	9							
30	3	400	9	1250						
20	2	400	6							
20	2	400	6							
20	2	400	6							
13.5	1.05		4.5							
13.5	1.05		4.5							
13.5	1.05		4.5							
20	3	400	6		18			15		
30	3	400	9	2500	27			15		
20	3	400	9		27			15		
30	3	400	9		27			15		
100	5		12		20	80	150	1.5	20	
100	6	400	18		18		150	15		
20	3	400	9		18	100	150	22.5	400	
20	3	400	6		18	100	150	15	162	125
20	2	400	6		18	100	150	15	129.6	100
20	2	400	6		18	100	150	15	162	109
20	2	400	6		18	40	150	15	108	50
20	2	400	6		18		150	15		
150	30	400	30		15			30		
100	2		7.5		15			1.5		
25	25	400	25		20			30		
20	3	400	6		18	100	150	15		
20	3	200	25		4	100	150	15	200	48
20	3	400	9		27	100	150	15	40	31
100	4.1		5							
100	4.1		5							

Name	Mfr	Vitamin A (5000 IU)*	Vitamin D (400 IU)	Vitamin E (30 IU)	Vitamin C (60 mg)	Thiamin (Vitamin B$_1$) (1.5 mg)	Riboflavin (Vitamin B$_2$) (1.7 mg)
PRENATAL VITAMINS							
Prenate 90	Bock	4000	400	30	120	3	3.4
Materna	Lederle	5000	400	30	100	3	3.4
Niferex-PN Forte	Central	5000	400	30	80	3	3.4
Pramilet FA	Ross	4000	400		100	3	2
Natalins RX	Mead Johnson	4000	400	15	80	1.5	1.6
Stuart-natal	Wyeth Ayerst	4000	400	11	100	1.8	1.7
SPECIALTY VITAMINS-RENAL							
Iberet Folic 500	Abbott				500	6	6
Tabron	Parke-Davis			30	500	6	6

Niacin (Vitamin B₃) (20 mg)	Pyridoxine (Vitamin B₆) (2 mg)	Folate (400 μg)	Vitamin B₁₂ (6 μg)	Beta carotene (IU)	Iron (18 mg)	Magnesium (400 mg)	Iodine (150 mcg)	Zinc (15 mg)	Calcium (1000 mg)	Phosphorus (1000 mg)
20	20	1000	12		90		150	25	250	
20	10	1000	12		60	25	150	25	250	
20	4	1000	12		60	10	200	25	250	
10	3	1000	3		40		100		250	
17	4	1000	2.5		60	100		25	200	
18	2.6	800	12		60			25	200	
30	5	800	25		105					
30	5	1000	25		100					

Index

WE WANT TO HEAR FROM YOU!

To help us publish the most useful materials, we would appreciate your comments on this book. Please take a few moments to answer the questions below, and E-mail us your comments. Thank you for your input.

Morgan: FUNDAMENTALS OF CLINICAL NUTRITION, 2e
nutrition.medtext@mosby.com

1. How are you using this book? Please be specific: for a first-year medical school course, as part of a clerkship rotation, to refresh the material before a Board examination, etc.

2. Was this book useful to you? Why or why not?

3. What features of textbooks are important to you?
   - -Color figures   -Self-assessment questions
   - -Summary tables and boxes   -Price
   - -Summaries   -What else?

4. What influenced your decision to buy this text?
   - -Required/recommended by instructor
   - -Recommended by student
   - -Bookstore display
   - -What else?

5. What other instructional materials did/would you find useful in this course?
   - -Computer-assisted instruction
   - -Slides
   - -What else?

Are you interested in doing in-depth reviews of our textbooks?
If so, please send us your name, address, and telephone number.

THANK YOU!